The Living Organ Donor as Patient

The Living Organ Donor as Patient

Theory and Practice

Lainie Friedman Ross, MD, PhD and
J. Richard Thistlethwaite, Jr., MD, PhD

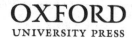

OXFORD
UNIVERSITY PRESS

OXFORD
UNIVERSITY PRESS

Oxford University Press is a department of the University of Oxford. It furthers
the University's objective of excellence in research, scholarship, and education
by publishing worldwide. Oxford is a registered trade mark of Oxford University
Press in the UK and certain other countries.

Published in the United States of America by Oxford University Press
198 Madison Avenue, New York, NY 10016, United States of America.

Library of Congress Cataloging-in-Publication Data
Names: Ross, Lainie Friedman, author. | Thistlethwaite, J. Richard, author.
Title: The living organ donor as patient : theory and practice /
by Lainie Friedman Ross and J. Richard Thistlethwaite.
Description: New York, NY : Oxford University Press, [2022] |
Includes bibliographical references and index.
Identifiers: LCCN 2021030802 (print) | LCCN 2021030803 (ebook) |
ISBN 9780197618202 (hardback) | ISBN 9780197618226 (epub) | ISBN 9780197618233 (online)
Subjects: MESH: Living Donors—ethics | Organ Transplantation—ethics
Classification: LCC RD120.7 (print) | LCC RD120.7 (ebook) | NLM WO 690 |
DDC 174.2/97954—dc23
LC record available at https://lccn.loc.gov/2021030802
LC ebook record available at https://lccn.loc.gov/2021030803

DOI: 10.1093/oso/9780197618202.001.0001

1 3 5 7 9 8 6 4 2

Printed by Integrated Books International, United States of America

We dedicate this book to our spouses:
John L. Ross
Susan B. Thistlethwaite

Contents

PART 5: DECISION-MAKING
AND RISK THRESHOLDS

Preface: In Memoriam

Lainie Friedman Ross

On November 16, 2020, as we were finishing our edits to this book, we learned of the death of our colleague, Robert M. Veatch, 1 week earlier. In 2001, I had the privilege of reviewing Bob's book *Transplantation Ethics* for the journal *Perspectives in Biology and Medicine*. I called the book a masterpiece and praised it loudly. I had one criticism:

> Despite its length, my major criticism of the book is what it does not cover. The section of organ procurement focuses almost exclusively on cadaveric transplantation, when in 2000 approximately 40 percent of all transplants use living organ sources, and living sources represent the faster growing supply of organs. Nevertheless, in the one chapter that Veatch discusses living donors, he accomplishes a lot.[1]

Little did I know that I would be Bob's coauthor for the book's second edition, and yet despite my criticisms in 2001, we would only slightly expand the discussion of living donor organ transplantation. In some ways, then, this book is an extension of the work that Bob began. It was a privilege to work with him and now to work with Dick Thistlethwaite. A memoriam can be found at: http://www.bioethics.net/2020/11/robert-m-veatch/

Note

1. Ross LF. *Transplantation Ethics* by Robert M Veatch. *Perspectives in Biology and Medicine*. 2001; 44:623–628, at p. 627.

Abbreviations

A2ALL	Adult to Adult Living Liver Study group
AAP	American Academy of Pediatrics
ADP	advance donor program
AIDS	acquired immune deficiency syndrome
aLDLT	adult living donor liver transplant
ALF	acute liver failure
ALFSG	Acute Liver Failure Study Group
ALS	amyotrophic lateral sclerosis
APOL1	apolipoprotein L1
APOLLO	*APOL1* Long-term Kidney Transplantation Outcomes Network
AST	American Society of Transplantation
BCAA	branched chain amino acid
BTS	British Transplant Society
CFR	Code of Federal Regulations
CI	confidence interval
CKD	chronic kidney disease
CMS	Centers for Medicare & Medicaid Services
CRC	colorectal carcinoma
CRLM	colorectal liver metastases
C-S	candidate-subject
DCD	donation after cardio-circulatory death
DDLT	deceased donor liver transplant(ation)
DDR	dead donor rule
DICG	Declaration of Istanbul Custodian Group
DILI	drug-induced liver injury
DOJ	Department of Justice
DONOR	Donor Nephrectomy Outcomes Research
DSA	donor specific antigen
ESRD	end-stage renal disease
FDA	Food and Drug Administration
Fed Reg	Federal Regulations
FHF	fulminant hepatic failure
GKE	Global Kidney Exchange
GKEP	Global Kidney Exchange Program
HCC	hepatocellular carcinoma
HIC	high-income country

HIV	human immunodeficiency virus
HLA	human leukocyte antigen
ICU	intensive care unit
IDD	imminent death donation
JRT	J Richard Thistlethwaite
KAS	Kidney Allocation System
KDIGO	Kidney Disease: Improving Global Outcomes (KDIGO)
KPE	kidney paired exchange
LDA	living donor advocate
LDAT	living donor advocate team
LDA(T)	living donor advocate or living donor advocate team
LDLT	living donor liver transplant(ation)
LFR	Lainie Friedman Ross
LL	left lateral lobe
LLC	life-limiting condition
LLS	left lateral segment
LMIC	low- to middle-income country
MELD	model for end-stage liver disease
MSUD	maple syrup urine disease
National Commission	National Commission for the Protection of Biomedical and Behavioral Research
NBAC	National Bioethics Advisory Committee
NEAD	never-ending altruistic donor
NIH	National Institutes of Health
NKR	National Kidney Registry
NOTA	National Organ Transplant Act
ODE	organ donation euthanasia
OHRP	Office of Human Research Protections
OPO	organ procurement organization
OPTN	Organ Procurement and Transplant Network
PL	prisoner liaison
pLDLT	pediatric living donor liver transplant
PRA	panel reactive antibodies
RAPID	resection and partial liver segment 2–3 transplantation with delayed total hepatectomy
RELIVE	renal and lung living donors evaluation
RL	right lobe
RTT	reverse transplant tourism
SCT	sickle cell trait
SECA-1	SEcondary CAncer Study 1
SEOPF	South-Eastern Organ Procurement Foundation
SEROPP	South-Eastern Regional Organ Procurement Program
SES	socioeconomic status

SRTR	Scientific Registry of Transplant Recipients
TBI	total body irradiation
UK	United Kingdom
UNOS	United Network for Organ Sharing
US	United States
WHO	World Health Organization

PART 1
SETTING THE STAGE

1

Introduction

This is a book about living solid organ donors as patients in their own right. This book is premised on the supposition that the field of living donor organ transplantation is ethical, even if some specific applications are not. Living donor organ transplantation is controversial at its core because it exposes 1 patient (the living donor) to clinical risks for the clinical benefit of another (the candidate recipient). It is different than obstetrics which also involves 2 patients—a pregnant woman and her fetus—because transplantation involves 2 physically individuated patients who, in most cases, individually consent to the medical interventions. And in many cases, the donor-recipient interdependence is optional because deceased donor organs provide an alternative option. So before one can begin, one must ask, even if only rhetorically: Is living donation ethical? The question is not new: one of the first to ask about the ethics of living donor transplantation was Joseph Murray, the surgeon credited with performing the first successful living donor kidney transplant, which paved the way for the broad adoption of kidney and other solid organ transplantation around the world.

1.1 History

Joseph Murray and colleagues at the Peter Bent Brigham Hospital in Boston successfully performed the first successful living donor kidney transplant between identical twin brothers in December 1954.[1] Identical twins were chosen to obviate the need for immunosuppression, which was in its infancy. Following this success and the success of other identical twin donor-recipient pairs, kidney transplants between nonidentical twins were attempted using total body irradiation (with and without prednisone) for immunosuppression. By the end of the decade, new immunosuppressive drugs like 6-Mercaptopurine and its analog, azathioprine, were being employed,[2] and by

The Living Organ Donor as Patient. Lainie Friedman Ross and J. Richard Thistlethwaite, Jr, Oxford University Press.
© Oxford University Press 2022. DOI: 10.1093/oso/9780197618202.003.0001

1960 both Murray's team in Boston and Jean Hamburger's team in Paris had successfully transplanted kidneys between fraternal twin brothers. However, there was "speculation that the donor and recipient, like twin cattle, had become chimeric by exchanging tolerogenic blood cells during gestation."[3] Between 1960 and 1962 Jean Hamburger and René Küss performed 4 successful transplants between nontwin recipients conditioned by total body irradiation.[4] Clyde Barker and James Markmann explain the significance of this achievement:

> This French experience was the principal (and perhaps the only) justification for continuing human kidney transplantation. Because bone marrow inocula were not used in these patients, it was assumed that chimerism was not necessary for success.[5]

Based on his own experience and the growing experiences across the United States (US), the United Kingdom (UK), and France, Murray had the forethought, in 1963, to establish the Human Kidney Transplant Registry, an international voluntary registry that documented all kidney transplants being performed around the world.[6] By March 1966, the registry included data about 672 primary transplants plus an additional 45 secondary and 2 tertiary transplants.[7] That month, the CIBA Foundation sponsored the first international, interdisciplinary transplant symposium focused on the "ethical, medical and legal difficulties which are now so dramatically accentuated by modern progress in medical research. . . ."[8] The attendees included not only physicians and surgeons, but also judges and legal scholars, a minister, and a science journalist.

At the CIBA Foundation symposium, Murray expressed reservations about living kidney donor transplantation: "we make a basic qualitative shift in our aims when we risk the health of a well person, no matter how pure our motives."[9] He urged the meeting attendants to view living donation as a temporary solution: "all clinicians working with kidney transplantation should strive for better organ procurement so that the day will come when even the identical twins will not require a living donor."[10]

Murray clearly pointed out the central ethical concern: why (or at least when) is it ethically permissible to electively expose one individual to harm for the clinical benefit of another? This question still needs examination.

1.2 Arguments Related to Harm

The primary objection to living donor organ transplantation rests on the claim that a physician's first responsibility is *primum non nocere*, or first not to do harm. Removing an organ from a healthy individual when it is not clinically indicated for the individual's own health puts the individual at risk for acute complications due to surgery and anesthesia, as well as postoperative complications and sequelae which may be short- or long-term.

What are the risks to the donor in living donor organ transplantation? The answer is that it depends on the organ. Since kidneys make up over 95% of all living donors reported in the US Organ Procurement and Transplant Network (OPTN) database (166,625 of 175,285 donors as of August 7, 2021) and livers account for another 8,075 (4.6%),[11] we will focus our discussion on these 2 organs.

Kidney donation has low peri-operative risks. The 90-day perioperative risk of mortality from living kidney donation is estimated to be about 3.1 per 10,000, and the risk of major short-term morbidity at < 1%.[12] Recent studies, however, document infrequent but serious long-term risks. Evidence suggests that living kidney donors in the US have an increased relative risk of end-stage renal disease, although overall this outcome remains uncommon (<0.5%) over 15 years.[13] The increased risk is more significant in Black donors, especially in young Black males.[14] Three retrospective cohort studies from Canada, Norway, and the US have examined pregnancy outcomes and found an increased risk of gestational hypertension and pre-eclampsia.[15] Whether there is an increased risk of cardiovascular disease is uncertain,[16] but at least 1 study has found increased risk of hypertension in Blacks post-donation.[17]

Contrast living kidney donation, which entails the removal of 1 of 2 kidneys, with living liver donation, where the amount of liver removed depends on many factors including donor and recipient size. When the recipient is a young child, the living liver donation usually involves the procurement of the left lateral segment (LLS) of the liver. When older (larger) minors and adults are recipients, the transplant requires either a full left liver lobe (LL) or right liver lobe (RL) from the living donor. Mortality and morbidity from living LLS donation from an adult to a young child is lower than adult to adult living liver donation. In a review of living donor hepatectomies performed at 46 centers in Japan, the morbidity rates after 1680 donor operations were 8.2% for 753 LLS donors, 12.0% for 484 LL donors, and 19.0% for 443 RL donors ($P < 0.01$).[18] Asian transplant centers have some of the lowest morbidity and mortality in the world.[19] In contrast, the largest study in the US to date, the A2ALL (Adult to Adult Living Liver Study group) found that approximately 40% of living liver donors experience morbidity, although the study did not distinguish by type of graft.[20] A small percentage of the patients (0.3%–1.8%) experienced serious (Clavien grade 3 or 4) complications, depending on era and center.[21] Acute morbidity in the A2ALL study included infections, pleural effusions, bile leaks, neuropraxia, re-explorations, and prolonged ileus.[22] However, as Abecassis and colleagues noted:

> a number of complications first occurred many months or even years after donation. Hernia, bowel obstruction and psychological complications first developed as late as 5 to 6 years following donation.[23]

Results in Europe and Canada are similar to US results.[24]

Since it cannot be accurately predicted which donors will develop complications, an absolute injunction not to cause harm would prohibit all living organ donation. However, the principle of nonmaleficence is not absolute, but rather only implies a *prima facie* obligation—one that can be overridden if there are compelling counter obligations. Many medical procedures cause harm, even as they benefit the patient. It is more accurate to understand the principle of nonmaleficence within the context of a harm-benefit ratio. That is, it is morally acceptable to permit an individual to serve as a donor if the benefits are expected to outweigh the harms. Thus, if the benefits to the donor (psychological) outweigh the risks to the donor (physical and possibly psychological), then the donation is morally permissible. Of course, it is also the case that the benefits to the recipient (medical and psychological) must outweigh the risks to the recipient (which includes peri-operative risks and longer-term risks of complications from both the procedure itself and, as importantly, those secondary to immunosuppression). Note that the calculation does not justify risks to the donor if only the recipient were to benefit. Rather, it requires that donor benefit:risk calculation and the recipient benefit:risk calculation are both positive. However, the benefit to the donor need not be solely self-serving. It is reasonable and legitimate for a donor to include other-regarding interests in her calculation. Thus, a prospective donor can judge that she stands to gain a great deal by promoting the well-being of the recipient. But a donor who fears undergoing the surgical procedure or has ambivalent feelings about her intended recipient may find that the risks outweigh the benefits, even in the exceptional case where the recipient is an identical twin who would require minimal to no immunosuppression.

The argument to prohibit all living donations on the basis of nonmaleficence fails because it assumes too narrow a notion of harm; it only addresses possible physical harm to the donor. Individuals can also suffer psychosocial and moral harms if they are prevented from serving as a donor. An individual who wants to donate an organ and is prohibited has her interests thwarted.[25] Although organ donation confers no physical benefits, studies have shown that most donors experience increased self-esteem and feelings of well-being.[26] To the extent that living donation is ethically permissible in some cases, the prohibition of donation can be psychologically harmful.[27] This is not to say that the potential donor has a right to serve as a donor, because the courts have made it clear that there is no such right.[28] In part, this is because donors require the aid of third parties to perform the operation and procure the organ, and surgeons have the right to refuse to do so if they feel the risks are too great or that the likelihood of significant recipient benefit is too low.

1.3 Arguments Based on Respect for Persons

The main moral argument to support living solid organ donation is based on the principle of respect for persons, which requires that individuals with decisional capacity should be treated as autonomous agents and that those with diminished autonomy should be protected. Since living donors have decisional capacity (with rare exception), the focus is on respect for autonomy. If a competent adult seeks to act altruistically by offering to donate a solid organ unconditionally, understands the risks and benefits of the procedure, and voluntarily consents to the procurement, then, assuming that she successfully passes medical and psychological screening and that there is an appropriate recipient, her autonomy should be respected.

Although the autonomy arguments are necessary to justify allowing some competent adults to serve as organ donors in some circumstances, the autonomy arguments are tempered by the fact that organ donation entails the participation of transplant personnel who are also autonomous moral agents and can refuse to help the subject achieve his or her goals:

> [A] doctor is in the position of deciding not simply whether a subject's choice is reasonable or morally justifiable, but whether *he* is morally justified in helping the subject accomplish it.[29]

And, in fact, all transplant personnel can and should refuse to proceed with organ donation if it would place the donor at significant risk of morbidity and mortality (as an extreme example, procuring both kidneys from a willing living donor[30]). Transplant teams need to decide for themselves whether (1) the donors must be genetically or emotionally related; (2) the organ procurement poses undue risks for the donor; and (3) the surgical and postoperative risks to the donor can be morally justified.

1.4 Why Focus on Living Donors?

We focus our project on living donors because the growing gap between the number of individuals needing transplants and the number of deceased donor organs available has led to numerous proposals to expand living donation, and these proposals need to be ethically evaluated. The deceased donor demand:supply gap continues to grow despite (1) the near universal legal acceptance of brain death, (2) the development of donation after cardio-circulatory death (DCD) policies, (3) higher rates of consent from families of deceased donors; (4) an increased number of potential deceased donors due to the opioid epidemic, (5) passage of first-person consent laws, and (6) the development of better immunosuppressive drugs and better immunosuppression regimens. Even if organs were recovered from all individuals dying under conditions that allowed for the recovery of transplantable organs, the gap would persist given a number of demand factors including an aging population and the option to expand the criteria for candidacy (eg, transplantation in the face of chronic candidate-recipient infection, such as human immunodeficiency virus [HIV]). As solid organ transplantation becomes more and more successful in reducing patient morbidity and mortality, even for conditions for which alternative treatments exist (eg, liver transplant for children with metabolic conditions who can alternatively be treated by a restrictive diet), previously excluded candidate recipients challenge current exclusion criteria because transplant offers a better option than the alternatives (eg, children with metabolic conditions who undergo liver transplantation are less likely to have an acute metabolic crisis due to illness or stress).[31]

In kidney transplantation, it is not only the wide gap between the number of deceased donor grafts and the number of transplant candidates, but also the superior clinical results from living donor kidney transplants that have resulted in increasing pressure for candidates to seek living kidney donors. The pressure to identify a living donor has been aided by (1) the move from only permitting donations from genetically related family members to the acceptance of emotionally related spouses and friends to current practice that permits donation by strangers; and (2) the trend of accepting less than ideal donors and less than ideal recipients including the very young, the very old, and those who are more medically complex.

The expansion has also been aided by the development of programs designed to increase the living kidney donor organ supply by educating and motivating candidates to actively find a live donor. Transplant programs that train potential kidney recipients on how to ask and attract living donors—whether by in-person engagement or through the use of social media—have been found to be effective.[32] Other research has found programs that encourage candidates to identify a family member or friend to become their "donor champion" who helps them identify and encourage family members, friends, and even acquaintances to consider becoming their living donor to be effective as well.[33] Whether these programs impose too much pressure on potential living donors has not been explored.

Our goal, then, is to explore the ethical issues raised by policies and practices proposed and/or implemented to expand living solid organ donation and transplantation to help define the moral limits of living donor organ transplantation. We argue that ethical practice requires the living donor always be treated and respected, first and foremost, as a patient in her or his own right.

1.5 Book Outline

Transplantation Ethics was recently revised by one of us (LFR) with Bob Veatch, the original author. Although *Transplantation Ethics, 2nd edition* does have a chapter on living donor organ transplantation, the main focus of the book is deciding (1) when human beings are dead; (2) when it is ethical to obtain organs for transplantation from deceased donors, and (3) how to allocate deceased donor organs, once obtained.[34] Living organ donation alsoasks when is it ethical to obtain organs from living donors for transplantation and how should these organs be allocated, but the issues are different in 3 important ways. First, in living organ transplantation, there are 2 living patients, the donor and the recipient, and both need to be treated as patients in their own right. Second, procuring organs from dead donors pose no risks to the donors whereas living donor procurement entails varying degrees of risk depending on the organ. Third, deceased donor organs are considered a public good to be allocated using an algorithm that balances equity and efficiency whereas living organ grafts are a private good that can be allocated at the discretion of the donor based on his or her sense of duty, altruism, and relational attachments.

1.5.1 Part 1: Development of an Ethics Framework and Exploration of Vulnerability

We begin this book focused exclusively on living donors by providing a short history of solid organ donor transplantation and some of the novel protocols proposed to expand living donor transplantation (chapter 2). In the next chapter, we develop an ethics framework for addressing the challenges raised by living donor solid organ transplantation (chapter 3). This living donor ethics framework has its origin in research ethics. Both living donor transplantation and human subjects research expose 1 set of individuals to clinical risks for the clinical benefits of others. In the *Belmont Report*, the National Commission for the Protection of Human Subjects of Biomedical and Behavior Research (National Commission) developed "an analytical framework that will guide the resolution of ethical problems arising from research involving human subjects."[35] The *Belmont Report* incorporated 3 principles: respect for persons, beneficence and justice.[36] The National Commission supported additional protections for vulnerable groups of potential research participants. In 2001, Kenneth Kipnis effectively argued that the concept of vulnerable groups failed to explore in what ways within particular groups of people vulnerability might vary thereby risking unnecessary protections for some and inadequate protections for others. He proposed a taxonomy that explored different types of vulnerabilities that all research participants may experience to provide a more robust framework for human subjects protections.[37]

In contrast, living donor transplantation lacks an overarching analytical framework to guide the resolution of ethical problems arising from transplantation involving living donors. In chapter 3 we adapt the 3 principles articulated in the *Belmont Report* to serve as the foundation for a living donor ethics framework, which we supplement with the principle of vulnerability using Kipnis' vulnerability taxonomy, and add a fifth principle, which holds that "special relationships create special responsibilities." The fifth principle derives from the work of Robert Goodin, who claims that health professionals, who stand in special relationship with patients, are responsible for promoting and protecting their well-being.[38] Application of this principle to transplantation ensures that the living donor is seen as a patient in her own right, not just as a means—a source of organs—for a recipient candidate.

The living donor transplant team consists of the health care providers who are responsible for the clinical work-up, surgery, and follow-up care of the living solid organ donor. The living donor team is responsible for getting an informed and voluntary consent from the prospective donor. Since 2007, all living donors in the US are required to have a living donor advocate (LDA).[39] We refer to the living donor team joined by an LDA as the living donor advocate team (LDAT). That is, the LDAT consists of 2 or more health care professionals responsible for donor well-being and promotes a shared decision-making process that allows donors to decide whether or not to donate by helping them explore their own values, needs, and interests. In living donor transplantation, then, the living donor transplant team is responsible for empowering prospective donors to make an authentic choice by helping them exercise their autonomy and address their vulnerabilities, and by protecting and disqualifying from donation those who cannot freely exercise their autonomy or adequately address their vulnerabilities.[40]

This fifth principle also acknowledges the moral agency of the transplant professionals to refuse to perform a living donor procurement even if the donor provides an informed and voluntary consent. As Carl Elliot argued in an article about living donor transplantation: "Thus a doctor is in the position of deciding not simply whether a subject's choice is reasonable or morally justifiable, but whether he is morally justified in helping the subject accomplish it."[41]

1.5.2 Part 2: Donor Demographics

In part 2, we explore how this 5-principle living donor ethics framework applies to various demographic categories of living donors. Chapter 4 examines who are the living donors and notes that there is an over-representation of women and an under-representation of Blacks. This raises the question of whether these differences are a reflection of mere preference or whether they reflect concerns of inequities. We examine these demographic differences using a vulnerability analysis. Chapters 5 and 6 examine 2 other historically vulnerable groups—children and prisoners. Chapter 5 explores the issue of children as living donors, which we first addressed in a policy statement for the American Academy of Pediatrics.[42] We now re-explore the issue considering what vulnerabilities children face and whether and how they can be addressed. Chapter 5 explores the specific vulnerabilities that prisoners face, whether and how they can be addressed, even if only in a limited number of cases.

1.5.3 Part 3: Expanding Living Donor Transplantation

Part 3 focuses on the ethical boundaries of expanding living donor transplantation (focused exclusively on the kidney and liver) as it moved from a solution of last resort to a preferred modality. Each of the 4 chapters begins with 1 or more cases to help shape the ethical discussion. In chapters 7 and 8, we explore creative attempts at expanding living donor kidney transplantation and the ethical limits of these attempts. These attempts derive from 2 distinct developments. First is the growing acceptance of donations by nonbiological relatives: from spouses to friends to strangers (also known as Good Samaritan donors or nondirected donors). Second is the development and adoption of kidney paired exchanges (see Figure 1.1). Since the publication of the ethical analysis of kidney paired exchanges in the *New England Journal of Medicine* in 1997,[43] many different modifications have been proposed and performed—some of which are ethically questionable.

Chapters 9 and 10 focus on living donor liver transplantation. Chapter 9 reviews the history of living donor liver transplantation, its rapid expansion, and its rapid decline due to a very public death of a living donor. Chapters 10 considers the role of living liver donation in acute liver failure (ALF).

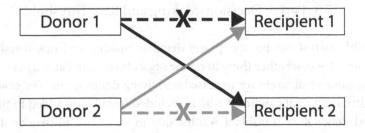

Figure 1.1   Paired Exchange of Organs Between Two Living Donor-Recipient Pairs Due to ABO- or HLA-incompatibility, Donor 1 cannot donate to Recipient 1, and Donor 2 cannot donate to Recipient 2, but Donor 1 can donate to Recipient 2, and Donor 2 can donate to Recipient 1. This is referred to as a kidney paired exchange.

1.5.4 Part 4: Moral Limits to Expanding Living Donors

Part 4 focuses on the moral limits to expanding the participation of living donors in organ transplantation. Using case studies, we discuss programs that we believe transgress ethical boundaries. Chapter 11 looks at the issue of the imminently dying donor. It examines challenges to the dead donor rule (DDR) which "is neither a law nor a regulation [but rather] —it is a description of an ethical norm."[44] It expresses the idea that all human life is valuable and that persons are treated and cared for as living patients until death is declared. Chapter 12 examines 2 practices that cross traditional (organ and global) boundaries: living liver-living kidney exchange programs (known as trans-organ or bi-organ transplant programs[45]) and global kidney exchange programs (originally described as reverse transplant tourism[46]) which involves a kidney paired exchange involving a donor-recipient pair from a low- to middle-income country (LMIC) who can participate in a kidney paired exchange with an incompatible donor-recipient pair from a high-income country (HIC). The underlying logic is that the costs of the surgeries for the donor and recipient from the LMIC would be paid for by the HIC because of the expected long-term savings that the HIC gains. In chapter 13, we consider the question of financial remuneration and payment to those who provide living organ grafts.

1.5.5 Part 5: Decision-Making and Risk Thresholds

The fifth part of our book explores decision-making and risk thresholds. Chapter 14 asks whether the criteria for organ transplant candidates should be the same or different for deceased and living donor grafts. For example, imagine a recipient candidate who is excluded from being added to the deceased donor liver transplant waitlist due to substance misuse or due to noncompliance but has a family member who is willing to donate an organ despite the concerns that the recipient will be a poor steward of the organ. While deceased donor organs are a public good and should be allocated according to a fair process, living donor grafts are often thought of as private goods that can be allocated according to the preferences of the living donor. And yet the infrastructure and resources needed for the living donor transplantation involves a large public investment, which justifies some public discussion of boundaries. We explore under what circumstances is it moral for transplant programs to allow different standards for living versus deceased donor organ transplantation and what changes in policy and practice are necessary to permit different standards.

In chapter 15 we examine the clinical use and disclosure of Apolipoprotein LI (APOL1), a multi-allelic gene that has 2 "high-risk" alleles (G1 and G2) found mainly in the Black community, that have potential adverse implications for kidney donors and their recipients. The association of APOL1 high risk alleles with kidney health and disease was only identified in 2010.[47] Over the next 10 years, APOL1 was found to have adverse impact on deceased donor kidney transplantation. Facts we know about Black deceased donors include: (1) On average, Black deceased donor kidneys have a decreased graft survival compared to deceased donor kidneys from other racial/ethnic groups and (2) Black deceased donor kidneys with 2 APOL1 risk alleles have an average decreased survival compared to deceased donor kidneys from Blacks who have 0 or 1 risk allele in relatively short-term studies.[48] Whether there is decreased survival for transplants with Black living donor kidneys with 2 APOL1 risk alleles is unknown.

When the donor is a living person, we need to assess not only the outcomes of the living donor graft for recipient kidney function and survival, but also the impact of donation on the living donor. Although our knowledge is limited, the potential impact of unilateral nephrectomy in individuals with 2 APOL1 risk alleles raises cause for concerns. While many Blacks with 2 APOL1 risk alleles do not develop kidney failure, Blacks with 2 APOL1 risk alleles have a greater risk of developing end-stage renal disease than Blacks who only have 1 or no APOL1 risk alleles. What is not known is whether uni-lateral nephrectomy may act as a "second hit" to exacerbate or accelerate the risk of end-stage renal disease in Black living kidney donors with 2 APOL1 alleles compared to other Black living donors.[49] Despite the unknowns, many transplant programs have implemented APOL1 testing of living donors in the clinical setting and many are excluding individuals with 2 APOL1 alleles.[50] We use APOL1 as an example of how a suspected but unproven risk should be discussed with potential living donors and their intended candi-date recipients under conditions of uncertainty.

Finally, in chapter 16, we return to the premise with which we began: the supposition that living donor transplantation can be ethical. We examine whether the premise would still stand if there were an adequate supply of "spare parts"[51] without living donors.

1.6 The Use of Case Studies

In this book we will examine actual and hypothetical cases gleaned from a variety of sources (medical journals, newspapers, and court rulings) in order to examine the ethical principles that morally justify or invalidate a partic-ular donation. We will use the pronouns associated with the actual cases described. When discussing donors and recipients hypothetically, we refer to donors as "she" because most living solid organ donors are women,[52] and we refer to candidates and recipients as "he" since men are more likely to be recipients,[53] except in this chapter where we have often used he or she. The only exception is in chapter 6 where we refer to prisoner donors as "he" since men are much more likely to be incarcerated than women.[54] In each chapter, we define our abbreviations when first used, but also provide a full abbreviations list at the back of the book.

The use of case studies is typical in medicine because they "bridge the gap between theory and practice and between the academy and the workplace."[55] Case studies also help ground the discussion "upon some of the stubborn facts that must be faced in real life situations."[56] Our aim is to achieve a "re-flective equilibrium" between judgments and principles, a concept popular-ized by John Rawls in A Theory of Justice.[57] The approach is to work back and forth between our moral intuitions and judgments with the particular-ities of the case to identify the principles or rules that explain our judgments, revising the judgments or principles whenever necessary in order to achieve an acceptable coherence among them.[58]

The use of case studies will also facilitate the engagement of the diverse stakeholders in the transplantation community as well as those in health policy and ethics in a bidirectional process in which intuitions and principles are applied to cases in order to determine when they collide and need to be modified.

Our approach, then, uses analytical moral philosophy in a way that is responsive to the clinical facts and the social and historical context with the aim of creating a morally sound, clinically useful book that provides guidance in transplant practice and policy development and refinement.

1.7 How to Read This Book

We have designed this book such that it can be read from cover to cover, but we also recognize that some will choose to read more selectively. We encourage the reader to start with part 1, in which we provide a broad history of living donor transplantation and its intersection with deceased donor organ transplantation (chapter 2) and then develop a living donor ethics framework that will guide the resolution of ethical problems arising from transplantation involving living donors, help establish the moral limits of transplantation involving living donors, and help clarify our moral responsibilities to the living donor as a patient in his or her own right (chapter 3). All the other chapters have been written in a way that readers can pick and choose the themes that they want to explore. This does lead to some degree of repetition as there are some arguments that hold steady across chapters, although we have tried to keep the redundancy to a minimum.

Notes

1. Merrill JP, Harrison JH, Murray J, Guild WR. Successful homotransplantation of the kidney in an identical twin. *Trans Am Clin Climatol Assoc.* 1956;67:166–173.
2. Starzl TE. History of clinical transplantation. *World J Surg.* 2000;24:759–782.
3. Barker CF, Markmann JF. Historical overview of transplantation. *Cold Spring Harb. Perspect Med.* 2013;3(4):a014977, at p. 9. doi:10.1101/cshperspect.a014977
4. Küss R, Legrain M, Mathe G, Nedey R, Camey M. Homologous human kidney transplantation: experience with six patients. *Postgrad Med J.* 1962;38:528–531.

5. Barker and Markmann, "Historical," at p. 9.

6. Human kidney transplant conference. *Transplantation*. 1964;2(1):147–165.

7. Murray JE, Barnes BA, Atkinson J. Fifth report of the Human Kidney Transplant Registry. *Transplantation*. 1967;5(4):752–774.

8. Wolstenholme GEW, O'Connor M, eds. *Ethics in Medical Progress: With Special Reference to Transplantation*. Boston, MA: Little, Brown and Company; 1966, at p. viii.

9. Wolstenholme and O'Connor, *Ethics in Medical Progress*, at p. 76.

10. Wolstenholme and O'Connor, *Ethics in Medical Progress*, at p. 59.

11. Organ Procurement and Transplantation Network. National Data. https://optn.tra nsplant.hrsa.gov/data/view-data-reports/national-data/. Hereinafter referred to as OPTN Database.

12. See, for example, Segev DL, Muzaale AD, Caffo BS, et al. Perioperative mortality and long-term survival following live kidney donation. *JAMA*. 2010;303:959–966; and Gaston RS, Kumar V, Matas AJ. Reassessing medical risk in living kidney donors. *J Am Soc Nephrol*. 2015;26:1017–1019.

13. See, for example, Muzaale AD, Massie AB, Wainwright J, McBride MA, Wang M, Segev DL. Long-term risk of ESRD attributable to live kidney donation: matching with healthy non-donors. *Am J Transplant*. 2013;13(suppl 5):204–205; Mjoen G, Hallan S, Hartmann A, et al. Long-term risks for kidney donors. *Kidney International*. 2014;86:162–167; and Maggiore U, Budde K, Heemann U, et al. Long-term risks of kidney living donation: review and position paper by the ERA-EDTA DESCARTES working group. *Nephrol Dial Transplant*. 2017;32:216–223.

14. See, for example, Gibney EM, King AL, Maluf DG, Garg AX, Parikh CR. Living kidney donors requiring transplantation: focus on African Americans. *Transplantation*. 2007; 84:647–649; Ross LF, Thistlethwaite JR. Letter to the editor: long-term consequences of kidney donation. *N Engl J Med*. 2009;360;2371; and Doshi MD, Goggins MO, Li L, Garg AX. Medical outcomes in African American live kidney donors: a matched cohort study. *Am J Transplant*. 2013;13:111–118.

15. See, for example, Ibrahim HN, Akkina SK, Leister E, et al. Pregnancy outcomes after kidney donation. *Am J Transplant*. 2009;9:825–834; Reisaeter AV, Roislien J, Henriksen T, Irgens LM, Hartmann A. Pregnancy and birth after kidney donation: the Norwegian experience. *Am J Transplant*. 2009;9:820–824; and Garg AX, Nevis IF, McArthur E, et al. Gestational hypertension and preeclampsia in living kidney donors. *N Engl J Med*. 2015;372:124–133.

16. See, for example, Garg AX, Prasad GV, Thiessen-Philbrook HR, et al. Cardiovascular disease and hypertension risk in living kidney donors: an analysis of health administrative data in Ontario, Canada. *Transplantation*. 2008;86:399–406; and Reese PP, Bloom RD, Feldman HI, et al. Mortality and cardiovascular disease among older live kidney donors. *Am J Transplant*. 2014;14(8):1853–1861.

17. Doshi et al., "Medical outcomes in African American".

18. Umeshita K, Fujiwara K, Kiyosawa K, et al. Operative morbidity of living liver donors in Japan. *Lancet*. 2003;362(9385):687–690.

19. See, for example, Umeshita et al, "Operative morbidity"; Lo CM. Complications and long-term outcome of living liver donors: a survey of 1,508 cases in five Asian centers.

Transplantation. 2003;75(suppl 3):S12–15; and Ng KK, Lo CM. Liver transplantation in Asia: past, present and future. *Ann Acad Med, Singapore*. 2009;38:322–331.

20. See, for example, Olthoff KM, Abecassis MM, Emond JC, et al. Outcomes of adult living donor liver transplantation: comparison of the Adult-to-adult Living Donor Liver Transplantation Cohort Study and the national experience. *Liver Transplant*. 2011;17(7):789–797; and Abecassis MM, Fisher RA, Olthoff KM, et al. Complications of living donor hepatic lobectomy—a comprehensive report. *Am J Transplant*. 2012;12(5):1208–1217.

21. See Olthoff et al, "Outcomes"; and Abecassis et al, "Complications."

22. See Abecassis et al, "Complications."

23. See Abecassis et al, "Complications," at p. 1212.

24. See, for example, Adcock L, Macleod C, Dubay D, et al. Adult living liver donors have excellent long-term medical outcomes: the University of Toronto liver transplant experience. *Am J Transplant*. 2010;10:364–371; and Azoulay D, Bhangui P, Andreani P, et al. Short- and long-term donor morbidity in right lobe living donor liver transplantation: 91 consecutive cases in a European Center. *Am J Transplant*. 2011;11(1):101–110.

25. Allen MB, Abt PL, Reese PP. What are the harms of refusing to allow living kidney donation? An expanded view of risks and benefits. *Am J Transplant*. 2014;14:531–537.

26. Clemens KK, Thiessen-Philbrook H, Parikh CR, et al. Psychosocial health of living kidney donors: a systematic review. *Am J Transplant*. 2006;6(12):2965–2977.

27. See Allen et al, "What are the harms?"

28. See, for example, *Lee v Quarterman*, No. C-07-476, 2008 WL 3926118 at *2 (SD Tex 2008); and *Campbell v Wainwright*, 416 F2d 949, 950 (5th Cir 1969).

29. Elliott C. Doing harm: living organ donors, clinical research and the tenth man. *J Med Ethics*. 1995;21(2):91–96.

30. Ross LF. Donating a second kidney: a tale of family and ethics. *Semin Dial*. 2000;13(3):201–203.

31. Mazariegos GV, Morton DH, Sindhi B, et al. Liver transplantation for classical maple syrup urine disease: long-term follow-up in 37 patients and comparative United Network for Organ Sharing experience. *J Pediatr*. 2012;160(1):116–121.e1.

32. Rodrigue JR, Cornell DL, Lin JK, Kaplan B, Howard RJ. Increasing live donor kidney transplantation: a randomized controlled trial of a home-based educational intervention. *Am J Transplant*. 2007;7:394–401; Waterman AD, Barrett AC, Stanley SL. Optimal transplants education for recipients to increase pursuit of living donation. *Prog Transplant*. 2008;18:55–56; Boulware LE, Hill-Briggs F, Kraus ES, et al. Effectiveness of educational and social worker interventions to activate patients' discussion and pursuit of preemptive living donor kidney transplantation: a randomized controlled trial. *Am J Kidney Dis*. 2013;61:476–486; and Waterman AD, Robbins ML, Paiva AL, et al. Measuring kidney patients' motivation to pursue living donor kidney transplant: development of stage of change, decisional balance and self-efficacy measures. *J Health Psych*. 2015;20:210–221.

33. Garonzik-Wang JM, Berger JC, Ros RL, et al. Live donor champion: finding live kidney donors by separating the advocate from the patient. *Transplantation*. 2012;93:1147–1150.

34. Veatch RM, Ross LF. *Transplantation Ethics.* 2nd ed. Washington, DC: Georgetown University Press; 2015.
35. The National Commission for the Protection of Human Subjects of Biomedical and Behavioral Research. *The Belmont Report: Ethical Principles and Guidelines for the Protection of Human Subjects of Research.* Washington, DC: Government Printing Office; 1978. http://www.hhs.gov/ohrp/humansubjects/guidance/belmont.html. August 7, 2021. Hereinafter referred to as the *Belmont Report.*
36. *Belmont Report.*
37. Kipnis K. Vulnerability in Research Subjects: A Bioethical Taxonomy. In: The National Bioethics Advisory Commission. *Ethical and Policy Issues in Research Involving Human Participants. Volume II: Commissioned Papers and Staff Analysis.* Bethesda, MD: National Bioethics Advisory Commission; 2001:G1–13; and Kipnis, K. Seven vulnerabilities in the pediatric research subject. *Theor Med.* 2003;24:107–120, at p. 110.
38. Goodin RE. *Protecting the Vulnerable: A Reanalysis of Our Social Responsibilities.* Chicago, IL: University of Chicago Press; 1985.
39. Department of Health and Human Services, Part II. Centers for Medicare and Medicaid Services. 42 CFR Parts 405, 482, 488, and 498. Medicare Program; Hospital Conditions of Participation: Requirements for Approval and Re-Approval of Transplant Centers to Perform Organ Transplants. *Fed Regist.* 2007;72(61):15198–15280
40. As we discuss in the next chapter, this is consistent with our modification of respect for persons to incorporate both relational autonomy as well as the more traditional autonomy described in bioethics textbooks. See, for example,Beauchamp TL, Childress JF. *Principle of Biomedical Ethics.* 3rd ed. New York, NY: Oxford University Press; 1989. Relational autonomy was first developed in the feminist ethics literature. See, for example, Mackenzie C, Sotljar N. *Relational Autonomy: Feminist Perspectives on Autonomy, Agency, and the Social Self.* New York, NY: Oxford University Press; 2000.
41. Elliott, "Doing harm," at p. 95.
42. Ross LF, Thistlethwaite JR, American Academy of Pediatrics Committee on Bioethics. Minors as living solid-organ donors. *Pediatrics.* 2008;122:454–461.
43. Ross, LF, Rubin D, Siegler M, Josephson MA, Thistlethwaite JR Jr, Woodle ES. Ethics of a paired-kidney-exchange program. *N Engl J Med.* 1997;336:1752–1755.
44. Sade RM. Brain death, cardiac death, and the dead donor rule. *J S C Med Assoc.* 2011;107:146–149, at p. 147.
45. Samstein B, de Melo-Martin I, Kapur S, Ratner L, Emond J. A liver for a kidney: ethics of trans-organ paired exchange. *Am J Transplant.* 2018;18(5):1077–1082.
46. Krawiec KD, Rees MA. Reverse transplant tourism. *Law Contemp Probl.* 2014;77:145–173.
47. See, for example, Genovese G, Friedman DJ, Ross MD, et al. Association of trypanolytic ApoL1 variants with kidney disease in African Americans. *Science.* 2010;329:841–845; and Tzur S, Rosset S, Shemer R, et al. Missense mutations in the APOL1 gene are highly associated with end stage kidney disease risk previously attributed to the MYH9 gene. *Hum Genet.* 2010;128:345–350.

48. See, for example, Genovese et al, "Association"; Reeves-Daniel AM, DePalma JA, Bleyer AJ, et al. The APOL1 gene and allograft survival after kidney transplantation. *Am J Transplant*. 2011;11:1025–1030; Foster MC, Coresh J, Fornage M, et al. APOL1 variants associate with increased risk of CKD among African Americans. *J Am Soc Nephrol*. 2013;24:1484–1491; Parsa A, Kao WH, Xie D, et al. APOL1 risk variants, race, and progression of chronic kidney disease. *N Engl J Med*. 2013;369:2183–2196; and Palanisamy A, Reeves-Daniel AM, Freedman BI. The impact of APOL1, CAV1, and ABCB1 gene variants on outcomes in kidney transplantation: donor and recipient effects. *Pediatr Nephrol*. 2014;29:1485–1492.

49. Olabisi O, Al-Romaih K, Henderson J, et al. From man to fish: what can Zebrafish tell us about ApoL1 nephropathy. *Clin Nephrol*. 2016;86(suppl 1):114–118; Mohan S, Iltis AS, Sawinski D, DuBois JM. APOL1 genetic testing in living kidney transplant donors. *Am J Kidney Dis*. 2019;74:538–543; and Shah S, Shapiro R, Murphy B, Menon MC. APOL1 high-risk genotypes and renal transplantation. *Clin Transpl*. 2019;33:e13582. https://doi.org/10.1111/ctr.13582

50. McIntosh T, Mohan S, Sawinski D, Iltis A, DuBois J. Variation of ApoL1 testing practices for living kidney donors. *Prog Transpl*. 2020;30:22–28.

51. The phrase "spare parts" was used by Joseph Murray at the CIBA symposium: "However, it is the kidney which is the current-day 'prototype' of the 'spare part' organ. Kidneys come in two's, and a person can live normally on one." As quoted in Wolstenholme and O'Connor, *Ethics in Medical Progress*, citing Murray at p. 61. Paul Ramsey in his classic work, *The Patient as Person* (New Haven, CT: Yale University Press; 1970) also used the phrase where he described "spart parts" transplant therapy as a challenge to our morality because it requires the sacrifice of one patient for the well-being of another (p. 194). The phrase was popularized in 1992 with the publication of *Spare Parts: Organ Replacement in American* Society, by Renée C Fox and Judith P Swazey (New York, NY: Oxford University Press; 1992), in which the authors assert that their disquietude (cynicism) has moved them to leave the field. Although Fox and Swazey wrote in the final chapter of *Spare Parts* about rereading Ramsey's *The Patient as Person*, they credit the sociologist Erving Goffman with proposing the phrase. They explain that Goffman proposed the phrase "spare parts" for their first book (which was ultimately entitled *The Courage to Fail*. Chicago, IL: Chicago University Press; 1974) because "at that time we considered it too cynical for us to adopt" (*Spare Parts*, at p. 205). That they chose the phrase for the title of their follow-up book emphasizes their disillusionment, their "increasingly troubled and critical reactions to the expansion organ replacement has undergone during the past decade" (*Spare Parts*, p. xv). We are more optimistic than Fox and Swazey given some greater attention by the transplant community to the risks that donors face in the last 2 decades. However, as we will discuss in forthcoming chapters, there are some trends and programs that raise serious red flags by seeking to solve the organ shortage by engaging more living organ donors without due consideration to the donor's status as a patient to whom we have special responsibilities.

52. As of August 7, 2021, women accounted for 104,760 and men accounted for 70,524 of all living solid organ donors in the US since 1988. Women were more likely to be living solid organ donors for all organs except lung (men accounted for 301 and women accounted for 177 living lung donors) and intestines (21 women and 23 men donors were living intestinal donors). See OPTN database. https://optn.transplant. hrsa.gov/data/view-data-reports/national-data/.

53. Between 1988 and August 7, 2021, men were the recipients of 105,071 living donor grafts whereas women were only the recipients of 70,013 living solid organ donor grafts in the United States. Men were more likely to be recipients for all living organ grafts except pancreas (men 10 and women 14), kidney/pancreas (men 20 and women 28), and lung (men 89 and women 164 living donor graft recipients). See OPTN database. https://optn.transplant.hrsa.gov/data/view-data-reports/national-data/.

54. Loesche D. The prison gender gap. *Statista*. October 23, 2017. https://www.statista.com/ chart/11573/gender-of-inmates-in-us-federal-prisons-and-general-population/

55. Barkley EF, Cross KP, Major CH. *Collaborative Learning Techniques: A Handbook for College Faculty*. San Francisco, CA: Jossey-Bass; 2005, at p. 182.

56. Lawrence P. The preparation of case material. In: Andrews KR, ed. *The Case Method of Teaching Human Relations and Administration*. Cambridge, MA: Harvard University Press; 1953, at p. 215.

57. Rawls J. *A Theory of Justice*. Cambridge, MA: Harvard University Press; 1971.

58. Daniels N. Reflective equilibrium. In: Zalta EN, ed. The *Stanford Encyclopedia of Philosophy*; 2003, rev. 2016. https://plato.stanford.edu/entries/reflective-equilibrium/

2

The History of Solid
Organ Transplantation

In this chapter we provide a brief history of solid organ transplantation. Although our focus is on the living donor, the history of living donor solid organ transplantation is intertwined with the history of deceased donor solid organ transplantation and so there is some detail on deceased donor transplantation. This is particularly important in the early years of solid organ transplantation because for some solid organs, the earliest success began with living donors (eg, kidney) and in other organs, the earliest success began with deceased donors (eg, liver).

2.1 Introduction

Between 1988 and 2020, over 160,000 individuals have served as living kidney donors in the United States (US) and over 8,000 individuals have served as living donors for other solid organs (> 90% of these other solid organ grafts are liver lobes, but individuals have also served as living donors for lung lobes, uterus, parts of pancreas, parts of intestine, and as living domino heart and liver donors).[1] A major benefit offered by living donors is flexibility in the timing of transplantation because one can often electively schedule a living donation which is not the case for deceased donor organ transplantation.[2] For some organs, living donor organs also offer improved long-term recipient outcomes.[3] The major disadvantage is the clinical risks to which the living donors are exposed (which we explored briefly in chapter 1).

Kidneys were the first (successful) living solid organ transplant and are the most frequent organs procured from living donors, so it makes sense that we begin the history of living donor solid organ transplantation with the history of living kidney donor transplants.

The Living Organ Donor as Patient. Lainie Friedman Ross and J. Richard Thistlethwaite, Jr, Oxford University Press.
© Oxford University Press 2022. DOI: 10.1093/oso/9780197618202.003.0002

2.2 Kidney Transplantation

The first deceased donor kidney transplant was performed in 1933 by the Soviet surgeon Yu Yu Voronoy. In writing about the historic experiment, Clyde Barker and James Markmann explain: "the kidney was not procured until 6 hours after the donor's death and . . . it was transplanted across a major blood group mismatch probably accounted for its prompt failure."[4] Voronoy performed fo4ur additional transplants over the following 16 years without success.[5]

In 1951, 2 teams working separately in Paris performed 9 kidney transplants.[6] The first 8 donors were deceased donors and all recipients died within days or weeks. The ninth transplant was a living donor kidney transplant (LDKT) that was performed by Drs. Louis Michon and Jean Hamburger at the Hospital Necker (Paris), where they transplanted a mother's kidney into her son.[7] The graft functioned well for 3 weeks despite the fact that the only immunosuppressive agent available was cortisone. Similar attempts were occurring in Boston, where David Hume performed 9 kidney transplants between 1951 and 1953 involving 6 deceased and 3 living donors.[8] Five kidneys did not function at all, 3 functioned briefly, and 1 functioned for 5.5 months before it was rejected.[9]

The first LDKT with long-term success is credited to Joseph Murray and colleagues at the Peter Bent Hospital (Boston) where, in 1954, they performed the first LDKT between identical twin brothers, obviating the need for immunosuppression.[10] The graft functioned for 8 years until Richard Herrick, the recipient, developed kidney problems unrelated to the surgery.[11] The donor, Ronald Herrick, died in 2010 at age 79 years from complications following heart surgery.[12]

By the early 1960s, more effective immunosuppression was actively being developed and the field of transplantation began to expand rapidly.[13] In 1963, Murray developed a voluntary registry for deceased and living donor kidney transplants. In the first published report, Murray cited global data about 244 kidney transplants.[14] The 13th and final report of the Human Renal Transplant Registry was published in 1977. At the time of the final report, 25,108 kidney transplants had been registered from 301 institutions, 165 of which were in the US.[15] An important factor in the expansion of kidney transplantation was the passage of an amendment to the Social Security Act in 1972, which was enacted in July 1973.[16] It provided national health insurance and coverage through Medicare to virtually all individuals in the US with end-stage renal disease (ESRD).[17]

Murray's registry included both living and deceased donor organs. Initially most donors were living: of the 374 donors reported in the registry as of March 1964, 275 (74%) were from living individuals and 99 (26%) from deceased donors.[18] But shortly thereafter the trend reversed. In 1967, 49% of transplants were deceased donor organs, and the percentage increased to 56% in 1968 and 62% in 1969.[19]

Although an organized system for procuring and allocating deceased donor organs was not needed in the earliest years, the increasing impor-tance of deceased donor transplantation, the development (and adoption) of brain death as an ethical and legal way to determine death in 1968, and better preservation techniques in the early 1970s made coordinated organ banks necessary.[20] These early organ banks transformed into organ procure-ment organizations (OPOs). While some only served 1 transplant program, others served as many as 10 nearby programs. Improved preservation and new advances in tissue typing led to greater cooperation between centers and several organ sharing programs such as the South-Eastern Regional Organ Procurement Program (SEROPP), the New England Organ Bank, and the Los Angeles Transplant Society formed.[21] Although originally co-ordinated at the Medical College of Virginia, in 1975 SEROPP incorporated as the South-Eastern Organ Procurement Foundation (SEOPF) with 18 charter member transplant programs. In January 1977, the SEOPF computer system was named United Network for Organ Sharing (UNOS) in response to requests from non-SEOPF transplant centers to use the SEOPF computer system for registering potential recipients and sharing kidneys.[22] By 1982, SEOPF's UNOS computer system was becoming a national transplant candi-date registry. Passage of the National Organ Transplant Act (NOTA) by the US Congress in 1984 led to the establishment of a "framework for a national organ recovery and allocation system in the private sector."[23] As M. Christian Williams and colleagues explain:

Although separate organizations, UNOS and SEOPF remained closely intertwined, sharing office space, computer hardware, and personnel. In 1986, UNOS was awarded a federal contract by the Health Resources and Services Administration of the U.S. Department of Health and Human Services to establish and operate the national OPTN [Organ Procurement and Transplantation Network]. UNOS separated from SEOPF in 1987, with SEOPF transferring to UNOS the Organ Center, computer facilities, office space, and personnel.[24]

While the main functions of UNOS was and continues to be the coordination of the procurement and allocation of deceased donor organs and the maintenance of deceased donor transplant registries, it has also collected limited data about living donors. With the ever-growing gap between demand and supply of deceased donors organs, transplant programs became more willing to accept living donors, and in 1994 the OPTN began collecting social security numbers of living donors making it feasible to track them.[25] Beginning in 2000, the OPTN required transplantation centers to collect 1 year of follow-up data for living donors, which was expanded to 2 years in 2006. In 2000, the number of living kidney donors (5511) surpassed the number of deceased donors (5489) for the first time, although the number of deceased donor kidney transplants (8126) was almost double the number of living donor kidneys because living donors can only provide 1 kidney whereas deceased donors can supply 2.[26] For the past 5 years, living kidneys donors have accounted for approximately 40% of all kidney donors annually.

Part of the reason for the growth of living donation between 1988 (1,817 living donors) and 2000 (5,511 living donors) was the growing acceptance of living kidney donors from non-genetically related living donors.[27] In the early years, non-genetically related living donors made up a significant percentage of living donors. In the first Report of the Registry in Human Kidney Transplantation,[28] Murray recorded 52 (29.5%) nonrelated donors out of 176 donors in September 1963, and 57 nonrelated donors and 9 spouses (66/275, or 24%) donors in the second report which ended in March 1964.[29] By the late 1960s, however, most surgeons stopped recruiting non-genetically related donors (spouses, volunteers who are now known as Good Samaritan or nondirected donors, and prisoners) because the results were no better than transplants using deceased donor grafts.[30] The recruitment of nonrelated donors only began to increase again in the late 1980s. Aaron Spital documented the changing recruitment practices of transplant programs. In 1989, he surveyed 169 transplant programs and received 100 responses. At the time, only 24 centers had performed a living donor transplant between spouses, although 76% stated they would consider it. Only 3 centers had used a friend donor, although 48% said they would consider it. None had performed a transplant using a kidney from a stranger (what is known today as a Good Samaritan or nondirected donor), although 8% stated they would consider it.[31] In 1994 and 1999, Spital repeated this survey documenting the greater acceptance of donations by spouses, friends, and strangers (see Table 2.1).[32]

What were the major concerns in expanding beyond the genetic relationship? The first was the potential for poorer results based on the greater chance for antigenic incompatibility between unrelated individuals, but improved immunosuppressive protocols reduced this concern. The second concern was the motivation of donors who were not genetically related. This concern was based on an idealistic view that "blood is thicker than water," meaning that family members have a greater vested interest in donating because of their genetic bonds. The scant data that exist suggest, in contrast, that family members may donate voluntarily to help a loved one, but also show that some donate less willingly—some feel subtle (or not so subtle) pressure, or choose to donate to avoid family conflict.[33] But acceptance of non-biological related donors took time, starting first with spouses on the basis of greatest emotional relationship. Acceptance was further strengthened by the data from Terasaki and colleagues, which showed that the results of transplants between spouses were as good as transplants between biological relatives.[34]

In 2000, Arthur Matas and colleagues at the University of Minnesota published an ethical evaluation of their experience with permitting living donation by non-directed donors.[35] Their center had been contacted by 98 persons, 18 of whom had been evaluated and 4 of whom had donated.[36] Their protocol addressed many important issues including, the evaluation process for the donor and recipient, the selection process of the recipient, the timing of the evaluation and surgery, and issues of privacy and confidentiality. A full

Table 2.1 US Transplant Centers' Willingness to Accept Non-Genetically Related Kidney Donors

Relation	Willingness	1987 (n=100)	1993 (n=127)	1999 (n =129)
Spouse	% centers had performed	24	46	n/a
	% would consider	76	88	n/a
Friend	% centers had performed	3	17	69
	% would consider	48	63	93
Stranger	% centers had performed	0	0	14
	% would consider	8	15	38

These data can be found in Spital A. Evolution of attitudes at US transplant centers toward kidney donation by friends and altruistic strangers. *Transplantation.* 2000;69:1728–1731.

discussion of the ethical issues raised by Good Samaritan donors can be found in chapter 7.

A second innovative expansion of living donors was the kidney paired exchange program. Imagine that Donor 1 cannot donate to her intended recipient (Recipient 1) because she is blood type A and he is blood type B. Now imagine that there is another Donor, Donor 2, who cannot donate to her intended Recipient (Recipient 2) because she is blood type B and he is blood type A. Donor 1, however, could donate to Recipient 2, and Donor 2 could donate to Recipient 1 in what is referred to as a kidney paired exchange (see Figure 2.1).

Although kidney paired exchange was first described by Rapaport in 1986,[37] the idea of kidney exchanges did not get traction in the US until we published an article in 1997 in *The New England Journal of Medicine* along with colleagues from the University of Chicago that addressed the ethical issues that such a program would need to address.[38] Although several exchanges had been performed by Kiil Park and colleagues in Korea in the 1990s,[39] the first US exchange took place at Rhode Island Hospital in October 2000[40] followed by a number of paired exchanges at Johns Hopkins.[41] Paired exchanges then expanded to 3-way exchanges and 4-way exchanges but were limited by the perceived need to perform all of the surgeries at the same time in order to ensure that no donor reneged, leaving his or her matched recipient without an organ.

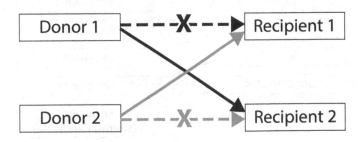

Dashed arrows with an X: Histo*incompatible* donations that *cannot* occur.
Solid arrows: Histocompatible donations that occur.

Figure 2.1 Paired Exchange of Organs Between Two Living Donor-Recipient Pairs Due to ABO- or HLA-incompatibility, Donor 1 cannot donate to Recipient 1, and Donor 2 cannot donate to Recipient 2, but Donor 1 can donate to Recipient 2, and Donor 2 can donate to Recipient 1. This is referred to as a kidney paired exchange.

In 2006, Robert Montgomery and colleagues at Johns Hopkins proposed a variation on kidney exchanges that they called "domino paired kidney donation."[42] Originally proposed as simultaneous operative procedures by Montgomery and colleagues, it was then modified by Rees and colleagues to an asynchronous chain performed over days to weeks.[43] An asynchronous chain involves allocating a kidney from a Good Samaritan donor to a candidate with an incompatible living donor, who then donates her kidney to another candidate with an incompatible donor, who "pays it forward"—that is, the donor donates to a candidate after her own intended recipient has received an organ (see Figure 2.2).[44] In Montgomery's first domino chain catalyzed by a nondirected living donor, the final recipient was a candidate from the waitlist ("1st eligible recipient from UNOS match run").[45]

In 2007, the National Kidney Registry (NKR), a private not-for-profit organization, was founded by Garet Hil to facilitate exchanges and chains.[46] NKR has been quite successful in coordinating paired exchanges and domino chains nationwide. In 2008, NKR facilitated 21 transplants, and that number has increased annually to 399 in 2016 and 760 in 2019.[47]

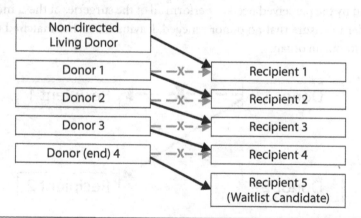

Dashed gray arrows with an X: Histo*incompatible* donations that *cannot* occur.
Solid black arrows: Histocompatible donations that occur.

Figure 2.2 Domino Chain Catalyzed by a Nondirected Living Donor
A domino chain involving multiple donor-recipient pairs is catalyzed by a nondirected or Good Samaritan donor. In this domino chain, all of the donors are incompatible with their paired recipients, but they are able to donate to other recipients. The domino chain ends with the end donor donating to a candidate on the deceased donor waitlist who does not have a paired living donor.

The original NKR design, however, was not to end chains with a waitlist candidate as proposed by Montgomery and colleagues, but instead to create a never-ending altruistic donor (NEAD) chain involving nonsimultaneous donation, with some donors waiting weeks to months to donate (so-called "bridge donors") until another incompatible donor-recipient pair was located.[48] But experience found that the longer the "bridge donor" had to wait, the less likely she was to donate. Some bridge donors became ineligible to donate while waiting or decided not to donate.[49] As such, NKR reversed course and began to end chains with candidates on the waitlist who did not have an available living donor. The ethics of ending a domino chain with a waitlist candidate versus employing a NEAD strategy is discussed in chapter 8.

One other change that has expanded living kidney donation has been the move from the very healthy living donor to the "medically complex" living donor. The term "medically complex" was coined by Peter Reese, who rejected "expanded living donor" and "marginal living donor" to avoid confusion with deceased donor organs that are called expanded (deceased) donors or marginal (deceased) donors.[50] Long-term donor and recipient outcomes for medically complex donors have not been adequately studied.[51]

Selection criteria as well as evaluation practices for donors have varied between centers from the beginning. In 1995, the Patient Care and Education Committee of the American Society of Transplant physicians (now the American Society of Transplantation (AST)) conducted a survey examining living donor evaluation procedures.[52] The study was repeated by Mandelbrot and colleagues in 2007.[53] In Table 2.2, we enumerate the changes in exclusion criteria.[54] For many conditions, the changes are minimal, although there is a movement to include less healthy individuals (eg, older individuals with well-controlled hypertension, individuals with higher BMIs, etc.).

A problem with both the variability and the "loosening" of criteria is summed up clearly by Peter Reese and colleagues: "The problem is one of decision making in the absence of sound medical data or consensus guidelines."[55] Long-term donor risks are difficult to ascertain when programs are still only required to collect 2 years' worth of follow-up outcomes. Nevertheless, in the last few years, several retrospective papers have been published that show both increased risk of ESRD as well as other long-term health problems including cardiovascular disease and all-cause mortality of living donors.[56] Niemi and Mandelbrot further note that the absence of sound data applies not only to the donor's risks for developing

Table 2.2 Living Kidney Donor Exclusion Criteria

	Bia (1985)	Mandelbrot (2007)
Age: older donor	27% no age exclusion; other programs have age exclusion from 55–75 years	59% no age exclusion; other programs have age exclusions from 55–75 years
Age: younger donors	11% have no age exclusion; 68% exclude those under 18 and 7% exclude those under 20	2% have no age exclusion; 77% exclude those younger than 18 and 19% have exclusions between 18–21
Diabetes	9% perform glucose tolerance testing on all donors	Most programs perform glucose tolerance testing
Hypertension	64% exclude a donor taking any antihypertensive agent	47% exclude a donor on any antihypertensive; 41% exclude if taking more than one medication
Kidney function	59% exclude donors with a creatinine clearance, 80ml/min/ 1.73m^2	67% exclude donors with a creatinine clearance $\leq$ 80ml/min/ 1.73m^2
Kidney stones	34% exclude if history of nephrolithiasis	23% exclude if history of nephrolithiasis
Hematuria	31% of centers exclude donors with persistent hematuria (10–15 RBCs per high powered field)	21% automatically exclude with persistent hematuria; others willing to consider if urological evaluation and renal biopsy are negative
Proteinuria	58% exclude if protein between 300–1000 mg/day	44% exclude if protein between 300–1000; and 36% use cut off of 150 mg/day
Obesity	16% exclude a donor with moderate obesity	52% exclude donors with BMI >35; 10% exclude donors with BMI >30

Data are derived from Bia MJ, Ramos EL, Danovitch GM, et al. Evaluation of living renal donors. The current practice of US transplant centers. *Transplantation*. 1995;60:322–327; and Mandelbrot DA, Pavlakis M, Danovitch GM, et al. The medical evaluation of living kidney donors: a survey of US transplant centers. *Am J Transplant*. 2007;7:2333-2343.

health problems, but also for consideration of recipient outcomes.[57] Making decisions under medical uncertainty is difficult; it is exacerbated in living donor transplantation by the fact that the clinical implications may accrue to both the donor and the recipient. In chapter 15 we discuss this specific issue with respect to Apolipoprotein L1 (APOL1).

Social scientists have also tried to expand LDKT by identifying and helping transplant programs overcome barriers to LDKT. Back in 1977, Roberta Simmons and colleagues noted that individuals with ESRD did not like to ask relatives for a kidney but instead would merely state that they needed a kidney.[58] The decision not to ask directly made it easier for the candidate who did not want to put pressure on potentially ambivalent relatives or have to face direct rejection. While it made it easier for the family member who did not want to donate to ignore the request, it also meant that some family members did not understand that the statement of need was actually a request and thus did not offer a kidney even though they may have been willing to do so.

To increase living donation, then, social scientists began to develop programs that teach candidates (or a designated "donor champion" or "donor coach") how to approach family members, friends, and even strangers by telling the story frequently in-person and/or on social media.[59] This is especially important for those of lower socioeconomic status and minority ethnicity who are more reluctant to share their story.[60] Transplant centers, however, are not only educating the candidates, but actively developing programs to educate potential donors and help them navigate the system.[61] A consensus conference was held in 2014 to identify best practices to overcome barriers to living donation as a means of expanding access to LDKT.[62] It included identifying best education practices both within and beyond the transplant center.[63]

2.3 Liver Transplantation

In contrast with kidney transplantation, which had its first successes with living donors, the first successful deceased donor liver transplants in the US were performed by Thomas Starzl in the 1960s,[64] but outcomes were poor and few were performed until the mid-1980s, when improvements in immunosuppression led to better results.[65] In 1983, a National Institutes of Health consensus conference on liver transplantation paved the way for deceased donor liver transplant to no longer be considered experimental,[66] and the number of liver transplant programs and the number of transplants performed increased significantly.

But even as deceased donor liver transplant gained traction, young children with congenital liver disease such as alpha-1-antitrypsin deficiency and biliary atresia had particularly high mortality rates because a satisfactory size-matched deceased donor liver was not available. It was estimated that 20%–30% of children with end-stage liver disease in the 1980s were dying waiting for a pediatric sized deceased donor organ.[67] Two deceased donor liver techniques—reduced-size and split-liver grafts from deceased liver donors—lowered but did not eliminate waiting list mortality for infants and children. The use of reduced-size grafts was devised by Henri Bismuth in France in 1984 and involved dissecting a deceased donor adult liver along intrahepatic segmental planes to create a smaller but anatomically intact functional liver appropriately sized for a small child (and the remaining portion of the liver discarded).[68] Split-liver transplants were pioneered by Rudolf Pichlmayr, who first performed this procedure in Germany in 1988.[69] The split-liver technique involves dividing the deceased donor liver in such a way that both halves can be allocated to recipients (the left lateral segment to the child; the extended right lobe to an adult). Even though the split liver procedure allows for 2 transplants—1 allocated to a child and the other to an adult—the larger (right lobe) split-liver grafts were found to have a lower survival rate than full-size (non-split) liver grafts.[70]

Both the reduced-size and split-liver procedures were controversial because it was felt that they solved the pediatric shortage by exacerbating the shortage for adults and/or by giving an adult a suboptimal partial graft even when the adult had allocational priority for the whole liver. However, recent data suggest that some centers with greater experience do have equivalent results with extended right lobe grafts when the second recipient is a child and is transplanted with a left lateral lobe segment.[71]

The split-liver technique, originally developed to increase deceased donor organs for children, was quickly attempted for use with 2 adult recipients. The first attempt was for 2 adults in acute liver failure by Bismuth and colleagues in 1988 (the same year Picylmayr first performed this for an adult and child recipient). Both died rather quickly (on day 20 and 45 respectively).[72] Since then, many have sought to improve the technique to maximize the number of deceased donor grafts available.[73] The main concern, however, is that split-liver transplantation "is technically demanding, may cause increased perioperative complications, and may potentially transform an excellent deceased donor organ into two marginal quality grafts."[74] While there have been some satisfactory results in selected centers, the complexities of the surgery and the risk of small-for-size grafts limits its widespread adoption.[75]

The split liver technique was quickly modified into a way of procuring living liver grafts. The idea of removing an anatomically intact portion of a liver to provide a living donor liver graft had actually been conceptualized as early as 1969.[76] In the 1980s, the first 2 attempts of living donor liver transplantation (LDLT) from an adult to a child in Brazil failed.[77] In 1989, Russell Strong and colleagues in Australia performed the first successful living adult left lateral segment (LLS) liver donor transplant into a child.[78] That same year, a team of transplant surgeons and clinical ethicists at the University of Chicago published a discussion of the process by which they decided to perform a prospective institutional review board-approved study of pediatric LDLT in the *New England Journal of Medicine*.[79] One of us was part of the team (JRT) that discussed the steps that needed to be taken by a surgical team before undertaking what was considered to be an experimental procedure. In the article, the authors described their protocol and consent form, the anticipated risks and benefits to the donors and recipients, the process by which donors and recipients would be selected, and the informed consent process for both the donors and recipients. This protocol was submitted to the institutional review board of the University of Chicago Hospital for approval and the manuscript was intentionally published well before the trial was begun to get feedback from the larger transplant and medical community.

The minimal feedback was positive and the study was performed. The results of the first 20 donor-recipient pairs that comprised the surgical trial were reported in the *Annals of Surgery* in 1991.[80] Because of concern for injury to the graft, the first 3 procedures were performed as full left lobe resections with transplantation of only the LLS after ex vivo reduction.[81] The procedure was then modified to only procure the left lateral segment, unless the recipient needed more liver mass (5 patients), in which cases the full left lobe was transplanted.[82] Patient survival was 91% at 6 months, 88% at 1 year, and 84% at 2 years, with graft survival 81% at 6 months and 73% at both 1 and 2 years.[83] The living donor graft survival was comparable to deceased donor transplants in all age groups at that time and better for children less than 1 year of age.[84] Living donor LLS liver transplant into pediatric patients was quickly adopted around the globe with excellent results.[85]

The first successful LDLT between 2 adults was performed in Japan in 1993 using the donor's left lobe.[86] It is not surprising that Asian countries were quick to develop adult LDLT given the dearth of deceased donor procurement systems in many of these countries and the high rate of infectious hepatitis causing liver failure.

The increasing awareness of the importance of graft volume and graft:recipient weight led to the introduction of right lobe LDLT. While a right lobe LDLT had been performed by the Kyoto group in 1992 for transplantation into a 9 year-old recipient because of a left lobe arterial anatomy variant not conducive to left lobe procurement and transplantation,[87] it was not until 1996 that the first right hepatic lobe LDLT between 2 adults was reported from Hong Kong.[88]

The first successful right hepatic lobe living liver transplant in the US was reported by the University of Colorado in 1998,[89] and its success led to rapid adoption of adult-to-adult living liver transplantation by many liver transplant programs throughout the US.[90] The rapid expansion of adult-to-adult living donor liver transplant (aLDLT) in the US and its unintended consequences will be discussed further in chapter 9.

The main concern about the rapid expansion is the donor morbidity associated with aLDLT using either a whole left lobe or right liver lobe. One proposal to reduce the risk in aLDLT in Asia was to experiment with 2 adult donors, both donating a LLS to a single adult candidate rather than removing a full lobe from 1 healthy donor.[91] While it reduces the risk to each donor, it does double the number of donors placed at risk. In a review of dual LLS graft adult LDLT at a single center in South Korea, Song and colleagues describe 400 dual LLS graft adult LDLT with excellent results (89.2%, 85.5%, and 80.2% patient survival at 1, 5, and 10 years respectively) although they acknowledge technical complexity and longer operative time limit as drawbacks.[92] Dual lobe segments from 2 different living liver donors have been performed around the world, although mainly in Asia.[93] It has not been performed in the US.

The low rate of deceased donor liver transplant in Asian countries and the high rate of end-stage liver disease secondary to viral hepatitis have led to the adoption of novel approaches like dual left lateral segment living liver donor transplants. Another novel approach is the living liver paired exchange programs, similar to kidney paired exchange programs, which have only been performed in Asia.[94] Unlike kidney paired exchanges, living liver paired exchanges raise ethical issues due to greater and more variable surgical risk for both the donor and recipient. For example, larger recipients may require an entire right lobe whereas a young child would only require a left lateral segment. The morbidity and mortality risks of these different procedures are discussed in chapter 1. Cronin and colleagues suggest that if this were to be adopted in the US, "candidates and donors would require prospective selection and matching for similar degrees of surgical intervention and expected outcomes."[95] At minimum, this would require a robust consent process with many opportunities for either donor to renege. It does not appear such lobar risk matching is done in Asia. The question of live donation between donor-recipient pairs involving different degrees of donor risk is discussed in the context of bi-donor paired exchange discussed in chapter 12.

2.4 Lung Transplantation

James Hardy and Watts Webb performed the first deceased donor lung transplant in June 1963, which functioned for 18 days before the patient died of renal failure and infection.[96] Over the next 15 years, 38 single lung, lung lobe, or heart-lung transplants were attempted without long-term success. Improvements in surgical techniques, candidate selection, and immunosuppression led to major improvements in deceased donor lung transplant outcomes in the 1980s, at which point supply became a problem.[97]

The first living donor lung donation was reported in 1990 and involved a mother who gave part of her right lung to her 12-year-old child who had been born premature and suffered from bronchopulmonary dysplasia.[98] Vaughn Starnes soon thereafter reported on 6 lung transplant candidates (including the original 12-year-old lung transplant recipient):

> Ages ranged from 17 days to 21 years. Transplant procedures were unilateral in the neonates and two of the children and bilateral in the child and adult who had cystic fibrosis. The donor lobes were from cadavers in the two neonates and living related donors in the children and the adult.[99]

The use of dual living donor lobar lung transplants, where a right and left lower lobe from 2 healthy donors are implanted in a recipient, became the norm. Describing 38 lung transplant recipients in 1996 involving 76 living donors, Starnes explained who the living donors were:

> Initially, as per our original institutional review board protocol at the University of Southern California and Children's Hospital Los Angeles, parents were the only donors used for living-donor lobar transplantation. This restriction limited the ability to offer this option to patients whose parents were not considered suitable donors because of results of diagnostic testing or age. Living-donor lobar transplantation was subsequently expanded to include all extended relatives and also unrelated donors. The evolution was gradual and in conjunction with the institutional review board.[100]

As of 2006, intraoperative complications were found to occur in 4% of donors and another 5% experience complications requiring surgical or bronchoscopic intervention without any reported deaths.[101] A national study group, RELIVE (Renal and Lung Living Donors Evaluation), did a retrospective analysis of lung transplantation in the US and was critical of the donor outcome data available:

> Due to a paucity of accurate, reliable and comprehensive outcomes data for live lung donors, potential donors do not have robust information on which to base an informed consent decision for undergoing donor evaluation and surgery. In addition to limited and inconsistent data regarding short-term donor morbidity, the long-term risk of pulmonary dysfunction and other adverse outcomes remains unknown. Investigators have not published results from large-scale and long-term studies of the effects of live lung donation on donor pulmonary function, health-related quality of life and psychological well-being. [102]

The main concern of living donor lung donation was the potential morbidity and mortality of 2 living donors for each candidate. Yusen and colleagues in the RELIVE study concluded that "the use of two live donors for each recipient and the risk of morbidity associated with live lung donation do not justify this approach when deceased lung donors are available."[103] Aided by "changes in the [deceased donor] lung allocation system and effects of medical management on transplant urgency," living donor lung transplantation became even less appealing.[104] Between 2005 and 2014, only 20 living donor lung transplants were performed in the US and none since.[105]

2.5 Pancreas Transplantation

The first deceased donor pancreas transplant was performed as a kidney-pancreas transplant in 1966 at the University of Minnesota by William Kelly and Richard Lillehei into a 28-year-old woman with diabetes and ESRD.[106] Since most pancreas transplants are performed for patients with Type 1 diabetes, it is not surprising that, even today, most deceased donor pancreas transplants are done either simultaneously with a kidney transplant or after a kidney transplant has already been performed.[107]

The first successful living donor non-renal transplant was a segmental pancreas transplant in 1979 (distal pancreas-body/tail) from a mother to her diabetic daughter at the University of Minnesota.[108] Initially, living donor pancreas transplants were not done in the same operation for diabetic patients with renal failure eligible for both pancreas and kidney. This meant that the donor (and recipient) were each exposed to 2 surgical procedures.[109] In 1994, the University of Minnesota began to perform simultaneous kidney and segmental pancreas transplants from live donors.[110] Live donor simultaneous segmental pancreas-kidney transplant has the advantage of being able to optimize timing of transplant over a deceased donor simultaneous pancreas-kidney transplant, but the procurement of 2 organs from a living donor is a major surgical procedure, and very few institutions in the US and internationally performed this procedure.[111]

In 2001, Rainer Gruessner and colleagues reviewed 115 living segmental pancreas donations performed at the University of Minnesota between January 1, 1978, and August 31, 2000, of which 51 were pancreas transplants alone, 32 were pancreas after previous kidney transplant, and 32 were simultaneous pancreas-kidney transplants. Of the 115 living donors, 111 were genetic relatives (10 identical twins, 39 HLA-identical siblings, 62 ≤ 1-haplotype-mismatched relatives) and 4 were living unrelated donors.[112] Eight years later, only an additional 40 living donor pancreas transplants were reported to the International Pancreas Transplant Registry from across the globe.[113]

There are at least 2 reasons why living donor pancreas transplantation did not expand in the US or globally. First were the risks to the donors. Of the 115 living donor pancreas transplants performed at Minnesota that were reported in 2001, Gruessner and colleagues were able to locate 67 (58%), and 46 responded to a follow-up questionnaire.[114] Forty-three (94%) said donation had been the correct decision despite the high risk of complications: "But the risk of elevated hemoglobin A1C levels were noted in 10 donors, 3 of whom required insulin for > 6 years postdonation."[115] The University of Minnesota then began to exclude donors with a history of gestational diabetes and obesity, and reported in 2001 that "all donors since September 1, 1996, have had normal hemoglobin A1C levels, ranging from 4.9% to 6.2%."[116] Of course, the timeline was still short and long-term follow-up was not available (and might never be obtained given the history of poor follow-up). Living donor pancreas transplants were also complicated by "a higher thrombosis rate, given the relatively small size of the splenic artery and vein."[117] Second, since the mid-2000s, the deceased donor allocation system in the US gives priority to candidates listed for simultaneous kidney and non-kidney organ transplants, including kidney-pancreas, kidney-liver, and kidney-heart.[118] This means that patients with diabetes in need of a simultaneous kidney-pancreas transplant are given priority over candidates in need of a kidney transplant alone, further reducing the need for living donor kidney-pancreas transplant in the US. UNOS/OPTN data show very few living donor pancreas transplants being performed in the past 2 decades in the US.[119]

2.6 Intestinal Transplantation

There were 8 reported attempts at intestinal transplantation performed in the 1960s, 5 using deceased donor grafts and 3 using living donor grafts in patients who previously had undergone massive bowel resection.[120] All died due to poor immunosuppression complicated by lack of means to provide nutritional support.[121] Total parental nutrition would not be developed until late 1960s and there was little activity or interest in intestinal transplant for almost 2 more decades.[122] Intestinal transplant resumed again in late 1980s, with the first successful combined deceased donor small bowel-liver grafts in Canada and Germany.[123] The peak of intestinal transplants were performed in 2007 with 198 deceased intestinal donor transplants and 1 living intestinal donor transplant. With the development of non-transplant surgical and metabolic approaches to small bowel lengthening in the past decade,[124] intestinal transplants have decreased in frequency. In 2019, there were 81 deceased donor intestinal transplants and 0 living donor intestinal donor transplants performed.[125]

2.7 Uterus Transplantation

The first human uterine transplants was performed in Saudi Arabia in 2000 using a living donor uterus from an unrelated donor and the second in Turkey in 2011 using a deceased donor.[126] The Saudi uterine allograft lasted for 3 months when inadequate structural support led to uterine prolapse and necrosis.[127] The Turkish uterine transplant lasted 18 months, and had a positive clinical pregnancy after in vitro fertilization. However, the gestational sac failed to develop on follow-up 7 days after the initial examination, and the patient began to have vaginal bleeding. The pregnancy was considered nonviable and was terminated by aspiration and curettage.[128] In 2012, Sweden became the first country to attempt living donor uterine transplant (from mothers and other female relatives), and newspaper stories reported 9 performed in the first 3 years.[129] The first infant of a transplant recipient was born October 4, 2014, and is well at 1 year of age.[130] Three other babies were born in 2015.[131] One of the women has since given birth to a second child.[132] Brazil was the first country in which a woman successfully gave birth to an infant after a deceased donor uterine transplant.[133]

In February 2016, Cleveland Clinic was the first US program to attempt uterine transplant. It used a deceased donor graft but the uterus had to be removed when the recipient developed a yeast infection.[134] Surgeons at Baylor attempted 4 living donor uterine transplants beginning in September 2016 with help from the Swedish surgeons. The first 3 failed and the uteri had to be removed, but the fourth uterine recipient gave birth to a healthy infant,[135] and 13 other infants have been born to women who have had a living donor uterine transplant, including a second child to one of these women.[136] At least some of these infants were born to women whose donors were not known to the recipients (Good Samaritan donors or nondirected donors).[137] In July 2019, the Cleveland Clinic announced the successful live birth in the US to a woman who received a deceased donor uterine transplant,[138] and a second success was reported in early 2020 at the hospital of the University of Pennsylvania.[139]

As of November 2020, 31 uterine transplants have been performed in the US: 19 with living donors and 12 with deceased donors.[140] It is still too early to know which has better recipient outcomes (live births).[141] Given that the availability of deceased donor organs should not be a limiting factor, an important ethical and policy question that has not been addressed in the US is how much higher the success rate of live births from living donor uterine transplants compared to deceased donor uterine transplants would have to be to justify the risks to the living donors. In the UK, that bar has not been reached and the Health Research Authority has only approved uterine transplants using deceased uterine donors due to the donor risks from living uterine donation.[142]

2.8 Domino Transplant

A domino transplant involves a candidate-recipient (most commonly the recipient of a deceased donor liver or heart) whose own organ is not discarded but is transplanted into another person.[143] Domino heart transplants may occur, for example, if a patient with cystic fibrosis receives a heart-lung transplant from a deceased donor. The patient with cystic fibrosis may have a healthy heart, but it is removed with their diseased lungs when a heart-lung transplant is thought to be a better option than a lung transplant alone.[144] The first reported domino heart transplant was performed in London's Harefield Hospital by Dr. Magdi Yacoub in 1987.[145] In 2020, Elizabeth Maynes and colleagues reported on 8 studies from across the globe.[146] In the US, between 1988 and 2020, 43 living donor (domino) heart transplants have been documented.[147]

The more common domino transplant involves a liver from a patient with a metabolic condition. Take maple syrup urine disease (MSUD) as an example.[148] The liver from a patient with MSUD provides all the functions of a healthy liver, except that it does not properly metabolize branched chain amino acid (BCAA) enzymes.[149] Non-MSUD individuals produce these BCAA enzymes in adequate quantity in other tissues (skeletal muscle, brain, kidney and pancreas). Since the patient with MSUD does not make the missing enzymes anywhere, they need a liver transplant to provide the needed enzymes. A review of UNOS domino liver data published in 2018 by Geyer and colleagues identified 126 such transplants.[150]

The potential risks to the domino liver donor who has MSUD are three-fold. The first set of risks occurs if there is any difference in the method of explanting the liver from a patient with MSUD which is to be transplanted into another recipient compared to explantation of a liver which would be discarded. For example, this may require a longer time in the operating room, which entails longer exposure to anesthesia with its attendant risks, or it might mean leaving slightly longer blood vessels with the explant to be retransplanted than if the liver were to be discarded. The second set of risks accrues due to potential changes in pre-operative management and any other changes to the medical care of the domino liver donor. For example, some programs anticoagulate all living donors and will anticoagulate the transplant candidate with MSUD who will serve as a domino donor, even though the patient with MSUD would not otherwise undergo anticoagulation during liver transplantation.[151]The third set of risks involves the outcome of the domino liver graft and the psychological impact that it may have on the domino donor (and her family). The potential domino donor must understand that (1) the explant may not actually be transplanted because of anatomy, timing, and/or other clinical and psychosocial factors; and (2) even if transplanted, the domino organ graft or recipient may do poorly.[152] Postoperatively, identification and disclosure of donor and recipient to each other may occur if permitted by institutional or country policies and if both parties agree to meet, usually after a specified time delay.[153]When the domino donor wants to meet the recipient, but the recipient does not, the donor may feel disappointed, even rejected. Still, when successfully attempted, they are one more way of expanding the organ donor pool.

2.9 Conclusion

The current success rate of organ and tissue transplantation has led to increasing indications for its usage, exacerbating the gap between demand and supply. Despite many policies to increase the procurement of deceased donor organs, the gap persists, and this has led to increased pressure to find living donors. Over the past 2 decades, over 90% of all living organ donors are kidney donors and approximately 4.5% are liver segment/lobe donors.[154] Transplant centers have been motivated to perform living donor organ transplantation both because of scarcity and the hope of better recipient outcomes. This has led to greater willingness to accept more medically complex donors, and to encourage candidates to be creative in their search for a living donor through the use of social media and advertising. Transplant programs have also been creative in addressing donor-recipient incompatibilities (see chapter 8) and in encouraging living donation from strangers (see chapter 7). The incentive to expand living donation raises major ethical issues. As Murray noted in 1963: "We make a basic qualitative shift in our aims when we risk the health of a well person, no matter how pure our motives."[155] It is in this spirit that we have undertaken the challenge of developing an ethics framework that can help us determine when living donation is and ought to be a permissible option.

Notes

1. Organ Procurement and Transplantation Network (OPTN) Data. https://optn.transplant.hrsa.gov/data/view-data-reports/national-data/. Last revision August 5, 2021. Last accessed 8/12/2021. Hereinafter cited as OPTN Data.
2. For an exception to elective timing, see the chapter on living donation for acute liver failure, chapter 10.

3. For example, living donor kidney grafts have better graft and patient survival than deceased donor kidney grafts. See, for example, the Scientific Registry of Transplant Recipients (SRTR). What do I need to consider to compare a living donor vs. a deceased donor? Published 2018; Accessed 8/12/2021. https://www.srtr.org/assets/media/Kidney_Transplant_Website/Living_vs_Deceased.html. Living liver grafts may also outperform deceased donor liver grafts. See Humar A, Ganesh S, Jorgensen D, et al. Adult living donor versus deceased donor liver transplant (LDLT versus DDLT) at a single center: time to change our paradigm for liver transplant. *Ann Surg.* 2019;270:444–451.

4. Barker CF, Markmann JF. Historical overview of transplantation. *Cold Spring Harb Perspect Med.* 2013;3:a014977, at p. 4 citing Voronoy.

5. Barker and Markmann, "Historical."

6. Barker and Markmann, "Historical."

7. Michon L, Hamburger J, Oeconomos N, et al. Une tentative de transplantation renale chez l'homme: aspects medicaux et biologiques. *Presse Med.* 1953;61:1419–1423.

8. Hume DM, Merrill JP, Miller BF, Thorn GW. Experiences with renal homotransplantations in the human: report of nine cases. *J Clin Invest.* 1955;34(2):327–382. Of note, there was a case report in 1945 when Charles Hufnagel (surgeon, Boston) and 2 residents treated a 29-year-old woman with acute renal failure by attaching her to a kidney extracorporally from an elderly individual who had just died. See Moore F. *A Miracle and a Privilege.* Boston, MA: Joseph Henry Press, 2001: at pp. 164–165. The kidney functioned long enough for her own kidney function to return. In 1950, Lawler and colleagues performed the first deceased donor intraabdominal kidney transplant in a patient with low renal function which lasted for at least 53 days. See Lawler RH, West JW, McNulty PH, Clancy EJ, Murphy RP. Homotransplantation of the kidney in the human. *J Am Med Assoc.* 1950;144:844–845. Barker and Markmann explain that when the kidney was removed "after several months, it was found to be shrunken. This procedure was of no scientific significance and of no benefit to the patient, who survived for several years with declining renal function of her own kidney . . . [and] was widely criticized." See Barker and Markmann, "Historical," at p. 5.

9. Hume et al, "Experiences."

10. Merill JP, Harrison JH, Murray J, Guild WR. Successful homotransplantation of the kidney in an identical twin. *Trans Am Clin Climatol Assoc.* 1956;67:166–173.

11. Murray JE. The kindest cut: commemorating the 50th anniversary of the first successful whole organ transplant. *Sci Am.* December 20, 2004. Last accessed 8/12/2021. https://www.scientificamerican.com/article/the-kindest-cut/

12. Missing from Murray's 50th anniversary account in which he talks about the Minnesota Transplant Games where Herrick and Murray were honored is the fact that Ronald Herrick (the donor) started dialysis in 2002 before he and Dr. Murray were honored at the Transplant Games (See, Murray, "The kindest cut"). It was included in an obituary that we had previously cited but was then removed from the web. We had cited it in Ross LF, Thistlethwaite JR. Outcomes after kidney donation. *JAMA J.* 2014;312:94. Ref 3: Crosby C. Transplant just one chapter of first organ

donor's life. Last accessed August 12, 2021. http://www.kjonline.com/news/transpl
ant-just-one-chapter-of-first-organ-donors-life   _2011-01-01.html?pagenum=full.
Accessed February 24, 2014. This link no longer works. The only mention we can find
on the web currently is in comments following an online obituary. See comments following: Obituary of first kidney donor—Ronald Herrick. December 30, 2010. Renal
Fellow Network. https://www.renalfellow.org/2010/12/30/obituary/

13. Starzl TE. The birth of clinical organ transplantation. *J Am Coll Surg.* 2001;192:431–446.
14. Human Kidney Transplant Conference. *Transplantation.* 1964;2(1):147–165.
15. Advisory Committee to the Renal Transplant Registry. The 13th report of the human renal transplant registry. *Transplant Proc.* 1977;9(1):9–26.
16. Social Security Amendments of 1972 (Pub L No. 92-603).
17. Hull AR. The legislative and regulatory process in the end-stage renal disease (ESRD) program, 1973 through 1997. *Semin Nephrol.* 1997;17:160–169.
18. Murray JE, Gleason R, Bartholomay A. Second report of Registry in Human Kidney Transplantation. *Transplantation.* 1964;2:660–667.
19. Murray JE, Barnes BA, Atkinson JC. Eighth report of the Human Kidney Transplant Registry. *Transplantation.* 1971;11:328–337, at p. 329.
20. Howard RJ, Cornell DL, Cochran I. History of deceased organ donation, transplanta-tion, and organ procurement organizations. *Prog Transplant.* 2012;22:6–16; quiz 17, at p. 10.
21. Williams MC, Creger JH, Belton AM, et al. The organ center of the United Network for Organ Sharing and twenty years of organ sharing in the United States. *Transplantation.* 2004;77(5):641–646, at p. 642.
22. Williams et al, "The organ center," at p. 642.
23. United Network for Organ Sharing UNOS. Improving Organ Procurement and Oversight. Last accessed August 12, 2021. https://unos.org/transplant/improving-organ-procurement-and-oversight/
24. Williams et al, "The organ center," at p. 643, citing UNOS. Improving Organ Procurement and Oversight. Last accessed August 12, 2021. https://unos.org/trans-plant/improving-organ-procurement-and-oversight/
25. Living Donor 101. Risks of Living Kidney Donation. http://www.livingdonor101.com/risks-of-living-kidney-donation/. Last accessed 8/12/21.
26. OPTN Data.
27. Levey AS, Hou S, Bush HL, Jr. Kidney transplantation from unrelated living donors. Time to reclaim a discarded opportunity. *N Engl J Med.* 1986;314:914–916.
28. Murray JE. Proceedings: Human Kidney Transplant Conference. *Transplantation.* 1964;2(1):147–165.
29. Murray et al, "Second report."
30. Opelz G, Michey MR, Terasaki PI. HLA matching and cadaver kidney transplant survival in North America: influence of center variation and presensitization. *Transplantation.* 1977;23:490–497; and Levey et al, "Kidney."
31. Spital A. Unconventional living kidney donors—attitudes and use among transplant centers. *Transplantation.* 1989;48:243–248.

32. These data can be found in Spital A. Evolution of attitudes at US transplant centers toward kidney donation by friends and altruistic strangers. *Transplantation*. 2000;69:1728–1731.

33. Tong A, Chapman JR, Wong G, Kanellis J, McCarthy G, Craig JC. The motivations and experiences of living kidney donors: a thematic synthesis. *Am J Kidney Dis*. 2012;60:15–26; and Simmons RG, Klein S, Simmons RL. *Gift of Life: The Social and Psychological Impact of Organ Transplantation*. New York, NY: John Wiley and Sons; 1977. Updated and reprinted as Simmons RG, Marine SK, Simmons RL. *Effect of Organ Transplantation on Individual, Family and Societal Dynamics*. New Brunswick, NJ: Transaction Books; 2002.

34. Terasaki PI, Cecka JM, Gjertson DW, Takemoto S. High survival rates of kidney transplants from spousal and living unrelated donors. *N Engl J Med*.1995;333:333–336.

35. Matas AJ, Garvey CA, Jacobs CL, Kahn JP. Nondirected donation of kidneys from living donors. *N Engl J Med*. 2000;343:433–436.

36. Matas et al, "Nondirected."

37. Rapaport FT. The case for a living emotionally related international kidney donor exchange registry. *Transplant Proc*. 1986;18(3 suppl 2):5–9.

38. Ross LF, Rubin D, Siegler M, et al. Ethics of a paired-kidney-exchange program. *N Engl J Med*. 1997;336:1752–1755.

39. Park K, Moon JI, Kim SI, Kim YS. Exchange donor program in kidney transplantation. *Transplantation*. 1999;67:336–338.

40. Veale J, Hil G. The National Kidney Registry: transplant chains—beyond paired kidney donation. *Clin Transpl*. 2009:253–364.

41. Montgomery RA, Zachary AA, Ratner LE, et al. Clinical results from transplanting incompatible live kidney donor/recipient pairs using kidney paired donation. *JAMA*. 2005;294:1655–1663.

42. Montgomery RA, Gentry SE, Marks WH, et al. Domino paired kidney donation: a strategy to make best use of live non-directed donation *Lancet*. 2006;368(9533):419–421.

43. Rees MA, Kopke JE, Pelletier RP, et al. Nonsimultaneous, extended, altruistic-donor chain. *N Engl J Med*. 2009;360:1096–1101.

44. Rees et al, "Nonsimultaneous."

45. Montgomery et al, "Domino paired," at p. 420.

46. Veale and Hil, "The National Kidney Registry."

47. National Kidney Registry. NKR Quarterly Reports. Paired Exchange Quarterly Reports. Q1 Results 2020. Published May 6, 2020. Accessed August 12, 2021. https://www.kidneyregistry.org/pages/p608/Q12020.php

48. Veale and Hil, "The National Kidney Registry."

49. Veale and Hil, "The National Kidney Registry."

50. Reese PP, Caplan AL, Kesselheim AS, Bloom RD. Creating a medical, ethical, and legal framework for complex living kidney donors. *Clin J Am Soc Nephrol*. 2006;1:1148–1153, at p. 1148.

51. See, for example, Niemi M, Mandelbrot DA. The outcomes of living kidney donation from medically complex donors: implications for the donor and the recipient.

Curr Transplant Rep. 2014;1:1–9. doi:10.1007/s40472-013-0001-6; and Iordanous Y, Seymour N, Young, A, et al. Recipient outcomes for expanded criteria living kidney donors: the disconnect between current evidence and practice. *Am J Transplant.* 2009;9:1558–1573. One study from Japan found similar results but only followed these donors for 1 year and acknowledged that the duration of follow-up needed to be expanded. Hiramitsu T, Tomosugi T, Futamura K. Preoperative comorbidities and outcomes of medically complex living kidney donors. *Kidney Int Reports.* 2020;5:13–27.

52. Bia MJ, Ramos EL, Danovitch GM, et al. Evaluation of living renal donors. The current practice of US transplant centers. *Transplantation.* 1995;60:322–327.

53. Mandelbrot DA, Pavlakis M, Danovitch GM, et al. The medical evaluation of living kidney donors: a survey of US transplant centers. *Am J Transplant.* 2007;7:2333–2343.

54. Table 2.2 is based on data from Bia et al, "Evaluation" and Mandelbrot et al, "The medical evaluation."

55. Reese et al, "Creating," at p. 1148.

56. See, for example, Ibrahim HN, Foley R, Tan L, et al. Long-term consequences of kidney donation. *N Engl J Med.* 2009;360:459–469; Mjøen G, Hallan S, Hartmann A, et al. Long-term risks for kidney donors. *Kidney Int.* 2014;86:162–167; Muzaale AD, Massie AB, Wang MC, et al. Risk of end-stage renal disease following live kidney donation. *JAMA.* 2014;311:579–586; Matas AJ, Hays RE, Ibrahim HN. Long-term non-end-stage renal disease risks after living kidney donation. *Am J Transplant.* 2017;17:893–900; and Lentine KL, Lam NN, Segev DL. Risks of living kidney donation: current state of knowledge on outcomes important to donors. *Clin J Am Soc Nephrol.* 2019;14:597–608.

57. Niemi M, Mandelbrot DA. The outcomes of living kidney donation from medically complex donors: implications for the donor and the recipient. *Curr Transplant Rep.* 2014;1(1):1–9.

58. Simmons et al, *Gift of Life.*

59. See, for example, Garonzik-Wang, JM, Berger JC, Ros RL, et al. Live donor champion: finding live kidney donors by separating the advocate from the patient. *Transplantation.* 2012; 93:1147–1150; and LaPointe Rudow D, Geatrakas S, Armenti J, et al. Increasing living donation by implementing the Kidney Coach Program. *Clin Transpl.* 2019;33:e13471.

60. Rodrigue JR, Cornell DL, Kaplan B, Howard RJ. Patients' willingness to talk to others about living kidney donation. *Prog Transplant.* 2008;18:25–31.

61. See, for example, Rodrigue JR, Pavlakis M, Egbuna O, Paek M, Waterman AD, Mandelbrot DA. The "House Calls" trial: a randomized controlled trial to reduce racial disparities in live donor kidney transplantation: rationale and design. *Contemp Clin Trials.* 2012;33:811–818; Rodrigue JR, Paek MJ, Egbuna O, et al. Making house calls increases living donor inquiries and evaluations for blacks on the kidney transplant waiting list. *Transplantation.* 2014;98:979–986;Kumar K, King EA, Muzaale AD, et al. A smartphone app for increasing live organ donation. *Am J Transplant.* 2016;16(12):3548–3553; Waterman AD, Robbins ML, Peipert JD. Educating prospective kidney transplant recipients and living donors about living

donation: practical and theoretical recommendations for increasing living donation rates. *Curr Transplant Rep.* 2016;3(1):1–9; Bramstedt KA, Cameron AM. Beyond the billboard: The Facebook-based application, donor, and its guided approach to facilitating living organ donation. *Am J Transplant.* 2017;17:336–340; and Reed RD, Hites L, Mustian MN, et al. A qualitative assessment of the living donor navigator program to identify core competencies and promising practices for implementation. *Prog Transplant.* 2020;30:29–37.

62. LaPointe Rudow D, Hays R, Baliga P, et al. Consensus conference on best practices in live kidney donation: recommendations to optimize education, access, and care. *Am J Transplant.* 2015;15:914–922.

63. See, for example, Tan JC, Gordon EJ, Dew MA, et al. Living donor kidney transplantation: facilitating education about live kidney donation—recommendations from a consensus conference. *Clin J Am Soc Nephrol.* 2015;10:1670–1677; and Waterman AD, Morgievich M, Cohen DJ, et al. Living donor kidney transplantation: improving education outside of transplant centers about live donor transplantation—recommendations from a consensus conference. *Clin J Am Soc Nephrol.* 2015;10:659–669.

64. Starzl TE, Groth CG, Brettschneider L, et al. Orthotopic homotransplantation of the human liver. *Ann Surg.* 1968;168(3):392–415; and Starzl TE, Marchioro TL, Vonkaulla KN, Hermann G, Brittain RS, Waddell WR. Homotransplantation of the liver in humans. *Surg Gynecol Obstet.* 1963;117:659–676.

65. Millard CE. The NIH Consensus Development Conference on liver transplantation. *R I Med J.* 1984;67(2):69–71.

66. Millard, "The NIH."

67. Emond JC, Whitington PF, Thistlethwaite JR, Alonso EM, Broelsch CE. Reduced-size orthotopic liver transplantation: use in the management of children with chronic liver disease. *Hepatology.*1989;10(5):867–872.

68. Bismuth H, Morino M, Castaing D, et al. Emergency orthotopic liver transplantation in two patients using one donor liver. *Br J Surg.* 1989;76(7):722–724. This was quickly adopted here in the US. See, for example, Broelsch CE, Emond JC, Thistlethwaite JR, Rouch DA, Whitington PF, Lichtor JL. Liver transplantation with reduced-size donor organs. *Transplantation.* 1988;45(3):519–524; Broelsch CE, Emond JC, Thistlethwaite JR, et al. Liver transplantation, including the concept of reduced-size liver transplants in children. *Ann Surg.* 1988;208:410–420; and Emond JC, Whitington PF, Broelsch CE. Overview of reduced-size liver transplantation. *Clin Transplant.* 1991;5 (2 part 2):168–173.

69. Pichlmayr R, Ringe B, Gubernatis G, Hauss J, Bunzendahl H. [Transplantation of a donor liver to 2 recipients (splitting transplantation)—a new method in the further development of segmental liver transplantation]. *Langenbecks Arch Chir.* 1988;373(2):127–130.

70. Emond JC, Whitington PF, Thistlethwaite JR, et al. Transplantation of two patients with one liver. Analysis of a preliminary experience with "split-liver" grafting. *Ann Surg.* 1990;212:14–22.

71. OPTN/UNOS Ethics Committee. Split Versus Whole Liver Transplantation. Published December 2016. Accessed August 12, 2021. https://optn.transplant.hrsa. gov/resources/ethics/split-versus-whole-liver-transplantation/

72. See, Bismuth H, Marino M, Castaing D. Emergency orthotopic liver transplantation in two patients using one donor. *Br J Surg.* 1989;76:722–724.
73. Colledan M, Segalin A, Andorno E, et al. Modified splitting technique for liver transplantation in adult-sized recipients. Technique and preliminary results. *Acta Chir Belg.* 2000;100(6):289–291.
74. Hacki C, Schmidt KM, Susal C, Dohler B, Zidek M, Schlitt HJ. Split liver transplantation: current developments. *World J Gastroenterol.* 2018;24:5312–5321, at p. 5312.
75. See, for example, Hacki et al, "Split liver"; and Lauterio A, Di Sandro S, Concone G, De Carlis R, Giacomoni A, De Carlis L. Current status and perspectives in split liver transplantation. *World J Gastroenterol.* 2015;21:11003–11015.
76. Smith B. Segmental liver transplantation from a living donor. *J Pediatr Surg.* 1969;4:126–132.
77. Raia S, Nery JR, Mies S. Liver transplantation from live donors. *Lancet.* 1989;2(8661):497–498.
78. Strong RW, Lynch SV, Ong TH, Matsunami H, Koido Y, Balderson GA. Successful liver transplantation from a living donor to her son. *N Eng J Med.* 1990;322:1505–1507.
79. Singer PA, Siegler M, Whitington PF, et al. Ethics of liver transplantation with living donors. *N Eng J Med.*1989;321:620–622.
80. Broelsch CE, Whitington PF, Emond JC, et al. Liver transplantation in children from living related donors. Surgical techniques and results. *Ann Surg.* 1991;214(4):428–437; discussion 437–429.
81. Broelsch et al, "Liver transplantation," at p. 429.
82. Piper JB, Whitington PF, Woodle ES, Newell KA, Alonso EM, Thistlethwaite JR. Living related liver transplantation in children: a report of the first 58 recipients at the University of Chicago. *Transpl Int.* 1994;7(suppl 1): S111–113.
83. Piper et al, "Living related."
84. Piper et al, "Living related."
85. See, for example, Rogiers X, Burdelski M, Broelsch CE. Liver transplantation from living donors. *Br J Surg.* 1994;81:1251–1253; Tanaka K, Uemoto S, Tokunaga Y, et al. Living related liver transplantation in children. *Am J Surg.* 1994;168:41–48; Chen CL, Chen YS, Liu PP, et al. Living related donor liver transplantation. *J Gastroenterol Hepatol.* 1997;12(9–10): S342–345; and Harihara Y, Makuuchi M, Kawarasaki H, et al. Initial experience with living-related liver transplantation at the University of Tokyo. *Transpl Proc.* 1998;30:129–131.
86. Hashikura Y, Makuuchi M, Kawasaki S, et al. Successful living-related partial liver transplantation to an adult patient. *Lancet.* 1994;343(8907):1233–1234.
87. Yamaoka Y, Washida M, Honda K, et al. Liver transplantation using a right lobe graft from a living related donor. *Transplantation.* 1994;57:1127–1130.
88. Lo CM, Fan ST, Liu CL, et al. Extending the limit on the size of adult recipient in living donor liver transplantation using extended right lobe graft. *Transplantation.* 1997;63:1524–1528.
89. Wachs ME, Bak TE, Karrer FM, et al. Adult living donor liver transplantation using a right hepatic lobe. *Transplantation.* 1998;66:1313–1316.

90. Brown RS Jr, Russo MW, Lai M, et al. A survey of liver transplantation from living adult donors in the United States. *N Engl J Med.* 2003;348(9):818–825.

91. Hwang S, Lee SG, Moon DB, et al. Exchange living donor liver transplantation to overcome ABO incompatibility in adult patients. *Liver Transpl.* 2010;16:482–490; and Chan SC, Lo CM, Yong BH, Tsui WJ, Ng KK, Fan ST. Paired donor interchange to avoid ABO-incompatible living donor liver transplantation. *Liver Transpl.* 2010;16(4): 478–481. This is not the only living solid organ transplant program involving 2 donors. Living lung transplant programs used 2 living lung donors in the early 1990s (see text corresponding to reference 100).

92. Song G-W, Lee S-G, Moon D-B, et al. Dual-graft adult living donor liver transplantation: an innovative surgical procedure for live liver donor pool expansion. *Ann Surg.* 2017;266:10–18.

93. Lee SG, Hwang S, Park KM, et al. Seventeen adult-to-adult living donor liver transplantations using dual grafts. *Transplant Proc.* 2001;33:3461–3463; Broering DC, Walter J, Rogiers X. The first two cases of living donor liver transplantation using dual grafts in Europe. *Liver Transpl.* 2007;13:149–153; Dayangac M, Taner CB, Akin B, et al. Dual left lobe living donor liver transplantation using donors unacceptable for right lobe donation: a case report. *Transpl Proc.* 2010;42:4560–4563; Nicoluzzi JE, Silveira F, Silveira FP, et al. [The first dual left lobe adult-to-adult liver transplantation in Brazil]. *Revista do Colegio Brasileiro de Cirurgioes.*2012;39:226– 229; and Lee S, Hwang S, Park K, et al. An adult-to-adult living donor liver transplant using dual left lobe grafts. *Surgery.* 2001;129:647–650.

94. Mirhra A, Lo A, Less GS, et al. Liver paired exchange: can the liver emulate the kidney? *Liver Transpl.* 2018;24: 677–686.

95. Cronin DC 2nd, Millis JM. Living donor liver transplantation: the ethics and the practice. *Hepatology.* 2008;47:11–13, at p. 12.

96. Hardy JD, Araslan S, Webb WR. Transplantation of the lung. *Ann Surg.* 1964;160:440–448.

97. Venuta F, Raemdonck DV. History of lung transplantation. *J Thorac Dis.* 2017;9:5458–5471, at p. 5461.

98. Goldsmith MF. Mother to child: first living donor lung transplant. *JAMA.* 1990;26:2724.

99. Starnes VA, Barr ML, Cohen RB. Lobar transplantation: indications, technique, and outcome. *J Thorac Cardiovasc Surg.* 1994;106:403–411, at p. 403.

100. Starnes VA, Barr ML, Cohen RG, et al. Living-donor lobar lung transplantation experience: intermediate results. *J Thorac Cardiovasc Surg.* 1996;12:1284–1290; discussion 1290–1291, at p. 1285.

101. Barr ML, Belghiti J, Villamil FG, et al. A report of the Vancouver Forum on the care of the live organ donor: lung, liver, pancreas, and intestine data and medical guidelines. *Transplantation.* 2006;81(10):1373–1385.

102. Yusen RD, Hong BA, Messersmith EE, et al. Morbidity and mortality of live lung donation: results from the RELIVE study. *Am J Transplant.* 2014;14: 1846–1852, at p. 1847. Hereinafter cited as the RELIVE study.

103. RELIVE study, "Morbidity and mortality," at p. 1851.

104. RELIVE study, "Morbidity and mortality," at p. 1846.

105. OPTN Data.

106. Kelly WD, Lillehei RC, Merkel FK, et al. Allotransplantation of the pancreas and duodenum along with the kidney in diabetic nephropathy. *Surgery.* 1967;61:827–837.

107. Laftavi MR, Gruessner A, Gruessner R. Surgery of pancreas transplantation. *Curr Opin Organ Transplant.* 2017;22:389–397

108. Sutherland DER, Goetz FC, Najarian JS. Living-related donor segmental pancreatectomy for transplantation. *Transplant Proc.* 1980;12:19–25.

109. Gruessner RWG. Chapter 35: Dual-Organ Donation. In: RWG Gruessner, ed, and E Benedetti, associate ed. *Living Donor Organ Transplantation.* New York, NY: McGraw Hill Medical. 2008:723–724.

110. Gruessner RWG, Sutherland DER. Simultaneous kidney and segmental pancreas transplants from living related donors—the first two successful cases. *Transplantation.* 1996;61:1265–1268.

111. Gruessner, "Dual-Organ Donation."

112. Gruessner RW, Sutherland DE, Drangstveit MB, Bland BJ, Gruessner AC. Pancreas transplants from living donors: short- and long-term outcome. *Transplant Proc.* 2001;33(1–2):819–820, at p. 819.

113. Reynoso JF, Gruessner CE, Sutherland DE, Gruessner RW. Short- and long-term outcome for living pancreas donors. *J Hepatobiliary Pancreat Sci.* 2010;17:92–96, at p. 92.

114. Gruessner, "Pancreas transplant."

115. Gruessner, "Pancreas transplant," at p. 820.

116. Gruessner, "Pancreas transplant," at p. 820.

117. Reynoso et al, "Short- and long-term outcomes," at p. 93.

118. Smith JM, Biggins SW, Haselby DG, et al. Kidney, pancreas, and liver allocation and distribution in the United States. *Am J Transplant.* 2012;12:3191–3212.

119. OPTN Data.

120. McAlister VC, Grant DR. Clinical small bowel transplantation. In: Grant DR, Wood RFM, eds. *Small Bowel Transplantation.* London, England: Edward Arnold, 1994:121–132

121. Pollard SG. Intestinal transplantation: living related. *Br Med Bull.* 1997;53(4): 868–878.

122. Dudrick SJ, Ignore DW, Vars HM, Rhoads JE. Long-term total parenteral nutrition with growth, development and positive nitrogen balance. Surgery. 1968;64:134–142; Wilmore DW, Dudrick SJ. Growth and development of an infant receiving all nutrients exclusively by vein. *JAMA.* 1968;203:860–864; and Kim J, Zimmerman MA. Technical aspects for live-donor organ procurement for liver, kidney, pancreas, and intestine. *Curr Opin Organ Transplant.* 2015;20:133–139.

123. Grant D, Wall W, Mimeault R, et al. Successful small-bowel/liver transplantation. *Lancet.* 1990;335:181–184; and Deltz E, Schroeder P, Gundlach M, Hansmann ML, Leimenstoll G. Successful clinical small bowel transplantation. *Transplant Proc.* 1990;22(66):2501.

124. See, for example, Cruz RJ Jr, McGurgan J, Butera L, et al. Gastrointestinal tract reconstruction in adults with ultra-short bowel syndrome: surgical and nutritional

outcomes. *Surgery.* 2020;168(2):297–304; and Mezoff EA, Minneci PC, Dienhart MC. Intestinal failure: a description of the problem and recent therapeutic advances. *Clin Perinatol.* 2020;47:323–340.

125. OPTN Data.

126. Brännström M, Diaz-Garcia C, Hanafy A, Olausson M, Tzakis A. Uterus transplantation: animal research and human possibilities. *Fertil Steril.* 2012;97:1269–1276.

127. Brännström et al, "Uterus transplantation."

128. Erman Akar M, Ozkan O, Aydinuraz B, et al. Clinical pregnancy after uterus transplantation. *Fertil Steril.* 2013;100:1358–1363.

129. Nine Swedish women receive womb transplants. *BBC News.* January 13, 2014. Last accessed August 12, 2021. http://www.bbc.co.uk/news/health-25716446

130. Orange R, MacRae F. Celebrating turning one. *The Daily Mail.* Published September 20, 2015. Updated September 21, 2015. Last accessed August 12, 2021. https://www.dailymail.co.uk/news/article-3242477/Celebrating-turning-one-baby-born-womb-transplant-Mother-speaks-fantastic-feeling-following-pioneering-project-saw-four-children-born.html

131. Orange and MacRae, "Celebrating turning one."

132. Kubista MG. Eight children born after uterus transplants. University of Gothenburg. ScienceDaily. Publication September 18, 2017, Last accessed August 12, 2021. www.sciencedaily.com/releases/2017/09/170918123535.htm

133. Associated Press. Brazilian baby is first using uterus from deceased donor. Published December 5, 2018. Last accessed August 12, 2021. https://www.nbcnews.com/health/health-news/brazilian-baby-first-born-using-uterus-deceased-donor-n944006

134. Kuehn BM. US uterus transplant trials under way. *JAMA.* 2017;317(10):1005–1007.

135. Sifferlin A. Exclusive: first U.S. baby born after a uterus transplant. *Time Magazine.* Publication December 1, 2017. Access August 12, 2021. https://time.com/5044565/exclusive-first-u-s-baby-born-after-a-uterus-transplant/

136. Castro B. Local Mom Is First in Country to Deliver 2 Babies After Uterus Transplant. 5NBCDFW. Published December 23, 2020, Updated on December 24, 2020. Last accessed August 21, 2021. https://www.nbcdfw.com/news/health/north-texas-mother-becomes-first-in-country-to-deliver-2-babies-after-uterus-transplant/2512851/

137. Warren AM, Testa G, Anthony T, et al. Live nondirected uterus donors: psychological characteristics and motivation for donation. *Am J Transplant.* 2018;18(5):1122–1128.

138. Flyckt R, Falcone T, Quintini C, et al. First birth from a deceased donor uterus in the United States: from severe graft rejection to successful cesarean delivery. *Am J Obstetr Gynecol.* 2020;223(2):143–151.

139. Rueb ES. Second U.S. baby to be born from a dead donor's uterus is delivered. *The New York Times.* January 9, 2020. Last accessed August 12, 2021.https://www.nytimes.com/2020/01/09/health/uterus-transplant-baby.html

140. OPTN Data.

141. Hur C, Rehmer J, Flyckt R, Falcone T. Uterine factor infertility: a clinical review. *Clin Obstet Gynecol.* 2019;62:257–270, at pp. 266–267.

142. BBC. Womb transplants given UK go-ahead. *BBC News Health.* September 30, 2015. Last accessed August 12, 2021. http://www.bbc.com/news/health-34397794; Hammond-Browning N. UK criteria for uterus transplantation: a review. *Br J Obstet Gynecol.* 2019;126:1320–1326

143. This section draws heavily from Schenck D, Mazariegos GV, Thistlethwaite JR, Jr and Ross LF. Ethical analysis and policy recommendations regarding domino liver transplantation. *Transplantation.* 2018;102(5):803–808.

144. See, for example, Khaghani A, Birks EJ, Anyanwu AC, Banner NR. Heart transplantation from live donors: "domino procedure." *J Heart Lung Transplant.* 2004;23:S257–259; Astor TL, Galantowicz M, Phillips A, Davis JT, Hoffman TM. Domino heart transplantation involving infants. *Am J Transplant.* 2007;11:2626–2629; Sutor S, Wieczorek P, DeMaio K, et al. Domino transplants. Sequential heart and heart-lung transplantation. *AORN J (Assoc of perioperative Registered Nurses J).* 1988;48: 876–889;and Anyanwu AC, Banner NR, Radley-Smith R, et al. Long-term results of cardiac transplantation from live donors: the domino heart transplant. *J Heart Lung Transplant.* 2002;21:971–975.

145. Smith JA, Roberts M, Mcneil K, et al. Excellent outcome of cardiac transplantation using domino donor hearts. *Eur J Cardiothorac Surg.* 1996;10:628–633.

146. Maynes EJ, O'Malley TJ, Austin MA, et al. Domino heart transplant following heart-lung transplantation: a systematic review and meta-analysis. *Ann Cardiothorac Surg.* 2020;9:20–28.

147. OPTN Data.

148. Kitchens WH. Domino liver transplantation: indications, techniques, and outcomes. *Transplant Rev.* 2011;25:167–177; Popescu I, Dima S. Domino liver transplantation: how far can we push the paradigm? *Liver Transpl.* 2012;18:22–28; and Schielke A, Conti F, Goumard C, Perdigao F, Calmus Y, Scatton O. Liver transplantation using grafts with rare metabolic disorders. *Dig Liver Dis.* 2015;47:261–270.

149. Barshop BA, Khanna A. Domino hepatic transplantation in maple syrup urine disease. *N Engl J Med.* 2005;353: 2410–2411; Khanna A, Hart M, Nyhan WL, Hassanein T, Panyard-Davis J, Barshop BA. Domino liver transplantation in maple syrup urine disease. *Liver Transpl.* 2006;12:876–882; and Badell IR, Hanish SI, Hughes CB, et al. Domino liver transplantation in maple syrup urine disease: a case report and review of the literature. *Transplant Proc.* 2013;45:806–809.

150. Geyer ED, Burrier C, Tumin D, Hayes D Jr, Black SM, Washburn WK, Tobais JD. Outcomes of domino liver transplantation compared to deceased donor liver transplantation: a propensity-matching approach. *Transpl Int.* 2018;31:1200–1206.

151. See, for example, Kim JD, Choi DL, Han YS. Is systemic heparinization necessary during living donor hepatectomy? *Liver Transpl.* 2015;21(2):239–247; and Lisman T, Porte RJ. Antiplatelet medication after liver transplantation: does it affect outcome? *Liver Transpl.* 2007;13(5):644–646.

152. Wray J, Whitmore P, Radley-Smith R. Pediatric cardiothoracic domino transplantation: the psychological costs and benefits. *Pediatr Transplant.* 2004;8:475–479.
153. Lennerling A, Fehrman-Ekholm I, Nordén G. Nondirected living kidney donation: experiences in a Swedish Transplant Centre. *Clin Transplant.* 2008;22:304–308.
154. OPTN Data.
155. Wolstenholme GEW, O'Connor M, eds. *Ethics in Medical Progress: With Special Reference to Transplantation.* Boston MA: Little, Brown and Company, 1966: citing Joseph Murry at p. 76.

3
Developing a Living Donor Ethics Framework

3.1 Introduction

Living donor transplantation has been controversial since its inception because it exposes 1 party to clinical risks for the clinical benefit of another. But it is not unique: research involving human participants exposes the participants to clinical risks for the benefit of others—in this case, future patients. This is not to deny that many living donors describe benefits to donation as do research participants about their participation.

Ethics frameworks are necessary to ensure the well-being and safety of both research subjects and living donors. In 1978, the National Commission for the Protection of Human Subjects of Biomedical and Behavioral Research (hereinafter "National Commission") published the *Belmont Report* in which it articulated 3 underlying principles for a research ethics framework: respect for persons, beneficence, and justice.[1] While a number of transplant organizations have developed standard of care guidelines regarding the evaluation and follow-up of the live kidney donor and the components required for a shared decision-making process,[2] to date, there has been no overarching living donor ethics framework. Given the analogies between living donor transplantation and human subjects research, we believe that the 3 principles enumerated in the National Commission's *Belmont Report* offer an excellent starting point for developing a living donor ethics framework.

3.2 Respect for Persons

In the *Belmont Report*, the principle of respect for persons incorporates at least 2 ethical convictions:

The Living Organ Donor as Patient. Lainie Friedman Ross and J. Richard Thistlethwaite, Jr, Oxford University Press.
© Oxford University Press 2022. DOI: 10.1093/oso/9780197618202.003.0003

first, that individuals should be treated as autonomous agents, and second, that persons with diminished autonomy are entitled to protection. The principle of respect for persons thus divides into two separate moral requirements: the requirement to acknowledge autonomy and the requirement to protect those with diminished autonomy.[3]

This principle is operationalized by the process of informed consent. The consent process contains 3 elements: information (the disclosure of risks, benefits, and alternatives), comprehension (the provision of information in a way that is understandable), and voluntariness (freedom from coercion and undue influence).[4]

The traditional conception of respect for persons as articulated in the *Belmont Report* incorporated a negative conception of autonomy: "To respect autonomy is to give weight to autonomous persons' considered opinions and choices while refraining from obstructing their actions unless they are clearly detrimental to others."[5] That is, (respect for) autonomy was traditionally understood as a negative right, a right to make health care decisions without interference. This approach reduces health care providers to individuals who merely provide information and then respect the choice (unless harmful to others) made by the autonomous individual, who is perceived to be an atomistic, asocial "self-made" man or woman.[6] In the 40 years since the publication of the *Belmont Report*, there have been a number of critics who have argued that autonomy should not be understood separate from our relationships and that health care providers specifically may have an obligation to help empower patients to exercise their autonomy more effectively. Feminist theorists call this construct of autonomy "relational autonomy." Marilyn Friedman expands on this concept:

> According to the relational approach, persons are fundamentally social beings who develop the competency for autonomy through social interaction with other persons. These developments take place in a context of values, meanings, and modes of self-reflection that cannot exist except as constituted by social practices. Also according to some theorists, autonomy is itself the capacity for a distinctive form of social and, in particular, dialogical engagement.[7]

Relational autonomy involves a more bidirectional approach in which health care providers go beyond the provision of mere facts and translate the information into concepts comprehensible and usable to the average patient. It entails providing support and structure in order for the patient (in this case, a potential living donor) to get a better grasp of the risks and benefits and to consider the psychosocial and emotional consequences of the decision in a safe and enabling environment. Through a shared decision-making process, potential living donors are empowered to move beyond pre-reflective preferences to exercise their autonomy and make an informed choice consonant with their considered values, beliefs, and interests that best reflect their deliberated judgment. As Susan Dodds explains:

> The physician standing as objective, neutral information source, is not necessarily an aide to autonomy. A health-care worker who has sufficient information; who can listen actively to the patients' identification of their concerns, desires, fears and so on; and who can ask them how much they want to know and why will often better promote autonomy both in decision making and in the patient's capacity to learn to accommodate or respond to the changes in their health. . . .[8]

In our living donor ethics framework, respect for persons incorporates this relational conception of autonomy. For prospective living organ donors with decisional capacity, respect for persons requires that the transplant team employ a shared decision-making process in which they empower patients to make decisions that best reflect their own interests and values, free from undue pressure or influence. It requires that the transplant team help enable living donors to act voluntarily; to ensure that they reflect upon and consider their own best interests, broadly construed; and that they remain aware of their right to renege (withdraw) up until the time of donation.[9] And for those who lack decisional capacity, respect for persons requires their protection, which almost always translates into non-donation.[10]

3.3 Beneficence

The *Belmont Report* is clear that obligations of beneficence extend both to particular research projects and to the entire enterprise of research. In the *Report*, beneficence refers to 2 different but complementary rules: "1) do not harm; and 2) maximize possible benefits and minimize possible harms,"[11] which are operationalized using a utilitarian calculation of benefits and risks.

Shifting the principle of beneficence from human subjects protections in the *Belmont Report* to the realm of transplantation ethics is complicated by the fact that living donor transplantation involves 2 separate persons: the donor and the recipient for whom the benefits and risks are both distinct and intertwined. The first step, then, is to calculate donor risk:benefit and to separately calculate recipient risk:benefit. This does not mean that recipient benefit is irrelevant to the donor's calculation. While some donors may define donor benefit to include only their own (psychological) benefit, most include not only their own psychological benefit but also the health benefits to the recipient as part of their donor benefit calculation. Donors also must decide which risks they balance against these benefits—to include only their own clinical and psychosocial risks or to include the potential clinical and psychosocial risks to the recipient.[12] In philosophical terms, donors may have both self-regarding and other-regarding interests and may define the benefits and the risks of donation not purely in self-regarding terms. The recipient also has self-regarding and other-regarding interests. Thus, the recipient must also agree that the medical benefits to him outweigh the risks, and the recipient may include not only his own risks but also the risks to the donor. An adult child who wants to donate to a parent may argue that his parent's survival is worth the physical risks of a living organ donation, but the parent (recipient) may reject the offer. That is, both donors and recipients must decide that the living donor transplant has a positive risk:benefit calculation for themselves as individuals, and each must voluntarily consent to the procedure.

Although risk:benefit calculations are necessary, they are not sufficient for determining the ethical permissibility of a transplant. Consider, for example, the actual case of Mr. Patterson, who donated a kidney to his daughter, Renada. The kidney failed and Mr. Patterson requested to donate his second kidney to his daughter, who was willing to accept it knowing that it would leave her father dialysis-dependent.[13] Some argue that if the potential donor and the potential recipient assert that the benefits outweigh the risks, then the living donation is ethically permissible.[14] While we agree that it is necessary that both donor and recipient judge the benefits to outweigh the risks, this calculation is not sufficient because it would allow serious harm to the donor—in this case, leaving Mr. Patterson anephric and therefore dialysis-dependent. The reason to reject the parent's offer to donate his second kidney is not that his calculation is wrong, but because there are limits to how much harm that transplant professionals, as moral agents, should be willing to voluntarily cause a potential living donor. As Carl Elliott eloquently explains:

Finally, it is important to realize that the doctor is not a mere instrument of the patient's wishes. Analyses of living organ donation and risky clinical research are often simplified needlessly by a failure to acknowledge outright that the doctor is also a moral agent who should be held accountable for his actions. If a patient undergoes a harmful procedure, the moral responsibility for that action does not belong to the patient alone; it is shared by the doctor who performs it. Thus a doctor is in the position of deciding not simply whether a subject's choice is reasonable or morally justifiable, but whether he is morally justified in helping the subject accomplish it.[15]

That is, the members of the transplant team are moral agents who must concur that the risks and risk:benefit to each party is reasonable or they should refuse to proceed with performing the living donor surgery. This position is clearly articulated in other documents focused on ethical issues in living donation. For example, Linda Wright and colleagues at the University of Toronto state:

If autonomy alone were the arbiter of living donation, then the donor and recipient could decide if they are agreeable and ask to proceed. However, members of the health care team are active participants in this process, with an obligation to maintain professional standards of practice. Thus, health care providers act as moral agents with rights to autonomy that must be respected in the decision-making process.[16]

The Ethics Committee of the Transplantation Society concluded similarly in a section entitled "Medical Judgement versus Donor Autonomy": "Donor autonomy does not overrule medical judgment and decision-making."[17] Similarly, the Live Organ Donor Consensus Group stated that "Transplant physicians must have decision making autonomy that prevents undue pressure on the medical team to perform a procedure that they do not believe is medically indicated."[18]

3.4 Justice

The *Belmont Report* acknowledges a variety of formulations of justice—ranging from various egalitarian conceptions of justice (eg, to each person an equal share; or to each person according to individual need) to conceptions of distributive justice based on effort or merit. But in the *Report*, justice is operationalized as the fair selection of subjects (social justice).[19]

The National Commission enumerated that certain groups are vulnerable and require extra protection. The list included:

> ... racial minorities, the economically disadvantaged, the very sick, and the institutionalized may continually be sought as research subjects, owing to their ready availability in settings where research is conducted. Given their dependent status and their frequently compromised capacity for free consent, they should be protected against the danger of being involved in research....[20]

The National Commission's reports serve as the basis for the *Code of Federal Regulations (CFR) for the Protection of Human Subjects* (45 CFR 46).[21] Subpart A is based on the *Belmont Report* and applies to all research participants. Other reports address research enrolling specific vulnerable populations including pregnant women, human fetuses and neonates,[22] prisoners,[23] and children,[24] and these reports serve as the basis for 45 CFR 46, Subparts B, C, and D respectively. Members of these groups would be considered vulnerable if they were solicited to be living donors as well.

The fair selection of subjects means ensuring fair opportunities for participation with additional safeguards for members of vulnerable groups to prevent over-reliance because they are convenient or because of a social perception of lower worth. For example, empirical data show that women are more likely to be living organ donors and yet less likely to be a recipient of a living donor organ (see chapter 3).[25] Fair selection also means not absolutely excluding donation by some members of vulnerable groups (eg, prisoners) if they can adequately address the threats that challenge their ability to give a voluntary and informed consent (see chapter 6).

3.5 Vulnerabilities

The National Commission's reports focusing on vulnerable groups were written in the late 1970s. Twenty years later, in a paper commissioned by the National Bioethics Advisory Committee, a successor to the National Commission, Kenneth Kipnis argued that the National Commission's concept of "vulnerable populations" failed to explore in what ways particular groups of people were vulnerable, thereby risking unnecessary protections for some and inadequate protections for others.[26] He proposed a taxonomy that explored the different types of vulnerabilities that research participants may feel. He offered an analytical approach to the concept of vulnerability, arguing that rather than focusing on groups, it would be more useful to consider 6 discrete types of vulnerability that an individual may face: cognitive, juridic, deferential, medical, allocational, and infrastructural.[27] In a later work focusing on why children may be vulnerable in research, Kipnis offers 7 discrete types of vulnerability—retaining the first 5 (cognitive, which he changed to incapacitational, and which we will refer to as capacitational); juridic, deferential, medical, allocational—and adding 2 more: social and situational.[28] We incorporate all 8 of Kipnis' vulnerabilities into a research taxonomy in Table 3.1, column 1. In Table 3.1, column 2, we show how they can be modified to apply to living donor transplantation.[29] We provide greater detail to show how these vulnerabilities are applied in the living donor context. It should be stressed that identification of 1 or more vulnerabilities in an individual potential donor is not, in and of itself, disqualifying for donation, but rather it presents an opportunity for the potential donor to explore with her transplant team whether these vulnerabilities can be adequately addressed such that the potential donor can exercise her autonomy and provide a voluntary and informed consent.

The first vulnerability is capacitational (previously described as incapacitational or cognitive). It refers to the vulnerability that would be experienced if a potential living donor lacked the capacity (decision-making ability) to give an informed consent for his or her own participation as a solid organ donor. A potential living donor may be cognitively vulnerable because of immaturity of age or because of intellectual disabilities or mental illness. Comparable to the research setting, one solution is to have a surrogate decision-maker. But there is a major difference: while it is important to do research on those who lack cognitive capacity if the research is to understand or reverse the inability or, in some other way, help those with a similar disability, there are few situations in which a person who is unable to make decisions for him- or herself should be considered for living donation. In general, it is not in a donor's medical interest to donate, and lack of capacity should be a strong (if not an absolute) contra-indication.[30]

The second vulnerability is juridic. It refers to whether a potential living donor is liable to the authority of others who may have an independent interest in that donation or, conversely, non-donation. The authority is meant

Table 3.1 Eight Vulnerabilities of Potential Living Donors

Trait	Research	Living donor transplantation
Capacitational (aka Incapacitational and Cognitive)	Does the C-S have the capacity to deliberate about and decide whether or not to participate in the study?	Does the potential living donor have the capacity to deliberate about and decide whether or not to participate as a living donor?
Juridic	Is the C-S liable to the authority of others who may have an independent interest in that participation?	Is the potential living donor liable to the authority of others who may have an independent interest in that donation?
Deferential	Is the C-S given to patterns of deferential behavior that may mask an underlying unwillingness to participate?	Is the potential living donor given to patterns of deferential behavior that may mask an underlying unwillingness to participate?
Social	Does the C-S belong to a group whose rights and interests have been socially disvalued?	Does the potential living donor belong to a group whose rights and interests have been socially disvalued?
Medical	Has the C-S been selected, in part, because of the presence of a serious health-related condition for which there are no satisfactory remedies?	Has the potential living donor been selected, in part, because of the presence of a serious health-related condition in the intended recipient for which there are only less satisfactory alternative remedies?
Situational	Is the C-S in a situation in which medical exigency prevents the education and deliberation needed to decide whether to participate in the study?	Is the potential living donor in a situation in which medical exigency of the intended recipient prevents the education and deliberation needed by the potential living donor to decide whether to participate as a living donor?
Allocational	Is the C-S or proxy lacking in subjectively important social goods that will be provided as a consequence of participation in research?	Is the potential living donor lacking in subjectively important social goods that will be provided as a consequence of participation as a donor?
Infrastructural	Does the political, organizational, economic, and social context of the research setting possess the integrity and resources needed to manage the study?	Does the political, organizational, economic, and social context of the donor care setting possess the integrity and resources needed to manage living donation process and follow-up?

This table, now modified, was first published in Ross LF, Thistlethwaite JR Jr. The Prisoner as Living Organ Donor. *Cambridge Quarterly of Healthcare Ethics*. 2018;27:93–108 at 97 at page 96, Table 1. Copyright © 2018 Cambridge University Press. Modified and reprinted with permission from Cambridge University Press.

Abbreviations: C-S: Candidate-Subject.

to be legal and can refer to prisoners and military personnel, although Kipnis does say that "the category also includes children (either juvenile or adult) under the authority of their parents, so for example, the juvenile whose parents seek for him to be a living donor to a twin sibling."[31]

The third vulnerability is deferential and refers to whether a potential living donor is given to patterns of deferential behavior that may mask an underlying unwillingness to participate. While similar to juridic vulnerability, it is less formal and more often self-imposed. It may be seen in the decision of an adult child who seeks to please his or her parents (or his or her grandparents), an employee who seeks to curry favor with their employer, or a woman who believes it is her role to make this type of personal sacrifice in a male-dominated culture. As Kipnis explains, the challenge is to devise a process that eliminates as much as possible the social pressures that the potential living donors "may feel even if, in reality, they are not being imposed."[32]

Persons may also express deferential vulnerability in their response to requests from transplant professionals. One can easily imagine the healthy individual asked to be a living donor for a family member finding it very hard to tell the members of the transplant team caring for the recipient candidate that she refuses to serve as a living donor. This is why it is critical that potential living donors have their own health care team focused on their own interests.

The fourth vulnerability is social. It refers to whether the potential living donor belong to a group whose rights and interests have been socially disvalued. For example, when families negotiate who should be the first to undergo screening, families may look to non-wage earners. It is also possible that the non-wage earners volunteer themselves, either because they view this as an opportunity to be an active contributor to the family's resources or because they have internalized the view that they are of lower worth. This vulnerability requires that the transplant team work with potential living donors to ensure that their participation is voluntary and that they are donating without "undue influence" (the language used in the *Belmont Report*[33]).

The fifth vulnerability is medical and focuses on the presence of a serious health-related condition in the intended recipient when a potential donor feels undue pressure to donate because only less satisfactory alternative remedies are available to the intended recipient. A remedy is less satisfactory when it is likely to lead to either worse outcomes (higher morbidity and/or mortality) or is not available in a timely fashion. Consider end-stage renal disease (ESRD). ESRD can be treated by dialysis or transplantation although data show that transplantation is better for virtually all patients.[34] The main stress is that demand greatly outpaces supply. The uncertainty of whether the intended recipient will receive a deceased donor organ in a timely fashion puts pressure, to varying degrees, on potential living donors. This is compounded by the fact that living donor grafts are superior (longer graft survival) to deceased donor grafts in most situations for most recipients.[35]

The sixth vulnerability is situational which refers to the medical exigency of the intended recipient that precludes adequate education of and deliberation by the potential living donor which are essential for the living donor's informed decision-making. That is, external circumstances may threaten donor voluntariness. Consider, for example, living donation in the setting of acute liver failure (ALF),[36] when an entire living donor work-up must be done in a matter of hours, rather than days or weeks. The potential living donor must grasp the risks and benefits and its implications for him- or herself in a very compressed time frame before a decision must be made. It is critical that health care provider(s) independent of the recipient's team be available to support and to empower the potential donor to make a voluntary decision that best reflects his or her own values and interests. This function can be achieved with an independent living donor advocate (LDA) as part of the living donor advocate team (LDAT) described in section 8 of this chapter.[37]

But even if the work-up is done expeditiously, the patient in ALF may deteriorate and become too ill to be transplanted. In fact, this can happen to any candidate on the waiting list for any organ. In such situations, the LDAT may decide that the potential recipient benefit is too low that it cannot justify exposing a living donor to risk, even if the living donor is willing to assume those risks. The potential living donor may experience situational vulnerability and find it very difficult, if not impossible, to deliberate rationally in such a situation because of the emotional stress of being "too late." Or the potential living donor may experience situational vulnerability in the form of denial or unrealistic hope and petition to donate on the grounds of "nothing ventured, nothing gained" without considering that a surgical attempt may increase or prolong pain and suffering without offering clinical benefit.

The seventh vulnerability is allocational and focuses on the potential living donor who is lacking in subjectively important social goods that she believes will be provided as a consequence of participation as a donor. Social goods can include, for example, improved community social status or improved intrafamilial relationships. It is important that living donors realize that these social goods may be transient or may never occur.[38]

The eighth vulnerability is infrastructural. Does the political, organizational, economic, and social context of the donor care setting possess the integrity and resources needed to manage living donation process and follow-up? This vulnerability examines the capacity of the transplant program and the institution to adequately perform living donor transplantation and follow-up care. This requires a wide range of skills: not just surgeons, but appropriate intensive care unit physicians as well as physician subspecialists to deal with both expected and unexpected complications of these procedures. Francis Moore, one of the pioneers of surgical innovation, described this as the "field strength" of the institution which, he stated must be complemented by the ethical climate of the institution.[39] Lacking either may create an infrastructural vulnerability for donors and/or recipients.

Infrastructural vulnerability can also be related to the social situation of potential donors themselves. Are they homeless? Do they live alone? Do they have an adequate support system to help them through recovery from surgery? Do they have adequate health literacy to be able to read and understand donor educational materials and the informed consent forms? Do they understand their need for life-long good health habits and follow-up and have the wherewithal, both financially and psychologically, to comply with this need? If they have low health literacy, do LDATs have the skills and resources to support and empower potential donors to fully evaluate the risks and benefits and make a decision consonant with their beliefs and values?

Another infrastructural vulnerability relates to the need for life-long living donor follow-up. It was only in 1994 that UNOS began to collect the Social Security numbers of living donors, which made any type of systematic follow-up possible. In 2000, UNOS/OPTN mandated 1-year follow-up, which it extended to 2 years in 2006, the cost being absorbed by the transplant programs. However, it is now known that complications may not develop for months or years, and yet many (~20%) living donors do not have health insurance and so may not get appropriate long-term evaluation and treatment to minimize their risks.[40] More worrisome is that a large percentage of donors are lost to follow-up despite the UNOS/OPTN mandatory 2 year follow-up.[41] Some donors may seek care elsewhere and not return to the transplant program so any health harms are not quantified. Other donors may not seek any care because either they assume themselves to be healthy or because they lack health insurance and fear that they will incur costs for which they will be responsible. Infrastructural vulnerability refers to both individual and institutional support systems both pre- and post-donation and over the long term.

3.6 Vulnerability Critiques

We have shown that, with minor modifications, Kipnis' model of vulnerabilities is useful for examining the ethical challenges raised by living organ donation. We now consider and reject 3 objections to his vulnerability analysis in order to further strengthen its adoption in a living donor ethics framework.

First, Kipnis' account of vulnerability has been criticized for being overreaching in that all of us will meet 1 or more of these vulnerabilities at some point in time.[42] Others contend, however, that this is a strength because it forces us to acknowledge that even completely healthy, adequately informed adult research subjects, not belonging to any identifiably vulnerable population enumerated in the *Belmont Report* may have vulnerabilities that lead them to participate.[43] The case of Ellen Roche shows how otherwise healthy cognitively normal adults may be vulnerable. Ms. Roche was a research technician at John Hopkins University Asthma and Allergy Center who volunteered to take part in a hexamethonium study in a proximate lab in April 2001. The study was "designed to provoke a mild asthma attack in order to help doctors discover the reflex that protects the lungs of healthy people against asthma attacks."[44] She became ill shortly thereafter, and was admitted to an intensive care unit in May 2001 but continued to worsen and died 1 month later.[45] Of primary importance in addressing Ms. Roche's death as a normal volunteer was the fact that inhalational hexamethonium was not approved by the Food and Drug Administration (FDA), and Hopkins was rebuked by the Office for Human Research Protections (OHRP) for failing to obtain sufficient information on the " 'source, purity, quality, and method of preparation and delivery' of the chemical before giving it to volunteers."[46] However, an external review committee also raised the additional concern about justice in the selection of subjects, pointing out that Ms. Roche and multiple other staff members who volunteered were exposed to the potential for "subtle coercive pressures," as these staff members were often given time off during the workday to participate in protocols.[47] So while laboratory staff may not be a "vulnerable group" per se, an "informal" expectation of participation would place these individuals at risk of deferential vulnerability (potentially juridic vulnerability), and the ability to collect additional financial rewards during work hours may raise further social vulnerability concerns as well.[48]

Likewise, we believe that adults with decisional capacity who are asked to serve as a living donor may be vulnerable in ways that may threaten the voluntariness of their consent even if they are not members of a traditional vulnerable group. For example, since many living donors are first-degree relatives with their recipient, they may be at risk of deferential and social vulnerability depending on family social structure, expectations, and the potential impact of non-donation on family relationships. Alternatively, in the case of ALF, a parent who is informed that their child may become too ill before a deceased donor liver graft is found, may be medically vulnerable and ignore or discount risks to herself. The parent may also be at risk of deferential vulnerability with respect to the transplant team who offered living donation as an option. Despite the limited time, it is critical that the team engage the parent in examination of these risks and the potential implications of an adverse event for him- or herself and other dependents in order to ensure that the consent is both informed and voluntary. These cases illustrate the utility of considering the entire taxonomy of vulnerabilities for each living donor to ensure that they can be adequately addressed.

Second, Kipnis has been criticized by Tricha Shivas for focusing on individuals and the process of informed consent and failing to consider how vulnerabilities impact justice or the fair selection of participants.[49] We disagree that Kipnis' vulnerability taxonomy fails to consider justice concerns because many of the vulnerabilities can be applied to entire groups. For example, prisoners as a class lack certain social goods (eg, freedom of movement) that would classify them as socially vulnerable. The social isolation of incarceration may also result in prisoners being deferentially and socially vulnerable to those family members who are often their only resource beyond the prison walls. This does not mean that prisoners should never be allowed to participate as living donors, but rather that it is critical that their vulnerabilities be explored and if these threats to a voluntary informed decision-making process cannot be adequately addressed, the individuals must be prevented from donating (see chapter 6).

A third criticism is that Kipnis fails to consider that vulnerability is a "relational concept." Shivas argues that Kipnis fails to acknowledge that "vulnerability cannot be defined independent of our understanding of the relationship, power dynamics, and social and political circumstances of the particular protocol."[50] We agree that vulnerability is relational, but so does Kipnis. For example, juridic and deferential vulnerabilities specifically focus on power dynamics, both those that are legally defined and those that are socially defined respectively.[51] In the following sections we show how understanding vulnerability as relational offers a way to protect and promote the interests of living donors.

3.7 Donors and Recipients as Distinct Patients

Robert Goodin, in his book *Protecting the Vulnerable*, starts from the premise that vulnerability is relational.[52] Goodin assigns special responsibilities for protecting the vulnerable to those with whom the vulnerable are in special relationships. Professionals such as doctors are 1 example that he examines.[53]

Consider, then, a patient who develops ESRD. The patient will be educated by his health care providers about treatment alternatives which include various types of dialysis as well as living and deceased donor transplantation. For most patients with ESRD, transplant offers an improvement in quality and quantity of life, and living donor kidney transplant has better outcomes than deceased donor transplant.[54] Thus the transplant team, focused on the candidate's medical needs, will encourage him to find a living donor.

Most patients in ESRD first look for a living donor within their own family.[55] However, asking a family member to serve as a living donor is not and should not be perceived as a benign request.[56] There are now data to show that kidney donation is not only associated with rare perioperative risks, but also increased risks of pre-eclampsia, kidney disease, and cardiovascular disease.[57] Most donors will be unaware of these risks at the time of the request and may commit to the process before they have adequate information, and may then feel obligated to continue even if they later develop feelings of ambivalence or downright objection to taking the risks being requested of them.[58] (Late development of ambivalence or concern about the level of risk to which they might subject themselves may be even greater for potential living liver donors.[59]) That is why it is critical for the potential donor to have her own health care team—a medical team focused on her own well-being—who can help her decide in favor of donating or, alternatively, against donating if that is what the potential donor decides is in her own best interest. In other words, it is critical that the potential donor be treated as a patient in his or her own right.

The donor has not always been regarded as a patient. Joseph Murray, the surgeon who performed the first successful living donor transplant between identical twins, recounts a discussion with the first successful living kidney donor:

> The donor, a 23-year-old intelligent person, asked a very pointed question: would the doctors at the Peter Bent Brigham Hospital be willing to take care of him medically for the rest of his life if he gave his kidney? We stated that we neither could nor desired to make a guarantee of that sort; we were there to help his brother and if he (the prospective donor) could help his brother, we felt that the chances of success were quite good.[60]

That is, from Murray's perspective, the donor was part of the transplant team engaged in helping the patient in ESRD. In fact, when Murray shared this anecdote at the CIBA symposium, the first international meeting on transplantation and ethics, David Daube, a British legal scholar, suggested that a way around the problem that the donor could be injured by the elective nephrectomy was to view the living donor transplant process "... from the start with the living donor to the finish—which, one hopes, is some relief at least for the recipient—as one composite, curative transaction";[61] that is, he proposed regarding "the two operations in the transplanting transaction as a unitary, positive, curative process."[62] In agreement, the Reverend Canon G.B. Bentley of Windsor Castle England elaborated:

> If the two operations were treated as a single action, the danger would be that the human rights of the donor might be overlooked. Unless perhaps he could be regarded as a member of the curative team: he would in a sense be a colleague of the surgeon.[63]

Likewise, in a 2002 update to their 1977 book on the social and psychological impact of organ transplantation, Roberta Simmons and colleagues described their original study which "follow[ed] patients, donors and nondonors up to a year post-transplant."[64] They then explain that they continued to follow these participants for another 5 to 9 years, and in their updated book, they describe the social-psychological effects of kidney transplantation on 3 sets of stakeholders:

1. upon the patients themselves (the transplant recipients) in order to determine whether their quality of life is high enough to warrant this expensive therapy
2. upon the living relatives who donate a kidney to the patient
3. upon the families involved in the decision to donate a kidney.[65]

In other words, the recipients are described as patients whereas the donors are not. Similarly, in describing the ambivalence experienced by all involved in the early days of organ transplantation, Renee Fox and Judith Swazey write in *The Courage to Fail*:

> Nowhere is this ambivalence more conspicuous than in the discoveries that physicians and patients, donors and their families have made about the dilemmas and paradoxes of the gift as they occur in the context of organ transplantation.[66]

Again, the word "patient" is used to describe organ recipients and not living kidney donors.[67]

What were the implications of not being perceived as a patient? It meant that there was minimal follow-up of living donors beyond removing the sutures and there was no systematic collection of data to determine if there were unknown long-term risks. In fact, it would not be until the mid-1990s when short-term living donor data were first collected and deposited in a national registry for possible retrospective analysis.

In 2000, the Live Organ Donor Consensus Report supported "an independent advocate for the donor. . . whose only focus is the best interests of the donor."[68] The donor advocate was conceived as an individual who would help empower the potential donor to understand the risks, benefits, and alternatives and then to freely decide whether or not to donate. The Live Organ Donor Consensus Group believed that the donor advocate should have the authority to veto the donation if the consent was not informed and voluntary.[69] This was given further support in 2002 when the Department of Health and Human Services Advisory Committee on Organ Transplantation recommended an independent donor advocate to ensure that informed consent standards were met.[70] In 2007 the Centers for Medicare and Medicaid Services mandated an independent donor advocate for all living donor organ transplants.[71] These independent donor advocates are now referred to as living donor advocates (LDAs).[72] Some programs involve a living donor advocate team (LDAT), which involves 2 or more persons who evaluate, educate, and advocate for the living donor.[73] Throughout this book, we refer to the donor's health care team which includes an LDA as a member of the LDAT. The LDAT approach acknowledges that all the skills needed to provide the appropriate medical and psychosocial care of a living donor may not reside in 1 individual and instead a multidisciplinary team is required to evaluate, educate, and advocate for the living donor.

We support the practice of treating potential living donors as patients from the moment that they begin a dialogue with the transplant center about possible donation. Given the potential conflicts of interest between the donor's own well-being with the recipient-candidate and the recipient-candidate's health team, it is critical that the donor has her own health care team that is independent of the recipient's team.[74] The LDAT must support and aid the potential donor to identify and address the vulnerabilities applicable to herself and to best address her values, needs, and interests. This is explored further in the next section.

3.8 Special Relationships Create Special Responsibilities

The central argument of Goodin's book is that "we bear special responsibilities for protecting those who are particularly vulnerable to us."[75] He begins with standard cases of family members, friends, and professionals. Specifically, for our purposes, Goodin argues that doctors (health care providers) "have special and especially strong obligations to protect the interests of their clients."[76]

In the transplant arena, the LDAT stands in special relationship with the potential living donor. Their role is to promote the best interest of the donor, to advocate for his or her rights, and to ensure that the donor obtains and understands information about the consent, evaluation, donation, and post-donation processes.[77] The LDAT may include a physician (usually a nephrologist or hepatologist), a surgeon, a social worker, and/or other health care professionals who are an integral component of the donor's health care team—a team dedicated exclusively to the donor's well-being and separate from the well-being of the potential recipient, even when the donor and recipient are family members, spouses, or close friends.[78] In the clinical setting, this means that the LDA and other members of the donor's transplant team not only ensure that the donor is physically, psychologically, and emotionally healthy enough to donate, but they also evaluate donor motivation and voluntariness. Using the language of Kipnis and Goodin, this means that the LDAT is responsible for evaluating all the different types of vulnerability threats that the potential donor may experience and ensuring that they are adequately addressed in order to empower the potential donor to give a voluntary and informed consent.

This does not mean that the LDAT should protect potential donors from all risks. The donor's transplant team should respect the donor's right to take health care risks if the donor perceives them to be outweighed by the benefits (which may include both self-regarding and other-regarding benefits). However, the LDAT is responsible not only for ensuring that the donor is acting voluntarily with adequate information but also that the donor's transplant team can morally justify enabling the donation.[79]

What does this mean in practice? It entails a reconception of autonomy and consent that empowers potential donors to address their vulnerabilities in a shared decision-making process. Using a relational autonomy approach as part of a shared decision-making process, the LDAT strives to empower the potential living donors to make decisions that reflect their own considered values. By providing information and examining the vulnerabilities that pertain to a particular living donor, the LDA and other members of the donor transplant team empower the potential donor to understand the risks and benefits tailored to the particular donor, acknowledge her particular vulnerabilities, and help determine whether these vulnerabilities can be adequately addressed or whether they overwhelm the donor's ability to give a voluntary and informed consent. In general, the LDAT should focus on employing a shared decision-making process in which the team goes beyond the provision of health information and engages in bidirectional discussion to enable the potential donor to determine what best reflects her interests, needs, and values. That is, the LDAT helps the donor address her vulnerabilities and promotes the development of a more reflective decision-making process. Such is what a relational autonomy approach entails:

[A] relational approach is committed to the view that the obligations arising from vulnerability extend beyond protection from harm to the provision of the social support necessary to promote the autonomy of persons who are "more than ordinarily vulnerable." A relational approach, then, provides a critical perspective from which some social policy responses to vulnerability can be identified as pathogenic: because they entrench or exacerbate existing vulnerabilities rather than scaffold the development and exercise of autonomy.[80]

If any member of the LDAT believes that the donor's vulnerabilities have not been adequately addressed, it is their responsibility to disqualify the donor, or at least to delay proceeding to donation until all the vulnerabilities are adequately addressed.[81]

Rarely, there are some cases where the team should protect the donor from him- or herself. Recall, then, the situation described above in which Mr. Patterson, who previously donated a kidney to his daughter Renada, wanted to donate his second kidney to her when the first one was rejected. Dr. Nancy Ascher, the transplant surgeon to whom the request was made, objected: "If you choose to walk through fire for your kid, that's great. But if you choose to take me with you, that's different."[82] That is, Ascher took ownership of her responsibility for deciding whether to procure an organ that would leave a donor dialysis-dependent. While a patient can decline to donate an organ or even refuse to accept life-saving treatment, "a competent patient does not have the right to demand a harmful medical intervention, even if her reasons for doing so . . . [are] admirable."[83] The transplant team, as moral agents in a special relationship with the potential living donor, accepted their responsibility to protect the father from his own seemingly autonomous decision because they perceived the outcome as too harmful. The ethics committee at the University of California at San Francisco rejected Mr. Paterson's request, and, instead, Renada received a living donor transplant from an uncle.[84]

3.9 Conclusion

Most living donors reflect very positively on their decision to donate and describe great benefit from donating for themselves and their recipients. An analytical framework to guide the resolution of ethical problems arising from transplantation involving living donors is necessary.

Research ethics principles are very useful for developing this living donor ethics framework. We have shown that a living donor ethics framework can be developed by adopting the 3 principles from the *Belmont Report*—respect for persons, beneficence, and justice—supplemented by 2 additional principles: vulnerability and responsibility. We believe these 5 principles provide the basis for a living donor ethics framework that can be used to explore the ethical challenges raised by current and evolving living donor transplantation practices and policies (see Table 3.2).

For ease of the reader, we end Part 1 with a full-page vulnerability typology which will be a guidepost for all discussions about vulnerabilities (see Table 3.3). In Parts 2, 3 and 4, the relevant vulnerabilities will be considered in each chapter when pertinent to the arguments offered and cases explored.

Table 3.2 Living Donor Ethics Framework

PRINCIPLE	APPLICATION
Respect for persons	Incorporates a relational conception of autonomy in which health care providers go beyond the provision of mere facts and translate the information into concepts comprehensible and usable to the average patient. Through a shared decision-making process, potential donors are empowered to move beyond pre-reflective preferences to exercise their autonomy by making an informed choice consonant with their considered values, beliefs and interests.
Beneficence	Risk:benefit calculation (of the living donor separately from the risks and benefits to the recipient, although the living donor can consider recipient factors in his or her calculation).
Justice	Fair selection of living donors.
Vulnerabilities	A comprehensive vulnerability taxonomy that enumerates the vulnerabilities that living donors may experience and that need to be addressed to ensure that potential living organ donors provide a voluntary informed consent.
Special relationships create special obligations	In the context of living donor organ transplantation, the living donor advocate team (LDAT) has the responsibility to ensure that the potential living donor gives an informed and voluntary consent, that the risks and benefits of living donation are medically appropriate, and that the LDAT is morally justified in performing the donor procurement.

Table 3.3 Eight Vulnerabilities of Potential Living Donors

Trait	Living donor transplantation
Capacitational	Does the potential living donor have the capacity to deliberate about and decide whether or not to participate as a living donor?
Juridic	Is the potential living donor liable to the authority of others who may have an independent interest in that donation?
Deferential	Is the potential living donor given to patterns of deferential behavior that may mask an underlying unwillingness to participate?
Social	Does the potential living donor belong to a group whose rights and interests have been socially disvalued?
Medical	Has the potential living donor been selected, in part, because of the presence of a serious health-related condition in the intended recipient for which there are only less satisfactory alternative remedies?
Situational	Is the potential living donor in a situation in which medical exigency of the intended recipient prevents the education and deliberation needed by the potential living donor to decide whether to participate as a living donor?
Allocational	Is the potential living donor lacking in subjectively important social goods that will be provided as a consequence of participation as a donor?
Infrastructural	Does the political, organizational, economic, and social context of the donor care setting possess the integrity and resources needed to manage living donation process and follow-up?

Notes

1. The National Commission for the Protection of Human Subjects of Biomedical and Behavioral Research. *The Belmont Report: Ethical Principles and Guidelines for the Protection of Human Subjects of Research*. Washington, DC: Government Printing Office;1978. Last accessed August 15, 2021. http://www.hhs.gov/ohrp/humansubje cts/guidance/belmont.html. Hereinafter referred to as the *Belmont Report*.
2. See, for example, Abecassis M, Adams M, Adams P, et al. Consensus statement on the live organ donor. *JAMA*. 2000;284:2919–2926; Ethics Committee of the Transplantation Society. The consensus statement of the Amsterdam Forum on the Care of the Live Kidney Donor. *Transplantation*. 2004;78:491–492; Wright L, Faith K, Richardson R, Grant D. Ethical guidelines for the evaluation of living organ donors. *Can J Surg*. 2004;47:408–413; Barr ML, Belghiti J, Villamil FG, et al. A report of the Vancouver Forum on the care of the live organ donor: lung, liver, pancreas and intestine data and medical guidelines. *Transplantation*. 2006;81:1373–1385; Pruett TL, Tibell A, Alabdulkareem A, et al. The ethics statement of the Vancouver Forum on the live lung, liver, pancreas, and intestine donor. *Transplantation*.

2006;81(10):1386–1387; and Lentine KL, Kasiske BL, Levey AS, et al. KDIGO clinical practice guideline on the evaluation and care of living kidney donors. *Transplantation*. 2017;101:(8S suppl 1):S1–S109.

3. *Belmont Report.*
4. *Belmont Report.*
5. *Belmont Report.*
6. Mackenzie C, Stoljar N. Introduction: Autonomy Refigured. In: Mackenzie C, Stoljar N, eds. *Relational Autonomy: Feminist Perspectives on Autonomy, Agency, and the Social Self.* New York, NY: Oxford University Press; 2000:3–31, at p. 6.
7. Friedman M. Autonomy Social Disruptions and Women. In: Mackenzie C, Stoljar N, eds. *Relational Autonomy: Feminist Perspectives on Autonomy, Agency, and the Social Self.* New York, NY: Oxford University Press; 2000:35–51, at pp. 40–41 (footnotes omitted).
8. Dodds S. Choice and Control in Feminist Bioethics. In: Mackenzie C, Stoljar N, eds. *Relational Autonomy: Feminist Perspectives on Autonomy, Agency, and the Social Self.* New York, NY: Oxford University Press; 2000: 213–235, at p. 232.
9. Abecassis et al, "Consensus statement."
10. Steinberg D. Kidney transplants from young children and the mentally retarded. *Theor Med Bioeth.* 2004;25:229–241.
11. *Belmont Report.*
12. See, for example, Spital A. Donor benefit is the key to justified living organ donation. *Camb Q Healthc Ethics.* 2004;13:105–109; and Glannon W, Ross LF. Motivation, risk, and benefit in living organ donation: a reply to Aaron Spital. *Camb Q Healthc Ethics.* 2005;14:191–194; discussion at pp. 195–198.
13. Ross LF. Donating a second kidney: a tale of family and ethics. *Semin Dial.* 2000;13:201–203.
14. Miller CM, Smith ML, Uso TD. Living donor liver transplantation: ethical considerations. *Mt Sinai J Med.* 2012;79:214–222.
15. Elliott C. Doing harm: living organ donors, clinical research and *The Tenth Man*. *J Med Ethics* 1995;21:91–96, at p. 95.
16. Wright et al, "Ethical guidelines," at p. 410 (references omitted).
17. Ethics Committee of the Transplantation Society, "The consensus statement," at p. 492.
18. Abecassis et al, "Consensus statement," at p. 2925.
19. *Belmont Report.*
20. *Belmont Report.*
21. Department of Health and Human Services. Code of Federal Regulations (CFR) Title 45 Public Welfare Part 46. Final Regulations Amending Basic HHS Policy for the Protection of Human Research Subjects. *Fed Regist.* 1981;46:8366–8391. Most recently revised *Fed Regist.* 2017;82:7259–7273. August 15, 2021. https://www.ecfr.gov/cgi-bin/retrieveECFR?gp=&SID=83cd09e1c0f5c6937cd9d7513160fc3f&pitd=20180719&n=pt45.1.46&r=PART&ty=HTML. Hereinafter referred to as 45 CFR 46.

22. National Commission for the Protection of Human Subjects of Biomedical and Behavioral Research. *Research on the Fetus: Report And Recommendations*. Washington, DC: Government Printing Office; 1975.

23. National Commission for the Protection of Human Subjects of Biomedical and Behavioral Research. *Research Involving Prisoners: Report and Recommendations*. Washington, DC: Government Printing Office; 1976.

24. National Commission for the Protection of Human Subjects of Biomedical and Behavioral Research. *Research Involving Children: Report and Recommendations*. Washington DC: Government Printing Office; 1977.

25. Kjellstrand CM. Age, sex, and race inequality in renal transplantation. *Arch Intern Med.* 1988;148:1305–1309; Jindal RM, Ryan JJ, Sajjad I, Murthy MH, Baines LS. Kidney transplantation and gender disparity. *Am J Nephrol* 2005;25:474–483; Gill J, Joffres Y, Rose C, et al. The change in living kidney donation in women and men in the United States (2005–2015): a population-based analysis. *J Am Soc Nephrol.* 2018;29:1301–1308.

26. Kipnis K. Vulnerability in Research Subjects: A Bioethical Taxonomy. In: The National Bioethics Advisory Commission. *Ethical and Policy Issues in Research Involving Human Participants. Volume II: Commissioned Papers and Staff Analysis.* Bethesda, MD: The National Bioethics Advisory Commission; 2001:G1–13, at G3.

27. Kipnis, "Vulnerability."

28. Kipnis K. Seven vulnerabilities in the pediatric research subject. *Theor Med.* 2003;24:107–120, at p. 110.

29. Ross LF, Thistlethwaite JR Jr. Prisoners as living donors: a vulnerabilities analysis. *Camb Q Healthc Ethics.* 2018;27:93–108, at p. 96, Table 1.

30. Steinberg, "Kidney transplants."

31. Kipnis, "Vulnerability," at p. G-7.

32. Kipnis, "Seven vulnerabilities," at p. 114.

33. *Belmont Report.*

34. Port FK, Wolfe RA, Mauger EA, et al. Comparison of survival probabilities for dialysis patients vs cadaver renal transplant recipients. *JAMA.* 1993;270:1339–1343; Tonelli M, Wiebe N, Knoll G, et al. Systematic review: kidney transplantation compared with dialysis in clinically relevant outcomes. *Am J Transplant.* 2011;11:2093–2109; and Vella J. Kidney Transplantation In Adults: Patient Survival After Kidney Transplantation. *UpToDate.* Last accessed August 15, 2021. https://www.uptodate.com/contents/kidney-transplantation-in-adults-patient-survival-after-kidney-transplantation?search=%20patient-survival-after-renal-transplantation&source=search_result&selectedTitle=1~150&usage_type=default&display_rank=1. Literature review current through April 2020. This topic last updated August 23, 2019.

35. Vella, *UpToDate.*

36. Lee WM, Squires RH Jr, Nyberg SL, Doo E, Hoofnagle JH. Acute liver failure: summary of a workshop. *Hepatology.* 2008;47:1401–1415.

37. Steele J. *Living Donor Advocacy: An Evolving Role Within Transplantation.* New York, NY: Springer; 2013; and Rudow DL. The living donor advocate: a team approach

to educate, evaluate, and manage donors across the continuum. *Prog Transplant.* 2009;19:64–70.

38. Jacobs C, Johnson E, Anderson K, Gillingham K, Matas A. Kidney transplants from living donors: how donation affects family dynamics. *Adv Ren Replace Ther.* 1998;5:89–97; Simmons RG, Klein S, Simmons RL. *Gift of Life: The Social and Psychological Impact of Organ Transplantation.* New York, NY: John Wiley and Sons; 1977; updated and with new material: Simmons RG, Marine SK, Simmons RL. *Gift of Life: The Effect of Organ Transplantation on Individual, Family, and Societal Dynamics.* New Brunswick, NJ: Transaction Books; 2002; and Saijad I, Baines LS, Salifu M, Jindal RM. The dynamics of recipient-donor relationships in living kidney transplantation. *Am J Kidney Dis.* 2007;50:834–854.

39. Moore FD. Three ethical revolutions: ancient assumptions remodeled under pressure of transplantation. *Transplant Proc* 1988;20(1 suppl 1):1061–1067.

40. Casagrande LH, Collins S, Warren AT, Ommen ES. Lack of health insurance in living kidney donors *Clin Transplant.* 2012;26(2):E101–104; and Gibney EM, Doshi MD, Hartmann EL, Parikh CR, Garg AX. Health insurance status of US living kidney donors. *Clin J Am Soc Nephrol.* 2010;5:912–916.

41. Schold JD, Buccini LD, Rodrigue JR, et al. Critical factors associated with missing follow-up data for living kidney donors in the United States. *Am J Transplant.* 2015;15;2394–2403; and Waterman AD, Dew MA, Davis CL, et al. Living-donor follow-up attitudes and practices in U.S. kidney and liver donor programs. *Transplantation.* 2013;95:883–888; and Henderson ML, Thomas AG, Shaffer A, et al. The National Landscape of Living Kidney Donor Follow-Up in the United States. *Am J Transplant.* 2017;17:3131–3140.

42. Levine C, Faden R, Grady C, Hammerschmidt D, Eckenwiler L, Sugarman J. The limitations of "vulnerability" as a protection for human research participants. *The Am J Bioeth.* 2004;4:44–49; and Schroeder D, Gefenas E. Vulnerability: too vague and too broad? *Camb Q Healthc Ethics.* 2009;18:113–121.

43. Rogers W, Mackenzie C, Dodds S. Why bioethics needs a concept of vulnerability. *Intl J Fem Approaches Bioeth.* 2012;5:11–38; and Rendtorff JD. Basic ethical principles in European bioethics and biolaw: autonomy, dignity, integrity and vulnerability—towards a foundation of bioethics and biolaw. *Med Health Care Philos.* 2002;5:235–244.

44. Savulescu J, Spriggs M. The hexamethonium asthma study and the death of a normal volunteer in research. *J Med Ethics.* 2002;28:3–4.

45. Savulescu and Spriggs, "The hexamethonium."

46. Marshall E. Most trials at Hopkins shut down. *Science.* July 19, 2001. Last accessed August 15, 2021. http://www.sciencemag.org/news/2001/07/most-trials-hopkins-shut-down

47. Keiger D, De Pasquale S. Trials & Tribulation. *Johns Hopkins Magazine.* February 2002. Last accessed August 15, 2021. http://pages.jh.edu/jhumag/0202web/trials.html

48. Keiger and De Pasquale, "Trials."

49. Shivas T. Contextualizing the vulnerability standard. *Am J Bioeth (AJOB)*. 2004;4:84–86.
50. Shivas "Contextualizing," at p. 85.
51. Kipnis, "Vulnerability."
52. Goodin RE. *Protecting the Vulnerable: A Reanalysis of Our Social Responsibilities*. Chicago, IL: University of Chicago Press; 1985, at p. 112.
53. Goodin, *Protecting*, at pp. 62–70.
54. See, for example, Vella, *UpToDate;* Collins BH. Kidney Transplantation. Medscape. Updated October 17, 2019. Last accessed August 15, 2021. https://emedicine.medscape.com/article/430128-overview
55. The presumption that family members have special obligations to each other is consistent with moral philosophy focused on relationships and partiality. See, for example, Williams B. *Ethics and the Limits of Philosophy*. Boston, MA: Harvard University Press; 1986; Keller S. *Partiality*. 1st ed. Princeton, NJ: Princeton University Press; 2013. The moral justification has been further developed by feminist ethicists and their focus on relationships and an ethics of care. See, for example, Held V. *The Ethics of Care: Personal, Political, and Global*. New York, NY: Oxford University Press; 2007.
56. Kane F, Clement G, Kane M. Live kidney donations and the ethic of care. *J Med Humanit*. 2008;29:173–188. This concern is also raised in the ethics of care literature.
57. See, for example, Ibrahim HN, Foley R, Tan L, et al. Long-term consequences of kidney donation. *N Engl J Med*. 2009;360:459–469; Muzaale AD, Massie AB, Wainwright J, McBride MA, Wang M, Segev DL. Long-term risk of ESRD attributable to live kidney donation: matching with healthy non-donors. *Am J Transplant*. 2013;13(suppl 5):204–205; and Mjoen G, Hallan S, Hartmann A, et al. Long-term risks for kidney donors. *Kidney Int*. 2014;86:162–167; and Maggiore U, Budde K, Heemann U, et al. Long-term risks of kidney living donation: review and position paper by the ERA-EDTA DESCARTES working group. *Nephrol Dial Transplant*. 2017;32:216–223; Garg AX, Prasad GV, Thiessen-Philbrook HR, et al. Cardiovascular disease and hypertension risk in living kidney donors: an analysis of health administrative data in Ontario, Canada. *Transplantation*. 2008;86:399–406; and Reese PP, Bloom RD, Feldman HI, et al. Mortality and cardiovascular disease among older live kidney donors. *Am J Transplant*. 2014;14:1853–1861.
58. Simmons et al, *Gift of Life,*1977, 2002; Franklin PM, Crombie AK. Live related renal transplantation: psychological, social and cultural issues. *Transplantation*. 2003;76:1247–1252; Halverson CME, Crowley-Matoka M, Ross LF. Unspoken ambivalence in kinship obligation in living donation. *Prog Transplant*. 2018;28(3):250–255.
59. Simpson, MA, Kendrick J, Vferbesey JE, et al. Ambivalence in living liver donors. *Liver Transpl*. 2011;17:1226–1233; and DiMartini A, Cruz RJ Jr, Dew MA, et al. Motives and decision making of potential living liver donors: comparisons between gender, relationships and ambivalence. *Am J Transplant*. 2012;12:136–151.
60. Wolstenholme GEW and O'Connor M, eds. *Ethics in Medical Progress: With Special Reference to Transplantation*. Boston, MA: Little, Brown and Company; 1966, citing Joseph Murray at pp. 17–18.

61. Wolstenholme and O'Connor, *Ethics,* citing David Daube at p. 194.

62. Wolstenholme and O'Connor, *Ethics,* citing David Daube at p. 208.

63. Wolstenholme and O'Connor, *Ethics,* citing the Reverend Canon G. B Bentley at p. 208.

64. Simmons et al, *Gift of Life,* 2002, at p. xxii.

65. Simmons et al, *Gift of Life,* 2002, at p. ix.

66. Fox RC, Swazey JP. *The Courage to Fail: A Social View of Organ Transplants and Dialysis.* Chicago IL: University of Chicago Press; 1978, at p. 381.

67. One of the few people to describe donors as patients was the Protestant theologian Paul Ramsey in his book, *The Patient as Person.* New Haven CT: Yale University Press; 1970. In a chapter in which he explores the ethical legitimacy of living donor transplantation, he wrote:

    > Physicians are rather more concerned about the integrity of the flesh—even when they adopt a procedure that makes a well person ill for the sake of making another well. They do this with ambiguity of conscience over the unmitigated conflict between the medical care both patients need. (p. 173)

    Later in the chapter he elaborates:

    > There is however no avoidance of measuring the costs/benefits. Moralists, meantime, should learn to follow the lineaments of the physicians' reasoning when they let themselves be the moralists they are while undertaking the unique medical procedure of impairing one patient in order to heal another. (pp. 196–197)

68. Abecassis et al, "Consensus statement," at p. 2920.

69. Abecassis et al, "Consensus statement," at p. 2921.

70. Department of Health and Human Services Advisory Committee on Organ Transplantation. Meeting archives: Full Consensus Recommendations, Recommendations 1–18. November 2002. https://www.hrsa.gov/advisory-com mittees/organ-transplantation/recommendations/1-18. Date last reviewed June 2021. Last accessed August 15, 2021. https://www.organdonor.gov/about-dot/acot/ acotrecs118.html

71. Department of Health and Human Services, Part II. Centers for Medicare and Medicaid Services. 42 CFR Parts 405, 482, 488, and 498. Medicare Program; Hospital Conditions of Participation: Requirements for Approval and Re-Approval of Transplant Centers to Perform Organ Transplants; *Fed Regist.* 2007;72:15198–15280. Of note, United Network for Organ Sharing (UNOS)/ Organ Procurement and Transplantation Network (OPTN) modified its bylaws the same year. Appendix B, Section XIII, 2007. Updated in current UNOS/OPTN policy handbook in section 14.2 Independent Living Donor Advocate Requirements. Accessed August 15, 2021. https://optn.transplant.hrsa.gov/media/1200/optn_policies.pdf

72. Hays RE, LaPointe Rudow D, Dew MA, Taler SJ, Spicer H, Mandelbrot DA. The independent living donor advocate: a guidance document from the American Society

of Transplantation's Living Donor Community of Practice (AST LDCOP). *Am J Transplant.* 2015;15:518–525.

73. Rudow DL, Brown RS Jr. Role of the independent donor advocacy team in ethical decision making. *Prog Transplant.* 2005;15:298–302; and Rudow DL. The living donor advocate: a team approach to educate, evaluate, and manage donors across the continuum. *Prog Transplant.* 2009;19:64–70.

74. McQuarrie B, Gordon D. Separate, dedicated care teams for living organ donors. *Prog Transplant.* 2003;13:90–93.

75. Goodin, *Protecting,* at p. 109.

76. Goodin, *Protecting,* at p. 62.

77. Steele, *Living Donor Advocacy*; and McQuarrie and Gordon, "Separate."

78. Steele, *Living Donor Advocacy*; and McQuarrie and Gordon, "Separate"

79. Elliott, "Doing harm."

80. Mackenzie and Stoljar, "Introduction," at p. 17.

81. Abecassis et al, "Consensus statement."

82. Ross, "Donating a second," at p. 201 (footnote omitted).

83. Ross, "Donating a second," at p 202.

84. Ross, "Donating a second," at p. 203.

PART 2
DONOR SELECTION DEMOGRAPHICS

4

Women and Minorities as Living
Organ Donors

4.1 Introduction

The first successful kidney transplant was performed in 1954 between iden-tical twin brothers,[1] and within the decade a voluntary international registry of kidney transplantation of both living and deceased donors was estab-lished. The actual data collected about the donors were quite sparse.

Historically, who were the donors? The first report of the Human Kidney Transplant Registry, published in January 1964, described 244 donors, 68 (28%) of which were deceased donors.[2] Of the remaining 176 kidney grafts, the donor's relationship to the recipients were 49 parents (28%), 39 non-twin siblings (22%), 33 twin siblings (19%), 3 other blood relatives (2%), and 52 nonrelated individuals (30%).[3] Neither gender nor race of the donors were reported. In fact, donor race would never be reported by this registry. Full gender breakdown was not provided until the fifth report, published in July 1967.[4] Males were more likely to be living donors in all categories of donor/recipient relationships except for parent-to-child donations, but because of the high frequency of mother-child donations, women were the majority of living donors (~54%).[5]

No further donor gender data were reported and donor race was never re-ported. A major demographic change, however, was occurring. In the sixth report, based on data through January 1, 1968, there was a trend toward increasing procurement of deceased donor organs and decreasing procure-ment of unrelated living donor grafts. Murray explains: "Presumably the fact that a kidney from an unrelated living donor has no better chances of success than a kidney from a cadaver accounts for this."[6] In the 12th and penultimate report published in August 1975, deceased donors now accounted for 70% of all donors.[7] Virtually all living kidney donors were first-degree relatives. Parents and siblings comprised 43% and 49% of all living donors respec-tively.[8] Again, neither the gender nor the race of the donors were reported.

The Living Organ Donor as Patient. Lainie Friedman Ross and J. Richard Thistlethwaite, Jr, Oxford University Press.
© Oxford University Press 2022. DOI: 10.1093/oso/9780197618202.003.0004

In 1988, the United Network for Organ Sharing (UNOS)/Organ Procurement and Organ Transplantation Network (OPTN) began the collection of systematic data on solid organ transplants in the United States (US).[9] In the first year of data collection, there were 5693 kidney donors of whom 1,817 (32%) were living donors (compared to 30% in 1975). The vast majority of the living donors were first-degree biological relatives: 513 (28%) parents, 977 siblings (54% including 1 identical twin and 5 half-siblings), and 158 (9%) children (mostly adults). Women accounted for 994 (55%) of all living donors and the racial/ethnic breakdown was White: 1384 (76%), Black: 210 (12%), and Hispanic: 166 (9%).[10]

In 2019, both the number and percentage of living kidney donors had increased. There were 18,018 kidney donors, 6866 (38%) of whom were living donors, most of whom were female (4472, 65%).[11] Most living donors were White (4852, 71%), with the percentage of Black (12%) and Hispanic donors (9%) unchanged from 1994. A major demographic change, however, had occurred over the 3 decades: whereas 91% of all living donors in 1988 were first-degree biological relatives, in 2019 they only accounted for 32% of all living donors.[12] The percentage decrease in living donation by first-degree biological relatives was more pronounced in the White community than in the Black community.[13]

Beginning March 2020, many living donor transplants were put on hold during the COVID-19 pandemic to avoid overtaxing hospitals that were inundated with COVID-19 patients and to avoid transmission of the SARS-CoV-2 infection. Only 5,238 living kidney donations occurred, a drop of 23.7% from 2019.[14] The percentage of Black living donors fell from 12% to 7.1% and Hispanic living donor increased from 9% to 14.7%,[15] but it remains to be seen whether these data represent a change in demographics or a one-time secondary effect of the pandemic.

In this chapter we examine the demographics of race and gender for living kidney donors. While deceased donor organs are a public good and are allocated using a transplant algorithm developed with broad stakeholder input, living donor grafts are a private resource and are allocated according to donor wishes. Most living donors who donate directly donate to a candidate of the same race and socioeconomic status (SES) such that the benefits of living donor transplantation are not evenly distributed across the kidney transplant candidate pool.[16] Specifically, we examine 2 demographic traits of living donors: the over-representation of women and the under-representation of Blacks.

A traditional bioethics approach would state that as long as living donors believe that the benefits of participation outweigh the risks and harms (beneficence) and they give a voluntary and informed consent (autonomy or, more accurately, respect for persons) free from undue influence, then the demographics reflect a mere difference in preferences. Such an analysis, however, ignores the social, economic, and cultural determinants as well as various forms of structural discrimination (eg, racism, sexism) that may imply that the distribution is less voluntary than may appear initially. The distribution also raises justice concerns regarding the fair recruitment and selection of living donors and their recipients. The justice concerns are asymmetrical since women are over-represented and Blacks (especially Black men) are under-represented.

So, should gender and racial differences in living donation be considered a disparity or a preference? We analyze this question by examining how the multiple vulnerabilities that an individual experiences—in contrast to the concept of a one-size-fits-all singular conception of vulnerability applied to groups as done in the *Belmont Report*[17]—can help explain why women tend to be over-represented as donors and under-represented as recipients, and why Blacks tend to be under-represented as both living donors and living donor recipients. Finally, we consider how our living donor ethics framework addresses 3 criticisms levied at Kipnis' vulnerability taxonomy raised in the previous chapter. The 3 criticisms are (1) that a vulnerability taxonomy is over-reaching, as everyone may have 1 or more vulnerabilities; (2) that a vulnerability taxonomy is too individualistic and cannot account for group concerns of justice; and (3) that a vulnerability taxonomy fails to consider vulnerability as a relational concept.

4.2 Gender Demographics 1956–Present

The limited gender data from the Human Transplant Kidney Registry (1963–1976) showed a slight predominance of women to men donors (54% to 46%).[18] In 1988, when UNOS/OPTN began to collect living donor data, the ratio of female-to-male living donors was 55% to 45%, although in the past 5 years men now comprise less than 40% of all living kidney donors.[19] The over-representation of female living donors over the past 30 years is not unique to the US. In all countries except Iran, women account for over 50% of living donors.[20]

Also noteworthy is that both women and men are more likely to be a living kidney donor to a male recipient. While part of this can be explained by the fact that men are more likely to have end-stage renal disease (ESRD),[21] there are data at all time points and in virtually all countries that women have reduced or delayed access compared to men for all steps of the transplantation process, in both living and deceased donor kidney transplantation.[22] As Anette Melk and colleagues explain:

> Potential reasons for reduced or delayed access to transplantation for women versus men have been described for all steps of the transplantation process, including a lower probability of discussing transplantation as a treatment option with women, fewer women completing the clinical workup needed for transplantation, and sex discrimination in waitlisting. Physicians may assess a woman's health differently.[23]

A striking example of gender difference in access to transplant is the female-to-male ratio of spousal donors. When Paul Terasaki and colleagues published their data to support non-biological relatives as living donors in 1995, they reported on 360 spousal donations of which 261 (72.5%) were wife-to-husband grafts and 99 (27.5%) were husband-to-wife grafts.[24] In 2019, the data are the same: of the 866 spousal and life partner living kidney donations, 229 (26%) were donations by men and 637 (74%) from women.[25] Some of the discordance may be due to the fact that men are more likely to develop ESRD, and/or that fewer men can donate to their spouses because of increased sensitization secondary to pregnancy. Others have postulated that the lower participation of men as living donors is that they are more frequently "excluded as donors as they are more likely to exhibit symptoms of hypertension and ischemic heart disease than their female counterparts."[26]

The lower participation of men may also be due to familial financial issues that are based on who works outside the home, who can afford to take time off from work, as well as the social value placed on men compared to women. In 1963, women who worked full-time, year-round made 59 cents on average for every dollar earned by men, which improved to 77 cents in 2010 and close to 80 cents to the men's dollar in 2018.[27] Recently, given the large number of households in which both spouses work, Adrianne Frech et al discussed the need for transplant teams to examine more closely kidney donation between couples:

Our findings suggest that transplant teams should consider household responsibilities and gender roles and should work with donor-recipient couples to identify the required social and economic support during recovery, as well as facilitating paid employment among couples facing the unique challenges of spousal kidney donation.[28]

4.3 Race/Ethnicity Demographics 1950s–Present

There are no race/ethnicity demographics of donors in the Human Transplant Registry Reports (1963–1977). In fact, race data are not provided until the 13th and final report,[29] when it was reported that Blacks represented 11.9% of the recipients.[30]With the passage of the 1972 Renal Replacement Act (Public Law 92-603), demand for kidney transplantation expanded rapidly with greater access as virtually all Americans with ESRD were covered by Medicare.[31] By 1977, Blacks accounted for ~24% of the transplant waitlist,[32] and today Blacks constitute over 30% of patients on the deceased donor waitlist.[33]

Overall, supply has not kept up with demand, and the waitlist is currently over 90,000 candidates.[34] In this book, we focus on only 1 part of the supply chain: grafts from living donors. Data from the UNOS/OPTN registry show an increasing number of living donors of all race/ethnicities from 1988 to 2004, at which time it begins to fall (see Figure 4.1).[35] This decrease in living donors continues for a decade (until 2014), varying across gender and race/ethnicity, with a greater percentage drop in males (see Figure 4.1) and in Blacks (see Figure 4.2).[36] In the past 3 decades, Black living donors account for 12.7% of all living donors—only slightly less than their percentage in the overall US population (13.4%),[37] but still underrepresented given their community's need. The absolute number of Black living donors peaked in 2004 when there were 927 Black donors (425 Black male donors), but there have been less than 600 living Black donors annually since 2014.[38] Of note, in 2018, there is a significant increase in total living donation in all racial and ethnic groups (White, Black, Hispanic, and Asian), except that the number of Black men continues to fall (from 228 men in 2014 to 205 men in 2018).[39]

Let us see how these gender and racial/ethnic differences can be understood using a vulnerability analysis.

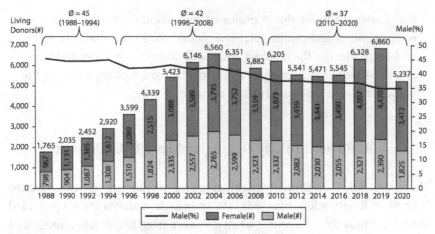

Figure 4.1 Gender of Living Kidney Donors 1998–2020

This graph depicts the number (left y-axis, bars) and percentage (right y-axis, line) of United States living kidney donors by gender from 1998 to 2020. The Φ at the top of the slide represents the average percentage of total donors during the time period who were male. Whereas men accounted for 45% of living donors between 1988 and 1994, the percentage dropped to 42% between 1996 and 2008, and to 37% between 2010 and 2020.

Legend: Left y-axis is number of living donors, right y-axis is percent male, and x-axis is year. The columns represent the number of male and female living donors in even years between 1988 and 2020. Dotted column = # of women and gray column = # of men; the black line depicts the percentage of male living donors over time.

Source: Based on OPTN data as of Jan 31, 2021.

4.4 Women as Living Donors: A Vulnerability Analysis (the complete vulnerability taxonomy can be found in Table 3.3)

The over-representation of women as living donors raises many vulnerability concerns. Let us begin by considering *juridic* and *deferential* vulnerabilities which refer to formal (juridic) and informal (deferential) power inequities in relationships that may lead to undue pressure to donate. In most US families, the vulnerability is better understood as deferential rather than juridic, and women may be more likely to be donors secondary to familial expectations that mothers, sisters, and wives care for, and therefore donate kidneys to, their male counterparts.[40] In their early groundbreaking study, Simmons and colleagues found that women were more likely to perceive donation as an extension of their obligation to their family whereas men were more likely

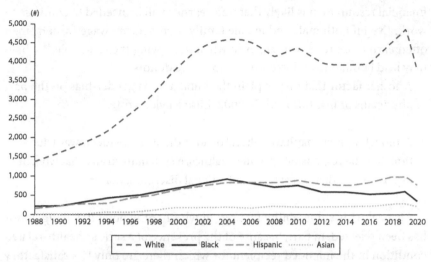

Figure 4.2 Living Kidney Donors by Race/Ethnicity and Year
This graph depicts the number of living kidney donors by race/ethnicity (White, Black, Hispanic, and Asian) by year. The number of living donors peaked in 2019 but fell in 2020 during the COVID-19 pandemic.
Legend: The y-axis is number of living donors; x-axis is year. The number of donors by race/ethnicity is depicted by different line colors and patterns: White = light gray dashed line; Black = black solid line; Hispanic = dark gray dotted line; and Asian = gray dotted line.
Source: Based on OPTN data as of January 31, 2021.

to express ambivalence.[41] This is despite the fact that women reported donation to be more stressful, although it is not clear if women donors were more stressed, were just more honest about feeling stressed, or received less emotional (and physical) support post-donation.[42]

Social vulnerability refers to whether the living donor belongs to a group whose interests have been socially disvalued. An important social vulnerability may be sexism, which can occur at the individual, societal/cultural, and institutional levels.[43] As we noted in chapter 3, when families negotiate intrafamilial donation, they may look to non-wage earners, who have traditionally been women who provide unpaid in-home family caregiving responsibilities to other household members. It is also possible that the non-wage earners volunteer themselves, either because they view this as an opportunity to be an active contributor to the family's resources or because they have internalized the view that they are of lower worth. It is also possible that financial issues, in and of themselves, are simply the driving social determinant. If there is only 1 wage earner and the family does not have alternative financial resources, it is likely that wage earner will be needed to continue to work. Even if both male and female family members are wage earners, men often earn more than women, even when occupying the same role,[44] which may lead families to endorse women to be the donors.

Another factor that may explain the imbalance is gender-bias on the part of physicians or institutions.[45] In 2002, Liise Kayler wrote:

> Although women may have cultural or attitudinal proclivities toward donation, it is the responsibility of the healthcare system to ensure that women experience neither active nor unintentional discrimination.[46]

Medical: This vulnerability focuses on whether the potential living donor has been selected, in part, because of the presence of a serious health-related condition in the intended recipient for which there are only less satisfactory alternative remedies. Clearly living donation is the best renal replacement treatment for most individuals with ESRD, and so all friends or relatives of an individual in ESRD face medical vulnerability because they may be asked to serve as a living kidney donor.

There are medical arguments to support encouraging male donors. Gender concordant donor-recipient pairs (particularly male donor-male recipient pairs) have better outcomes than gender discordant donor-recipient pairs, with the worst graft survival seen with female donors to male recipients.[47] Thus, men in ESRD should be encouraged to find male rather than female living donors whose kidneys achieve better outcomes than grafts from a female living donor.

Allocational: Is the potential living donor lacking in subjectively important social goods that will be provided as a consequence of participation as a donor? In many cultures where male dominance within the family is the norm, there can be a relative lack of self-esteem of female family members. Living donation may increase women's self-esteem as their family members praise and or socially reward them for their donation.[48]

Infrastructural: Does the political, organizational, economic, and social context of the donor care setting possess the integrity and resources needed to manage living donation process and follow-up? Consider, first, economic vulnerability. After the economic recession in 2008, the number of living donors of both genders decreased, suggesting economic infrastructural vulnerability of both men and women. However, the decline in living donation was most marked in men from lower income groups.[49] It is also important to note that financial barriers to donation are not limited to out-of-pocket expenses and lost wages, but also concerns that an interruption in employment or loss of employment may lead to loss of work-related benefits, including health insurance.[50]

A second concern is the need for both short- and long-term medical follow-up of donors to mitigate the short- and long-term medical risks that unilateral nephrectomy entails.[51] However, our current system only guarantees living donors short-term follow-up related to the kidney procurement itself. Approximately 20% of donors lack health insurance,[52] exposing them to lack of long-term health care access. As women tend to utilize more health care services, lack of adequate insurance may be even more problematic for them.[53]

A particular health issue relevant to premenopausal women is that women who donate are at increased risk of developing complications during pregnancy. Data show that women who become pregnant post-donation are at increased risk of pre-eclampsia, premature birth, and low birth weight infants] What impact pregnancy post-donation has on whether these women developing ESRD or other medical co-morbidities (eg, hypertension, cardiac disease) is unknown.[54] It is critical that adequate gynecological and obstetrical infrastructure be in place for women post-donation especially if they are premenopausal when they donate. This will require ensuring that transplant programs counsel female donors about reproductive risks of pre-eclampsia, low birthweight, and preterm birth and what actions they can take to reduce these risks. Clearly, obstetricians and gynecologists also need to be familiar with these risks, and a means for long-term data collection shared with the transplant team should be developed.

In sum, while all donors have vulnerabilities, there are reasons to believe that women may experience greater deferential, social, and allocational vulnerabilities with respect to their relationship to their recipients and wider social circle (family), and these vulnerabilities may lead to their over-representation. They may also be more deferential to transplant teams and feel unable to say no. It is important for the living donor advocate (LDA) or the living donor advocate team (LDAT)—a required component of living donor transplant programs since 2007[55]—ensure that the donation is voluntary and that women donors are not experiencing undue pressure.

However, it may be that women are donating at a rate consistent with their autonomous preferences and that the real problem is that men are underrepresented. Male under-representation may express a male preference not to donate due to greater ambivalence about donating, which shifts the burden to women. Alternatively, male under-representation as living donors may be due to the social pressures and expectations of being the major bread winner, which deprives men of the psychosocial benefits of serving as a living donor. Justice then would require attempts to promote donation among potential male donors: to remove barriers (such as out-of-pocket expenses and paid medical leave) and to promote more education about why donation is safe. Furthermore, explaining the benefits of gender concordance in graft outcomes may encourage male candidates with ESRD to preferentially seek out male donors both within and outside their family when more than 1 potential donor is available to a candidate. And yet, such programs should proceed with caution, as it may be that male under-representation is appropriate since the medical data show that some male donors, particularly young Black male donors, are at greater risk of ESRD post-donation than older donors and White donors.[56]

That women are more likely to be living donors is only part of the issue. As important is that women are less likely to be a living donor transplant recipient.[57] The reasons are multifactorial including cultural, social, economic, and personal factors. It is from this more holistic perspective that the over-representation of women as living donors raises justice concerns.

4.5 Blacks as Living Donors: A Vulnerability Analysis (again, the complete vulnerability taxonomy can be found in Table 3.3)

A vulnerability analysis also helps explain why Blacks are under-represented as living donors. However, before we undertake this analysis, several caveats should be enumerated.

First, Blacks donate kidneys comparable to their representation in the population. Of the 163,664 living donors listed on the UNOS website between 1988 and 2020, 19,169 (11.7%) are classified as Black,[58] and Blacks account for 13.4% of the US population.[59] Similarly, 115,335 (70.4%) of the living donors on the UNOS website are White,[60] and Whites account for 76.3% of the population.[61] However, of the 99,060 candidates on the UNOS deceased donor kidney waitlist, Blacks account for 31.9% (31,587) and Whites 35.2% (34,950) of the waitlist.[62] Since most living donors donate within their ethnic group,[63] Black candidates in ESRD are disadvantaged in receiving a living kidney donor compared to White candidates. Purnell and colleagues showed that from 1995 to 2014, of the 453,162 first-time adult candidates on the Scientific Registry of Transplant Recipients (SRTR), receipt of a kidney from a living donor within 2 years on the waiting list increased from 7.0% to 11.4% among White candidates and decreased from 3.4% to 2.9% among Blacks candidates.[64] That is, although Blacks donate at a similar rate as Whites, Black candidates are less likely to get a living donor transplant. More research is needed to understand whether this is driven by recipient factors (such as a reduced willingness to seek out potential donors), donor factors (such as the lower rate of Good Samaritan donors among Blacks), or a combination of both. Unfortunately, most of the available studies focus on recipient-related factors that contribute to decreased identification of potential living donors by ethnic minorities and less research on donor-related factors.[65]

Second, part of the under-representation of Black living donors may be due to greater health comorbidities within the Black community, including obesity, hypertension, and diabetes,[66] making fewer Blacks eligible to be living donors such that candidates may be less likely to find medically acceptable living donors within their social networks.[67]

Third, the interplay between race and SES is complex, and efforts to understand the under-representation of Black living donors must account for these effect.[68] The data suggest that racial disparities in access to living donor transplantation may be more related to SES factors rather than to cultural differences.[69] Many of the obstacles attributed to living donation in the Black community may be more accurately attributed to lower SES rather than race/ethnicity.[70] A study by Gill found that the incidence of living kidney donation was lower in Blacks than Whites in the lowest income quintile (incidence rate ratio, 0.84; 95% confidence interval, 0.78 to 0.90), but higher in Blacks in the 3 highest income quintiles.[71] Thus potential financial barriers for prospective Black donors are both their capacity to absorb the financial consequences of donation and/or the limited capacity of their recipients to reimburse allowable expenses.[72]

Now let us look at the relevant vulnerabilities and examine whether they explain why Blacks are under-represented as living donors.

Juridic and *deferential* vulnerabilities refer to formal and informal power inequities in relationships that may lead to undue pressure. While this may lead women to be over-represented, it may lead potential minority donors *not* to donate. Kimberly Harding explains:

Prospective living donors may be challenged with barriers created by their own friends, family, and even the intended recipients. Many potential donors have reported having to defend themselves from friends and family who persistently question their wisdom in donating. Negative responses from everyone involved can deter living donation.[73]

The negative responses of friends and family coupled with a potential donor's respect and/or dependence on them may create an influence that the potential donor cannot overcome. The lack of support for donation among family and social networks may explain, at least in part, why Blacks are less likely to complete living donor work-up and are less likely to be living donors.[74]

Social vulnerability refers to whether the living donors belong to a group whose interests have been socially disvalued. Given that donors and recipients are usually of the same race/ethnicity and SES group, potential donors and recipients may share social vulnerabilities that exacerbate their negative impact. For example, the lack of awareness by the health care providers of the racial disparities in kidney transplantation may result in failure to provide the necessary supports that minority patients in ESRD may need to overcome personal and structural barriers toward seeking kidney transplantation.[75] Multiple studies confirm that Black patients, older patients, obese patients, uninsured patients, and Medicaid-insured patients are less likely to receive education about transplantation,[76] despite the 2005 and 2008 Centers for Medicare & Medicaid Services' (CMS') Conditions for Coverage for ESRD facilities that required education about transplantation.[77] As Amy Waterman et al point out:

> Transplant educators in dialysis centers (predominantly nurses and dialysis social workers) themselves report having limited time and knowledge to successfully educate patients about transplantation, with educators at for-profit dialysis centers less likely to administer high-quality, more intensive transplant educational strategies (*e.g.*, one-on-one discussions) compared with nonprofit centers.[78]

Part of the reason for Blacks being under-represented as living donors, then, may be that they are not being asked to be living kidney donors by their loved ones in ESRD. Recipient candidates may not ask because (1) they did not receive adequate education about the benefits of living donor transplantation, and the low knowledge of living donation in their social networks reinforces their silence; (2) they fear the potential donor may refuse; (3) Black recipients and Black donors worry about long-term health of Black donors; (4) cultural attitudes about not sharing health problems makes it difficult for potential Black donors to know that they are needed; and (5) the implicit bias of some transplant professionals that Black patients with ESRD would not want a transplant and that they do as well on dialysis as with transplants.[79] How much of these are environmental and modifiable, and what interventions may be effective, need to be explored.

Medical: Has the potential living donor been selected, in part, because of the presence of a serious health-related condition in the intended recipient for which there are only less satisfactory alternative remedies? Virtually all patients in ESRD would do better with a transplant compared with dialysis, and survival of a living donor graft is, on average, far better than a deceased donor graft.[80] Friends and relatives of candidates face medical vulnerability in that the candidates may ask them to serve as a living donor. However, any attempt to increase Black living donation must confront the fact that multiple studies have shown that Black living donors are at greater risk for ESRD, particularly young Black male donors.[81]

Infrastructural: Does the political, organizational, economic, and social context of the donor care setting possess the integrity and resources needed to manage living donation? First, living kidney donation may be a bigger barrier for those of lower SES, especially for those who have physical requirements for employment (lifting heavy boxes for example) requiring longer recuperation periods before work activity can be resumed.[82] Since donors often "look like" recipients in terms of SES, the financial barriers may be tougher on those of lower income, consistent with the greater drop off in living donation among Blacks of lower SES after the financial crisis of 2008.[83] This has led many to talk about reimbursement of wages, health insurance for donors, and other financial resources to make it possible for all to be able to donate.[84] The transplant community has been fighting for legislation for years to permit some donor reimbursement to make donation financially neutral. On July 10, 2019, then-President Trump issued an executive order entitled Advancing American Kidney Health which included a provision to remove financial disincentives.[85] On December 29, 2019, a proposed rule was published in the *Federal Register* entitled "Removing Financial Disincentives to Living Organ Donation."[86] Final rule was published September 22, 2020 and went into effect on October 22, 2020.[87] Its actual impact remains to be seen.

Concern about income loss for living donors may affect decision-making by both transplant candidates and potential donors. In a study of 2 centers with over 450 candidates and transplant recipients, James Rodrigue et al found:

> One-third (32%) were told by a family member/friend that they were willing to donate but were concerned about potential lost income. The majority of those who expressed financial concern (64%) did not initiate donation evaluation. Many patients (42%) chose not to discuss living donation with a family member/friend due to concern about the impact of lost income on the donor. In the multivariable model, lower annual household income was the only statistically significant predictor of both having a potential donor expressing lost income concern and choosing not to talk to someone because of lost income concern.[88]

As noted previously, the financial barriers to donation are not limited to lost wages and out-of-pocket expenses, but also include potential for loss of work-related benefits, including health insurance. Approximately 20% of donors lack health insurance, and this is more common in ethnic minorities,[89] which exposes them to less access to needed life-long care post-nephrectomy.

A second potential infrastructural barrier is health literacy.[90] While health illiteracy is an issue for all racial and ethnic groups, Hispanics and Blacks have a higher rate of health illiteracy.[91] At the systems (infrastructural) level, health care professionals may be unwilling to promote potential donor understanding by taking more time, using simpler language, and/or employing decision aids to improve comprehension and overcome literacy barriers that exist. This may be complicated by poor communication skills, lack of cultural awareness, or implicit bias of health care professionals, which may contribute to the current under-representation of Black living donors, particularly those of lower educational and lower SES.[92] Whether and to what extent health illiteracy may be surmountable by an LDAT needs to be determined.

Third, some of the barriers to living donor transplantation by Blacks may also reflect structural racism.[93] Racial disparities can result from clinicians' misinterpretation of patients' indecision or passivity as lack of interest.[94] Clinician complacency about referring Blacks for transplantation because they are reported to have a high quality of life on dialysis also leads to referral delays.[95] For example, in a survey of 278 nephrologists and 606 patients, John Ayanian and colleagues asked about quality of life and survival for Black and White patients undergoing renal transplantation and reasons for racial differences in access to transplantation. They found that:

> [p]hysicians were less likely to believe transplantation improves survival for blacks than whites (69% versus 81%; P < 0.001), but similarly likely to believe it improves quality of life (84% versus 86%). Factors commonly cited by physicians as important reasons why blacks are less likely than whites to be evaluated for transplantation included patients' preferences (66%), availability of living donors (66%), failure to complete evaluations (53%), and comorbid illnesses (52%). Fewer physicians perceived patient-physician communication and trust (38%) or physician bias (12%) as important reasons.[96]

How to address these infrastructural vulnerabilities needs to be studied.

In sum, while all donors are at risk for a variety of vulnerabilities, there are reasons to believe that Black donors may be at greater social and infrastructural vulnerabilities due to lack of awareness of the benefits, misconceptions of the risks, and racism at the individual, social/cultural and institutional levels. To increase living donation in the Black community, we need culturally tailored educational resources to increase knowledge and awareness, social support provided by transplant programs, and reduced financial disincentives. Since living kidney donation may require costs to travel, costs of meals, as well as the need to take time off from work, potential Black living donors without adequate financial flexibility may not be able to donate. Ensuring that these costs are covered for living donors would likely increase the number of Black living donors.

There are also reasons, however, why some level of lower donation rate in the Black community may be appropriate, given that living kidney donation does have health risks to donors and the risks are greater for Black living donors. Data show that, post-donation, Blacks have an even greater risk than other donors for developing hypertension, cardiovascular disease, diabetes, and ESRD and that their risk of developing these conditions is increased over their non-donor Black counterparts.[97]

4.6 Re-Examination of the Criticisms Aimed at Kipnis' Vulnerability Analysis

A vulnerability analysis can help understand the demographics of living donation. It also effectively addresses the 3 criticisms levelled against Kipnis in chapter 3.

The first criticism was that a vulnerabilities account is over-reaching, as everyone may have 1 or more vulnerabilities. For living donor transplantation, the issue is not whether everyone has vulnerabilities, but whether these vulnerabilities interfere with an individual's ability to decide about donation. While everyone may have 1 or more vulnerabilities, our analysis shows that there are some systemic issues regarding both gender and race that make women and Blacks more vulnerable than other donors.

The second criticism was that a vulnerability account is too individualistic and cannot account for group concerns of justice. By examining why females are over-represented as donors and Blacks under-represented, we found both individual and systemic factors that can explain these group differences. The selection of non-wage earners (more commonly women) by families threatens fairness (justice) in donor selection by downplaying the importance of voluntary self-selection. The concern that a significant number of Black candidates and their potential donors may find the out-of-pocket expenses of living donation prohibitive is also a group justice concern.

Another justice concern at the group level is the need for better education and training of staff in dialysis units, particularly those centers in lower SES neighborhoods, to ensure that all candidates are educated about the benefits of living donation and are encouraged to talk about donation with both male and female members of their families. The family members of patients with ESRD who are unaware of the possibility of living donation cannot offer to be a living donor and may be distressed by learning about this option when it is too late.

But it is also important to look past group labels to determine the individual vulnerabilities of potential donors. This will help identify individuals within groups traditionally labeled as vulnerable for whom serving as a living donor would provide significant benefit, and it will help identify individuals within groups traditionally considered not vulnerable who are vulnerable and should be precluded from donating.

Finally, the third criticism was that a vulnerability account fails to consider vulnerability as a relational concept. The relational character of vulnerability is why Goodin argued that health care professionals have special responsibilities to their patients.[98] It is why the transplant community requires that donors and candidates have separate health care teams. The LDAT focuses on the well-being of the donor patient as a patient in her own right. The LDAT is responsible for engaging potential donors in a robust consent process that empowers them to make an informed decision that reflects not just their pre-reflective preferences but, rather, their informed choices free of undue influence.[99] The LDAT helps to achieve this by employing a richer conception of autonomy (relational autonomy) that engages potential donors to more fully consider whether donation is in their best interests and is consistent with their goals. Employing a shared decision-making process, the LDAT helps the potential donor address all the different types of vulnerability threats that the potential donor may experience—even if neither the donor nor the LDAT frame it in such language. This process enables the living donor to make a decision that best reflects her informed preferences, to ensure the voluntariness of her consent, and to serve as a buffer from families that may exert undue pressure.

4.7 Conclusion

There are many reasons why women may be over-represented and Blacks under-represented as living donors. Our vulnerability analyses show that these differences may not be mere individual preferences but may reflect serious justice concerns that need to be addressed at both the individual and systems levels. At the individual level, the LDAT must help living donors identify and address their various vulnerabilities in a shared decision-making process that allows them to decide whether or not the benefits of donation outweigh the risks and harms. At the systems level, the transplant community needs to take a more proactive role in addressing structural challenges (eg, inadequate education at for-profit dialysis centers) and work to remove or at least reduce the institutional and systemic inequities (structural racism and sexism) that may inhibit Black and female potential donors from making decisions that best reflect their own preferences, interests, and needs.

Notes

1. Merrill JP, Harrison JH, Murray J, Guild WR. Successful homotransplantation of the kidney in an identical twin. *Trans Am Clin Climatol Assoc.* 1956;67:166–173.
2. Murray JE. Proceedings: human kidney transplant conference. *Transplantation.* 1964;2(1):147–155.
3. Murray, "Proceedings"; and Murray JE, Gleason R, Bartholomay A. Second Report of Registry in Human Kidney Transplantation. *Transplantation.* 1964;2:660–7.
4. Murray JE, Barnes BA, Atkinson J. Fifth report of the Human Kidney Transplant Registry. *Transplantation.* 1967;5:752–774.
5. Murray, "Fifth report."
6. Advisory Committee of Human Kidney Transplant Registry. Sixth Report of the Human Kidney Transplant Registry. *Transplantation.* 1968;6(8):944–955, at p. 945.
7. Advisory Committee to the Renal Transplant Registry. The 12th Report of the Human Renal Transplant Registry. *JAMA.*1975;233:787–796.
8. Advisory Committee, "The 12th Report."
9. OPTN (Organ Procurement and Transplantation Network) National Data. https://optn.transplant.hrsa.gov/data/view-data-reports/national-data/. Hereinafter referred to as OPTN Data.
10. OPTN Data.
11. OPTN Data.
12. OPTN Data. These numbers may underestimate the number of donor-recipient pairs who are first-degree relatives because the current national database classifies a donor as a non-biologically related donor if donating to a stranger through a kidney paired exchange or kidney domino chain mechanism, even though the intended recipient was a first-degree relative, and almost 10% of all living donors participate in exchanges or chains. Even still, the trend away from biological relatives is significant.
13. OPTN Data.
14. OPTN Data.
15. OPTN Data.
16. See, for example, Gill J, Dong J, Rose C, Johnston O, Landsberg D, Gill J. The effect of race and income on living kidney donation in the United States. *J Am Soc Nephrol.* 2013;24:1872–1879; and Gill JS, Gill J, Barnieh L, et al. Income of living kidney donors and the income difference between living kidney donors and their recipients in the United States. *Am J Transplant.* 2012;12:3111–3118.
17. The National Commission for the Protection of Human Subjects of Biomedical and Behavioral Research, *The Belmont Report: Ethical Principles and Guidelines for the Protection of Human Subjects of Research.* Washington, DC: Government Printing Office; 1978. http://www.hhs.gov/ohrp/humansubjects/guidance/belmont.html. Hereinafter referred to as the *Belmont Report.*
18. Murray et al, "Fifth report."
19. OPTN Data.

20. Carrero JJ, Hecking M, Chesnave NC, Jager KJ. Sex and gender disparities in the epidemiology and outcomes of chronic kidney disease. *Nat Rev Nephrol.* 2018;14:151–164, at p. 157.
21. Goldberg I, Krause I. The role of gender in chronic kidney disease. *Eur Med J.* 2016;1(2):58–64.
22. See, for example, Melk A, Babitsch B, Borchert-Mörlins B, et al. Equally interchangeable? How sex and gender affect transplantation. *Transplantation.* 2019;103(6):1094–1110; and Antlanger M, Noordzij M, van de Luijtgaarden M, et al. Sex differences in kidney replacement therapy: initiation and maintenance. *Clin J Am Soc Nephrol.* 2019;14:1616–1625.
23. Melk et al, "Equally interchangeable," at p. 1097 (references omitted).
24. Terasaki PI, Cecka JM, Gjertson DW, Takemoto S. High survival rates of kidney transplants from spousal and living unrelated donors. *N Engl J Med.* 1995;333:333–336.
25. OPTN Data.
26. Jindal RM, Ryan JJ, Sajjad I, Murthy MH, Baines LS. Kidney transplantation and gender disparity. *Am J Nephrol.* 2005;25:474–483, at p. 474.
27. The New York Times Editorial Staff, ed. *The Gender Pay Gap: Equal Work, Unequal Pay (In the Headlines).* 1st ed. New York, NY: The New York Times Educational Publishing, the Rosen Publishing Group, Inc; 2019.
28. Frech A, Natale G, Tumin D. Couples' employment after spousal kidney donation. *Soc Work Health Care.* 2018;57(10):880–889, at p. 888.
29. Advisory Committee to the Renal Transplant Registry. The 13th report of the Human Renal Transplant Registry. *Transplant Proc.* 1977;9:9–26.
30. Social Security Amendments of 1972 (Pub L No. 92-603), also known as the Renal Replacement Act, which provided health insurance for virtually all US residents in end-stage renal disease (ESRD).
31. Evans RW, Blagg CR, Bryan FA. Implications for health care policy: a social and demographic profile of hemodialysis patients in the United States. *JAMA.* 1981;245:487–491, citing End-Stage Renal Disease Medical Information System, Medicare Bureau. Chronic Renal Disease, Table 50. Baltimore, MD, Health Care Financing Administration, 1979.
32. Huang E, Danovitch G. Kidney transplantation in adults: the kidney transplant waiting list in the United States. UpToDate. Literature review current through July 2021. Topic last updated January 6, 2020. Last accessed August 15, 2021. https://www.uptodate.com/contents/kidney-transplantation-in-adults-the-kidney-transplant-waiting-list-in-the-united-states.
33. Huang and Danovitch, "Kidney."
34. Huang and Danovitch, "Kidney." Of note, at its peak, there were over 100,000 kidney transplant candidates but it now hovers in the mid-90,000s.
35. OPTN Data.
36. United States Census Bureau. Quick Facts. https://www.census.gov/quickfacts/fact/table/US/PST045219. Hereinafter referred to as Census Bureau.
37. OPTN Data.

38. OPTN Data.

39. Tong A, Chapman JR, Wong G, Kanellis J, McCarthy G, Craig JC. The motivations and experiences of living kidney donors: a thematic synthesis. *Am J Kidney Dis.* 2012;60:15–26.

40. Simmons RG, Marine SK, Simmons RL. *Gift of Life: The Effect of Organ Transplantation on Individual, Family, and Societal Dynamics.* New Brunswick, NJ: Transaction Books, 2002.

41. Jacobs C, Johnson E, Anderson K, Gillingham K, Matas A. Kidney transplants from living donors: how donation affects family dynamics. *Adv Ren Replace Ther.* 1998;5:89–97.

42. Norris K, Nissenson AR. Race, gender, and socioeconomic disparities in CKD in the United States. *J Am Soc Nephrol.* 2008;19(7):1261–1270.

43. The New York Times Editorial Staff, *The Gender Pay Gap.*

44. See, for example, Jindal et al, "Kidney"; and Kayler LK, Meier-Kriesche H-U, Punch JD, et al. Gender imbalance in living donor renal transplantation. *Transplantation.* 2002;73:248–252.

45. Kayler et al, "Gender," at p. 252.

46. Oh C-K, Kim SJ, Kim JH, Shin GT, Kim HS. Influence of donor and recipient gender on early graft function after living donor kidney transplantation. *Transplant Proc.* 2004;36:2015–2017; Kwon OJ, Kwak JY. The impact of sex and age matching for long-term graft survival in living donor renal transplantation. *Transplant Proc.* 2004;36:2040–2042; Kayler LK, Armenti VT, Dafoe DC, Burke JF, Francos GC, Ratner LE. Patterns of volunteerism, testing and exclusion among potential living kidney donors. *Health Care Women Int.* 2005;26:285–294; and Ashby VB, Leichtman AB, Rees MA, et al. A kidney graft survival calculator that accounts for mismatches in age, sex, HLA, and body size. *Clin J Am Soc Nephrol.* 2017;12(7):1148–1160.

47. Simmons et al, "The Gift"; and Tong, "The motivations."

48. Gill J, Joffres Y, Rose C, et al. The change in living kidney donation in women and men in the United States (2005–2015): a population-based analysis. *J Am Soc Nephrol.* 2018;29:1301–1308.

49. See, for example, Clarke KS, Klarenbach S, Vlaicu S, Yang RC, Garg AX. The direct and indirect economic costs incurred by living kidney donors—a systematic review. *Nephrol Dial Transplant.* 2006;21:1952–1960; Gaston RS, Danovitch GM, Epstein RA, Kahn JP, Matas AJ, Schnitzler MA. Limiting financial disincentives in live organ donation: a rational solution to the kidney shortage. *Am J Transplant.* 2006;6:2548–2555; Sickand M, Cuerden MS, Klarenbach SW, et al. Reimbursing live organ donors for incurred non-medical expenses: a global perspective on policies and programs. *Am J Transplant.* 2009;9:2825–2836; and LaPointe Rudow D, Hays R, Baliga P, et al. Consensus conference on best practices in live kidney donation: recommendations to optimize education, access, and care. *Am J Transplant.* 2015;15:914–922.

50. See for example, Muzaale AD, Massie AB, Wainwright J, McBride MA, Wang M, Segev DL. Long-term risk of ESRD attributable to live kidney donation: matching with healthy non-donors. *Am J Transplant.* 2013;13(suppl 5):204–205; and Mjoen G, Hallan S, Hartmann A, et al. Long-term risks for kidney donors. Kidney International.

2014;86:162–167; and Maggiore U, Budde K, Heemann U, et al. Long-term risks of kidney living donation: review and position paper by the ERA-EDTA DESCARTES working group. *Nephrol Dial Transplant.* 2017;32:216–223.

51. See, for example, Casagrande LH, Collins S, Warren AT, Ommen ES. Lack of health insurance in living kidney donors. *Clin Transplant.* 2012;26(2):E101–104; Gibney EM, Doshi MD, Hartmann EL, Parikh CR, Garg AX. Health insurance status of US living kidney donors. *Clin J Am Soc Nephrol.* 2010;5(5):912–916.

52. Bertakis KD, Azari R, Helms LJ, Callahan EJ, Robbins JA. Gender differences in the utilization of health care services. *J Fam Pract.* 2000;49(2):147–152.

53. Reisaeter AV, Roislien J, Henriksen T, Irgens LM, Hartmann A. Pregnancy and birth after kidney donation: the Norwegian experience. *Am J Transplant.* 2009;9:820–824; Ibrahim, HN, Akkina SK, Leister E, et al. Pregnancy outcomes after kidney donation. *Am J Transplant.* 2009;9:825–834; Garg AX, Nevis IF, McArthur E, et al. Gestational hypertension and preeclampsia in living kidney donors. *N Engl J Med.* 2015;372(2):124–133; and Davis S, Dylewski J, Shah PB, Holmen J, You Z, Chonchol M, Kendrick J. Risk of adverse maternal and fetal outcomes during pregnancy in living kidney donors: a matched cohort study. *Clin Transplant.* 2019;33(1):e13453.

54. See, for example, Josephson MA. Transplantation: pregnancy after kidney donation: more questions than answers. *Nat Rev Nephrol.* 2009;5(9):495–497; Nevis IF, Garg AX. Donor Nephrectomy Outcomes Research (DONOR) Network. Maternal and fetal outcomes after living kidney donation. *Am J Transplant.* 2009 9(4):661–8; and Reese PP, Boudville N, Garg AX. Living kidney donation: outcomes, ethics and uncertainty. *Lancet.* 2015;385(9981):2003–2013.

55. Department of Health and Human Services, Part II. Centers for Medicare and Medicaid Services 42 DFR Parts 405, 482, 488, and 498. Medicare Program; Hospital Conditions of Participation: Requirements for Approval and Re-Approval of Transplant Centers to Perform Organ Transplants; *Fed Regist.* 2007;72:15198–15280.

56. Lentine KL, Patel A. Risks and outcomes of living donation. *Adv Chronic Kidney Dis.* 2012;19(4):220–228; Lentine KL, Segev DL. Understanding and communicating medical risks for living kidney donors: a matter of perspective. *J Am Soc Nephrol.* 2017;28(1):12–24; Cherikh WS, Young CJ, Kramer BF, et al. Ethnic and gender related differences in the risk of end-stage renal disease after living kidney donation. *Am J Transplant.* 2011;11:1650–5.

57. See, for example, OPTN Data; Schaubel DE, Stewart DE, Morrison HI, Zimmerman DL, Cameron JI, Jeffrey JJ, Fenton SS. Sex inequality in kidney transplantation rates. *Arch Intern Med.* 2000;160:2349–54; and Carrero et al, "Sex and gender"; and Peracha J, Hayer MK, Sharif A. Gender disparity in living-donor kidney transplant among minority ethnic groups. *Exp Clin Transplant.* 2016;14:139–145.

58. OPTN Data.

59. Census Bureau.

60. OPTN Data.

61. Census Bureau.

62. OPTN Data.

63. Gill, "The effect of race."
64. Purnell TS, Luo X, Cooper LA, et al. Association of race and ethnicity with live donor kidney transplantation in the United States from 1995 to 2014. *JAMA.* 2018;319:49–61.
65. See, for example, Institute of Medicine (IOM). *Unequal Treatment: Confronting Racial and Ethnic Disparities in Health Care.* Washington, DC: The National Academies Press; 2003. Hereinafter referred to as IOM, *Unequal*; and more recently, Harding K, Mersha TB, Pham P-T, et al. Health disparities in kidney transplantation for African Americans. *Am J Nephrol.* 2017;46:165–175.
66. Harris MI, Flegal KM, Cowie CC, et al. Prevalence of diabetes, impaired fasting glucose, and impaired glucose tolerance in U.S. adults. The Third National Health and Nutrition Examination Survey, 1988–1994. *Diabetes Care.* 1998;21:518–524; Carson AP, Howard G, Burke GL, et al. Ethnic differences in hypertension incidence among middle-aged and older adults: the multi-ethnic study of atherosclerosis. *Hypertension.* 2011;57:1101–1107; and Kato N. Ethnic differences in genetic predisposition to hypertension. *Hypertens Res.* 2012;35:574–581.
67. Ladin K, Hanto DW. Understanding disparities in transplantation: do social networks provide the missing clue? *Am J Transplant.* 2010;10(3):472–476; Weng FL, Reese PP, Mulgaonkar S, Patel AM. Barriers to living donor kidney transplantation among black or older transplant candidates. *Clin J Am Soc Nephrol.* 2010;5(12):2338–2347; Lunsford SL, Simpson KS, Chavin KD, et al. Racial disparities in living kidney donation: is there a lack of willing donors or an excess of medically unsuitable candidates? *Transplantation.* 2006;82:876–881; Harding et al, "Health disparities"; and Garg AX. Helping more patients receive a living donor kidney transplant. *Clin J Am Soc Nephrol.* 2018;13(12):1918–1923.
68. IOM, *Unequal*; Purnell et al, "Association"; Gill et al, "The effect of race"; Gill "Income"; and Reese PP, Nair M, Bloom RD. Eliminating racial disparities in access to living donor kidney transplantation: how can centers do better? *Am J Kidney Dis.* 2012;59:751–753.
69. IOM, *Unequal*; Harding et al, "Health disparities."
70. IOM, *Unequal*; Harding et al, "Health disparities"; Patzer RE, McClellan WM. Influence of race, ethnicity and socioeconomic status on kidney disease. *Nat Rev Nephrol.* 2012;8:533–541; and Reed RD, Sawinski D, Shelton BA, et al. Population health, ethnicity, and rate of living donor kidney transplantation. *Transplantation.* 2018;102:2080–2087.
71. Gill et al, "The effect of race."
72. Gill et al, "The income."
73. Harding et al, "Health disparities," at pp. 166–167.
74. Reed et al, "Population"; Alexander G, Sehgal A. Why hemodialysis patients fail to complete the transplantation process. *Am J Kidney Dis.* 2001;37:321–328; Clark CR, Hicks LS, Keogh JH, Epstein AM, Ayanian JZ. Promoting access to renal transplantation: the role of social support networks in completing pre-transplant evaluations. *J Gen Intern Med.* 2008;23:1187–1193; and Davis LA, Grogan TM, Cox J, Weng FL.

Inter- and intrapersonal barriers to living donor kidney transplant among black recipients and donors. *J Racial Ethn Health Disparities.* 2017;4:671–679.

75. Kim JJ, Basu M, Plantinga L, et al. Awareness of racial disparities in kidney transplantation among health care providers in dialysis. *Clin J Am Soc Nephrol.* 2018;13:772–781; and Lipford KJ, McPherson L, Hamoda R, et al. Dialysis facility staff perceptions of racial, gender, and age disparities in access to renal transplantation. *BMC Nephrol.* 2018;19(1):5. doi:10.1186/s12882-017-0800-6

76. See, for example, Waterman AD, Peipert JD, Hyland SS, McCabe MS, Schenk EA, Liu J. Modifiable patient characteristics and racial disparities in evaluation completion and living donor transplant. *Clin J Am Soc Nephrol.* 2013;8:995–1002; Balhara KS, Kucirka LM, Jaar BG, Segev DL. Disparities in provision of transplant education by profit status of the dialysis center. *Am J Transplant.* 2012;12:3104–3110; and Gander JC, Zhang X, Ross K, et al. Association between dialysis facility ownership and access to kidney transplantation. *JAMA.* 2019;322:957–973.

77. Department of Health and Human Services. Centers for Medicare and Medicaid Service. Medicare and Medicaid Programs; Conditions for Coverage for End-Stage Renal Disease Facilities. *Fed Regist.* 2008;73:20369–20484. https://www.federalregister.gov/articles/2008/04/15/08-1102/medicare-and-medicaid-programs-conditions-for-coverage-for-end-stage-renal-disease-facilities

78. Waterman AD, Peipert JD, Goalby CJ, Dinkel KM, Xiao H, Lentine KL. Assessing transplant education practices in dialysis centers: comparing educator reported and Medicare data. *Clin J Am Soc Nephrol.* 2015;10:1617–25, at pp. 1617–1618 (references omitted).

79. Patzer and MacClellan, "Influence"; Harding et al, "Health disparities"; Davis et al, "Intra- and inter"; and Ayanian JZ, Clearly PD, Keogh JH, Noonan SJ, David-Kasdan JA, Epstein AM. Physicians' beliefs about racial differences in referral for renal transplantation. *Am J Kidney Dis.* 2004;43(2):350–357.

80. Chadban SJ, Ahn C, Axelrod DA, et al. Summary of the Kidney Disease: Improving Global Outcomes (KDIGO) clinical practice guideline on the evaluation and management of candidates for kidney transplantation. *Transplantation.* 2020;104:708–714; and Vella J. Kidney transplantation in adults: patient survival after kidney transplantation. UpToDate. Literature review current through May 2020. This topic last updated August 23, 2019. Literature review current through July 2021. Topic last updated June 21, 2021. Last accessed August 15, 2021.https://www.uptodate.com/contents/kidney-transplantation-in-adults-patient-survival-after-kidney-transplantation?search=kidney%20transplantation&topicRef=7309&source=see_link

81. Lentine KL, Lam NN, Segev DL. Risks of living kidney donation: current state of knowledge on outcomes important to donors. *Clin J Am Soc Nephrol.* 2019;14:597–608; and Muzaale AD, Massie AB, Wang MC, et al. Risk of end-stage renal disease following live kidney donation. *JAMA.* 2014;311:579–586.

82. Rodrigue JR, Schold JD, Mandelbrot DA, Taber DJ, Phan V, Baliga PK. Concern for lost income following donation deters some patients from talking to potential living donors. *Prog Transplant.* 2016;26:292–298; and Clarke et al, "The direct and indirect."

83. Gill et al, "The effect,"
84. Przech S, Garg AX, Arnold JB, et al. Financial costs incurred by living kidney donors: a prospective cohort study and on behalf of the Donor Nephrectomy Outcomes Research (DONOR) Network. *J Am Soc Nephrol.* 2018;29:2847–2857; and Bailey P, Tomson C, Risdale S, Ben-Shlomo Y. From potential donor to actual donation: does socioeconomic position affect living kidney donation? A systematic review of the evidence. *Transplantation.* 2014;98:918–926.
85. Health and Human Services. HHS Launches President Trump's "Advancing American Kidney Health" Initiative. July 10, 2019. Last accessed August 15, 2021.https:// www.hhs.gov/about/news/2019/07/10/hhs-launches-president-trump-advancing-american-kidney-health-initiative.html
86. Health Resources and Services Administration (HRSA). Proposed rule: Removing Financial Disincentives to Living Organ Donation. 42 CFR 121. *Fed Regist.* 2019;84:70139–70145. Rule was proposed December 20, 2019. Last accessed August 15, 2021. https://www.federalregister.gov/documents/2019/12/20/2019-27532/removing-financial-disincentives-to-living-organ-donation
87. Health Resources and Services Administration (HRSA), Health and Human Services Department (HHS). Removing Financial Disincentives to Living Organ Donation. 42 CFR 121. *Fed Regist.* 2020;85:59438–59445. The rule was published September 22, 2020. The rule became effective on October 22, 2020. Last accessed August 15, 2021.https://www.federalregister.gov/documents/2020/09/22/2020-20804/removing-financial-disincentives-to-living-organ-donation
88. Rodrigue et al, "Concern for lost income," at p. 292.
89. See, for example, Casagrande et al, "Lack"; and Gibney et al, "Health insurance."
90. United States Department of Health and Human Services, Office of Disease Prevention and Health Promotion. *National Action Plan to Improve Health Literacy.* Washington, DC: United States Department of Health and Human Services; 2010; and Institute of Medicine. *Promoting Health Literacy to Encourage Prevention and Wellness: Workshop Summary.* Washington, DC: The National Academies Press; 2011.
91. Nielsen-Bohlman L, Institute of Medicine Committee on Health Literacy. *Health Literacy: A Prescription to End Confusion.* Washington, DC: National Academies Press; 2004.
92. See, for example, IOM, *Unequal;* Harding et al, "Health disparities"; Patzer and McClellan, "Influence"; and Norris and Nissenson, "Race, gender."
93. Harding et al, "Health disparities"; and Norris and Nissenson, "Race, gender."
94. Ayanian et al, "Physicians' beliefs"; and Humi AM, Sullivan CM, Pencak JA, Sehgal AR. Accuracy of dialysis medical records in determining patient interest in and suitability for transplantation. *Clin Transplant.* 2013;27(4):10.1111/ctr.12147.
95. IOM, *Unequal;* Purnell et al, "Association"; Harding et al, "Health disparities."
96. Ayanian et al, "Physicians' beliefs," at p. 350.
97. Lentine KL, Lam NN, and Segev DL. Risks of living kidney donation: current state of knowledge on outcomes important to donors. *Clin J Am Soc Nephrol.* 2019;14:597–608.

98. Goodin RE. *Protecting the Vulnerable: A Reanalysis of Our Social Responsibilities.* Chicago, IL: University of Chicago Press; 1985.
99. Hays R, LaPointe Rudrow D, Dew MA, Taler SJ, Spicer H, Mandelbrot DA. The independent living donor advocate: a guidance document from the American Society of Transplantation's Living Donor Community of Practice. *Am J Transplant.* 2007;15:518–525.

5
Minors as Living Organ Donors

5.1 Introduction

We begin with 2 not well-known facts about children as organ donors. First, for the past 2 decades, a child is more likely to become a solid deceased organ donor than a solid deceased organ recipient.[1] Second, while approximately one-third of all kidney transplants for children involve living donor grafts, children rarely serve as living solid organ donors (although they frequently do serve as living tissue donors—bone marrow or stem cell donors).[2]

Although minors rarely serve as living organ donors, minors were some of the first living donor-recipient identical twin transplants. In 1957, 3 years after the first successful kidney transplant between 23-year-old identical twin brothers, the Supreme Judicial Court in Massachusetts authorized kidney transplantation between 3 sets of identical twin minors (ages 14, 14, and 19; at the time, the age of majority was 21 years old)[3] and approved another 2 dozen minor donor transplants over the next 20 years.[4] The United Network for Organ Sharing (UNOS)/Organ Procurement and Transplantation Network (OPTN) data reveal that at least 60 children below the age of 18 years served as living kidney donors between 1987–2000.[5] Another 8 children have been recorded as kidney donors on the UNOS/OPTN website since 2000.[6] Although children younger than 10 rarely serve as living organ donors, there is a case report in the literature of a 7-year-old identical twin serving as a kidney donor.[7] There are also case reports of minors donating outside the United States (US): Webb and Fortune report 3 cases of minors as kidney donors in the United Kingdom between 1986 and 2005, 23 minors donating in Italy between 1987 and 2000, and 1 donation from a 17-year-old Canadian to his identical twin in early 2000s.[8] There is also a report of a 15-year-old Canadian donating to her twin sibling in 1958.[9] There are also a handful of case reports of minors serving as living donors for other organs.[10] However, for this chapter, we will focus only on the child as a potential living kidney donor. We will also only focus on the unemancipated minor, meaning that

The Living Organ Donor as Patient. Lainie Friedman Ross and J. Richard Thistlethwaite, Jr, Oxford University Press.
© Oxford University Press 2022. DOI: 10.1093/oso/9780197618202.003.0005

we will not address the older adolescent who may be a parent seeking to serve as a living donor for her child.[11]

Although minors have served as living donors, that does not answer whether it is ethical for them to do so. The ethics question was raised quite early on. At the first international symposium on transplantation and ethics sponsored by the CIBA Foundation in 1966, opinions were voiced on both sides.[12] Joseph Murray, a US surgeon, and Robert Platt, a British physician, argued in favor of allowing adolescent identical twins to be donors.[13] Jean-Pierre Revillard, a French surgeon, and David Daube, a British legal scholar, said it should always be forbidden.[14]

Today, the attitudes of transplant professionals regarding the minor serving as a living donor differ widely around the globe,[15] leading to conflicting policies. In 2005, an International Forum on the Care of the Live Kidney Donor was held in Amsterdam and recommended an absolute prohibition of living solid organ donation by minors (those younger than 18 years).[16] This contrasts with the US Live Organ Donor Consensus Group, which argued 5 years earlier that minors under 18 years could ethically serve in exceptional circumstances.[17] In 2008, we were the lead authors of the American Academy of Pediatrics (AAP) statement on children as living donors in which we also concluded that "minors may ethically serve as living donors in specific, limited circumstances."[18] An international review of living solid organ donor policy statements in 2013 reviewed 39 documents written in English, French, German, Spanish, Italian, Dutch, or Danish and found that being a minor was an absolute contraindication in 27 and a relative contradiction in 12 countries.[19] No country permitted minors to donate freely. Similarly, an online survey sent to 1128 members of the European Society of Transplantation in August 2014 yielded 331 (29.3%) survey responses from all over the globe. It found that only 3.6% of respondents stated that their institution allowed minors to donate.[20]

The US Live Organ Donor Consensus Group offered 4 conditions, all of which should be satisfied for a minor to serve as an organ donor.[21] We adopted these conditions for the AAP statement and added a fifth condition.[22] A decade later we further clarify the fourth criterion (see Box 5.1). Three of the conditions focus on beneficence and risk:benefit analysis: (1) donor and recipient are both highly likely to benefit, (2) surgical risk for the donor is extremely low, and (5) emotional and psychological risks to the donor are minimized. The other 2 conditions focus on respect for persons: (4) the minor freely agrees (and has the cognitive capacity to provide an affirmative assent)

Box 5.1   When Children May Ethically Serve as Solid Organ Donors

---

Children may serve as solid organ donors if:

  (1) donor and recipient are both highly likely to benefit
  (2) surgical risk for the donor is extremely low
  (3) all other deceased and living donor options have been exhausted
  (4) the minor freely agrees (*has the cognitive capacity to provide an affirmative assent*) to donate without coercion (established by an independent advocacy team)
  (5) emotional and psychological risks to the donor are minimized.

This table, now modified, was originally printed in Ross LF, Thistlethwaite JR, Jr, and the American Academy of Pediatrics Committee on Bioethics. Policy Statement: Minors as Living Solid Organ Donors. *Pediatrics.* 2008; 122: 454–461 at p. 457, Table 1. (Modifications are in italics). With permission from the American Academy of Pediatrics.

---

to donate without coercion (established by an independent advocacy team), and on justice: (3) all other deceased and living donor options have been exhausted. That is, the conditions are consistent with the traditional bioethics framework as delineated in the *Belmont Report*: respect for persons, beneficence, and justice.[23]

In this chapter, we consider whether minors should participate as living donors using our living donor ethics framework that was specifically developed for living donor transplantation. As described in chapter 3, the 5 principles include the 3 Belmont principles and 2 additional principles: vulnerabilities and special relationships creating special obligations.

5.2 Living Donor Ethics Framework

5.2.1 Respect for Persons

The first principle is respect for persons which, in the *Belmont Report*, focuses on respect for autonomy for those who have decisional capacity and protection for those who have diminished autonomy.[24]

Legally all children are presumed to lack decisional capacity for health care decision-making. There are exceptions (eg, married minors) and there are exceptional circumstances (eg, emergencies) but neither of these addresses the question of whether some minors have the cognitive ability to make an autonomous decision. This question was not addressed in the early years of transplantation (1950s to 1970s). Rather, judicial review was sought whenever children were considered for organ donation, and the courts affirmed parental authority to authorize an invasive medical procedure on a healthy child that does not promote the child's own medical well-being provided that the family demonstrated that the donation was in the donor's best interest.[25] Later courts would not require that parents prove that living donation was in the child's best interest but only that the parents had considered all the risks and benefits and had determined that the benefits outweighed the risks.[26] This frequently entailed that the family show that the donor would experience psychological benefit from helping his sibling and psychological harm if not allowed to help. The courts did prohibit some donations by minors or others who lacked cognitive capacity when, for example, there was lack of intimacy (eg, the donor was institutionalized).[27]

Recent neurocognitive data show that the human brain continues to mature into the late twenties, which challenges the concept of adolescents having full cognitive capacity,[28] although empirical studies have also shown that some adolescents, particularly older adolescents, may have cognitive capacity comparable to adults.[29] But even if adolescents do have the cognitive capacity to donate a solid organ, a transplant program would not (and should not) empower them to make this decision alone, as parents still have ultimate responsibility for their children, even if their children have decisional capacity.[30] As such, parental permission is necessary for organ donation by minors.

However, what if the adolescent has decisional capacity (understands the risks, benefits, and alternatives) and his or her parents agree? Does the principle of respect for persons require the transplant team to perform the organ procurement? Here again the answer is "no." The transplant team, as moral agents, should almost always refuse to permit the work-up and procurement due to other principles that we will explore vide infra. But in exceptional circumstances (eg, a sibling with lack of venous and peritoneal access and no other potential live donor due to parental and other potential adult living donor comorbidities), the parents' permission and the child's assent might be necessary and sufficient. By assent we mean that the minor has good comprehension; understands the risks, benefits, and alternatives; and is actively agreeing to participate, not merely failing to object. This assent requirement disqualifies all young children and those with cognitive disability who are unable to give a meaningful assent.

In sum, the principle of respect for persons presumes that children lack decisional capacity and require protection, which means that minors should rarely be considered for living donation except in exceptional situations. In the rare case where minors are considered, respect for persons requires both parental permission and the child's assent.

5.2.2 Beneficence

Beneficence is represented in 3 of the conditions enumerated by the AAP that must be fulfilled for ethical donation by minors. Condition 2 from the AAP policy statement requires that surgical risk for the donor is extremely low. In the AAP statement, we noted that the mortality risks of unilateral nephrectomy and anesthesia are rare (approximately 2 in 10,000). Other surgical risks enumerated in the AAP statement are

> risks of postoperative bleeding and infections. All donors experience acute pain, and some develop chronic pain. The risks of serious or significant morbidity to kidney donors are often quoted at <5% regardless of the surgical method of procurement (e.g., laparoscopic versus open).[31]

However, condition 2 from the AAP statement should be modified to focus not only on the short-term surgical risks, but on the long-term risks as well. Since the publication of our original AAP report, much has been learned about the long-term risks of living donors. Medical risks include an increased risk of end-stage renal disease (ESRD), hypertension, and gout,[32] and these risks increase over time, suggesting that minors may be at greater risk than older adults given that they are expected to live many decades post-donation. While it is reassuring that 1 study of minor donors found that the long-term health risks in individuals who donated as adolescents are no different than the risks for those who donated as young adults,[33] long-term continued follow-up is needed. Young female donors also need to know that if they become pregnant, they are at greater risk for gestational hypertension, prematurity, and low birth weight.[34]

Even with our greater awareness of the long-term risks of unilateral ne-phrectomy, we believe that condition 2 can be met.

Condition 1 from the AAP statement requires that donor and recipient are both highly likely to benefit in order to justify permitting a minor to serve as a living donor. The benefit to the recipient is that living donor transplant is the best form of renal replacement therapy. The benefit to the donor is more psychological. As we wrote in the AAP statement:

> Although serving as an organ donor is not in the donor's medical best interest, it may be in the donor's best interest, all things considered. For example, there are potential psychological and emotional benefits that a minor donor may experience. The child may develop greater self-esteem and be seen as a hero by his or her family, friends, classmates, and larger community. There are also the potential benefits that a child accrues when his or her family is relieved of the burden of caring for a seriously ill family member. For example, the donor may now receive more parental time and energy and more intrafamilial companionship and may benefit from improved financial resources. The psychological benefits may even accrue if the transplant fails because the donor and his or her family can take solace in the fact that everything possible was done.[35]

However, there are also psychological risks. In the AAP we enumerated a few:

> lower self-esteem, a sense of neglect, and lack of appreciation after the do-nation as the attention refocuses on the recipient. The donor may experi-ence guilt and blame if the transplant fails and/or the recipient dies.[36]

Condition 5 from the AAP policy statement requires that emotional and psychological risks to the donor be minimized. To do this, the AAP statement requires a person with pediatric psychological expertise to be a member of a living donor advocate team (LDAT)—a team that is focused on the donor's clinical and psychological well-being and is separate from the recipient's transplant team. (The role of the LDAT will be discussed further under the principle of special relationships creating special obligations.) Thus condi-tion 1—that donor and recipient are both highly likely to benefit—is met if (1) the LDAT and the donor believe that the psychological benefits to the donor are significant and they outweigh the short- and long-term risks (condition 2); and (2) the psychological and emotion risks are minimized (condition 5).

5.2.3 Justice

The principle of justice requires the fair selection of living donors. Our third condition requires that "all other opportunities for transplantation have been exhausted, no potential adult living donor is available, and timely and/or effective transplantation from a cadaver donor is unlikely."[37] We believe that justice requires that children serve only as donors of last resort because of their inability to give an independent informed consent and because of their vulnerabilities (discussed in 5.2.4 Vulnerabilities). In this vein, we argued that children should not be worked up until other potential living donors are evaluated and found to be unable to donate.

In the AAP statement we considered whether to bypass condition 3 when the donor and recipient are identical twins because of the additional benefit provided to the potential recipient, who will not require immunosuppression. This issue was addressed at the 1966 CIBA symposium where Lord Kilbrandon, the chair of the meeting, rejected the twin exception: "You are implying that identical twins are something less than two personalities."[38] Daube agreed with Lord Kilbrandon:

> Children should on no account be donors and there should be no cheating by maintaining, for example, that the child would suffer a trauma if he were not allowed to give his twin a kidney or whatever it might be. . . . the likelihood of a trauma incidentally will be greatly lessened if the law leaves not the shadow of a doubt that a transplantation is here out of the question.[39]

The AAP statement also rejected the identical twin exception: "Although such a transplant provides great benefit to the recipient and, by extension, to the family, the benefit does not significantly alter the risks to the donor."[40] And in 1 survey, most US physicians also rejected it.[41] Moreover, living donors who are identical twins may be at greater risk of serious health problems as they share the same genetic risk factors as the recipient.[42] A recent analysis showed identical twin donors were at greater risk of developing ESRD than donors with any other relationship to their recipient.[43] While virtually all of the data involved adult identical twins, the data are not reassuring given that the risk for ESRD continues as the donors aged, and minor donor twins would need to live with only 1 kidney for an even longer period of time. As such, we continue to reject a twin exception that would permit a minor to donate to his or her identical twin unless the 5 criteria (including the search for an alternative adult donor) are not fulfilled.

5.2.4 Vulnerabilities

What makes children vulnerable? Again, we return to the vulnerability taxonomy developed by Kipnis that we modified for living donor transplantation (see Table 3.3). Children are at risk for having multiple vulnerabilities.

Capacitational: As we explored in the principle of respect for persons, young children are vulnerable because they lack cognitive capacity to understand the risks, benefits, and alternatives. For example, in *Hart v Brown* (involving a 7-year-old donating to her identical twin sister), the psychiatrist noted that the donor admitted that she was not sure what a kidney was.[44]

Older children may also be cognitively vulnerable. Even as they gain cognitive capacity to understand the risks and benefits and alternatives of renal replacement therapies, they often fail to appreciate long-term consequences and lack the experience to make an informed judgment.

Minors are at risk for *juridic* vulnerability because they are answerable to the authority of others who may have an independent interest in that donation. First, parents have the authority to make decisions on behalf of their children. Second, since minors are mainly considered as donors for first-degree relatives (siblings or parents), their parents almost always have a significant conflict of interest in the well-being of the potential recipient. Thus, even if minors are asked to provide assent, the parental support for the donation makes it difficult for the minor to say no, even if she does not want to donate. On the flip side, a minor who wants to donate would also be juridically vulnerable because she would be unable to do so without parental permission.

Deferential: Minors are often deferentially vulnerable to their parents. This is well-described in the bone marrow literature where parental expectations led many children to state that they did not feel that they had a choice.[45]

Social: Minors are also socially vulnerable because they belong to a group whose rights and interests have been socially disvalued. Minors cannot vote, cannot make decisions for themselves, and are dependent on their parents for many of their needs. As a group, the preferences of minors are often overridden or even ignored, sometimes for cause but at other times seemingly arbitrarily. Thus, a concern regarding living donation is that the minor may be seeking social status (parental approval) and be willing to take risks to achieve it.

Medical: This vulnerability considers whether the potential living donor been selected, in part, because of the presence of a serious health-related condition in the intended recipient for which there are only less satisfactory alternative remedies. Recall condition 5, which requires that "all other deceased and living donor options have been exhausted." This may have justified Dr. Murray going to court in 1957 because the lack of chronic dialysis made transplant necessary and the lack of immunosuppression meant that any kidney transplant from anyone other than an identical twin had a short life expectancy. In the US since 2005, minors have priority for a high-quality deceased donor organ (first under Share 35 and now under the new Kidney Allocation System [KAS]),[46] further reducing the need to permit donation by individuals younger than 18 years of age.

Situational: This vulnerability refers to whether the potential living donor is in a situation in which medical exigency of the intended recipient prevents the education and deliberation needed by the potential living donor to decide whether to participate as a living donor. A minor is situationally vulnerable because they may not have the cognitive ability to discern whether a medical exigency actually exists for the intended recipient. While they may be able to grasp that the intended recipient is very sick, even an adolescent with age-appropriate cognitive function may not be able discern whether their being a donor is an urgent necessity or only a perceived preferred treatment modality for the intended recipient. For an identical twin, the possibility that the recipient can avoid immunosuppression may also make the pediatric donor think that their donation is a necessity when the principle would limit the twin's donation to a last-resort situation when no other donor is available.

Allocational: This vulnerability examines whether the potential living donor is lacking in subjectively important social goods that will be provided as a consequence of participation as a donor. In the AAP statement, we noted that there are potential psychological and emotional benefits that may accrue to a minor donor including (1) greater self-esteem, (2) greater status within the family or community, and (3) potentially more parental time and companionship, given that the ill sibling may require less energy and resources post-transplantation.[47] While these are benefits that may entice the adolescent to assent to donation, it is critical that the adolescent understand that these benefits may not accrue: (1) the transplant may fail and the recipient may do poorly, which may cause lower donor self-esteem; (2) even if the transplant is successful, the parents may still consider the donor to be the healthy child, needing less of their attention especially if the sibling recipient has typical post-transplant complications (eg, rejection episodes or immunosuppression-related infections); (3) the parents may limit the donor's participation in group activities that increase exposure to communicable infections in order to protect the sibling recipient from common childhood viral communicable diseases; and (4) unilateral nephrectomy may prohibit the adolescent from participating in some sports and from some professions (eg, military). That is, it is critical that the LDAT ensure that the adolescent understands that the donation does not guarantee allocational benefits and may even reduce the opportunities to engage in certain activities (ie, restrictions on certain social goods).

Infrastructural: Does the political, organizational, economic, and social context of the donor care setting possess the integrity and resources needed to manage living donation process and follow-up? If a pediatric living donor has the same longevity as a healthy non-donor, she would be anticipated to live many decades after her donation. While the UNOS/OPTN database started to document living donors 25 years ago, UNOS/OPTN regulations only require 2-year follow-up data on living donors. No systematic long-term outcome data have been collected. In 2017, a voluntary living donor registry was established, but whether there will be long-term resources and whether participation will be adequate for understanding long-term donor health will depend on the willingness of the transplant community and living donors to provide the necessary data voluntarily.[48] The failure of the transplant community, through its institutional structure (eg, UNOS/OPTN in the United States), to have long-term registries to answer questions about long-term risks makes it even harder to justify allowing minors to serve as living donors. Since minors have the greatest life expectancy of all age groups, unknown long-term risks are most crucial to this population.

Infrastructural vulnerability can also be related to the social situation of children. Children may be at infrastructural vulnerability due to low health literacy.[49] Although many adults also have low health literacy,[50] attempts to promote health literacy in childhood will be important as children and adolescents develop their health behavior habits.[51] Low health literacy may interfere with their understanding of the short- and long-term risks of nephrectomy. Children are at additional infrastructural vulnerability because it is not known whether they will have health insurance or access to quality health care as adults. Thus, these individuals, who are at risk from the unilateral nephrectomy for decades, may not have access to adequate health care to ensure that their risks are minimized.

5.2.5 Special Relationships Create Special Obligations

In living donor kidney transplantation, there are 2 patients—the potential donor and the potential recipient. Each patient should have his or her own medical team focused on his or her well-being. At the time we were writing the AAP statement, the concept of an independent advocate (or advocate team) was just being developed and adopted.[52] In our AAP statement, we argued that when the potential donor is a minor, there needs to be an LDAT with special pediatric expertise including:

(1) training and education in child development and child psychology,
(2) skills in communicating with children and understanding children's verbal and non-verbal communication, and (3) working knowledge of transplantation and organ donation.[53]

We thought this might require supplementing the membership of the standard LDAT with 1 or more pediatric professionals with specific pediatric skills and expertise. At minimum, this will include an appropriate mental health professional with pediatric expertise to ensure that the adolescent has the cognitive capacity and maturity to grasp the risks and benefits and to make a voluntary decision free of undue influence.

Again, as we noted in the AAP statement:

Although there have been few studies that explored the minor's psychological response to serving as an organ donor, the adult literature shows that individuals may have unexpected reactions to donation. The minor needs to understand that the donated organ may fail or may be rejected by the recipient; or that the original cause of the organ failure may recur; and that the outcome is beyond his control.[54]

To promote the minor's ability to freely assent (or to have the space in which to dissent), we further argued that it was necessary for the LDAT to meet independently with the potential pediatric donors: that "[a]t least some of the conversations between the potential minor donor and the independent advocacy team should be held in the absence of other family members,"[55] and that the minors must be "counseled at various junctures that it is permissible to say no or to withdraw at any time prior to the procedure."[56] If the minor is unwilling to serve or is emotionally or cognitively unable to appreciate at some level the risks and benefits of the procedures involved, we argued that the LDAT should recommend against the donation.

5.3 Conclusion

In the AAP statement, we concluded that it is morally permissible for minors to serve as living donors in exceptional circumstances provided that 5 criteria are met (see Box 5.1). A similar position has been taken by several US commentators,[57] whereas others have argued for more leniency,[58] and others for an absolute prohibition.[59]

If we were to revise the AAP statement today, we would argue that the donation must meet not only the 5 conditions enumerated in the AAP statement but also that the LDAT ensure that all of the vulnerabilities are fully addressed. It is also worth noting that many of the reasons that an adult may have been excluded from donating in the past have been eliminated (eg, ABO incompatibility, donor-specific antibodies, or positive crossmatch) because of donor paired exchange programs, domino chain programs (catalyzed by a Good Samaritan donor), and/or desensitization protocols. As such, the likelihood that a minor is the only potential donor in a family who can donate should be incredibly rare. We believe that an adult donor who can donate through a paired exchange or domino chain should be preferred over a minor donor who can donate directly. We emphasize that minors should be donors as last resort both because of their vulnerabilities but also because in the 15 years since we wrote the statement, there is greater awareness of the potential long-term risks of living donation. Data showing that younger donors are at greater risk than older donors provide even more reasons to support very restrictive policies regarding pediatric solid organ donation, although we still support exceptions in exceptional circumstances.

Notes

1. UNOS/OPTN National Data. Last updated August 15, 2021. Last accessed August 16, 2021. https://optn.transplant.hrsa.gov/data/view-data-reports/national-data/. Hereinafter referred to as OPTN Data.

2. Data about children as living donor kidney transplant recipients can be found at OPTN Data. For data about children as tissue donors, see Bitan M, van Walraven SM, Worel N, et al. Determination of eligibility in related pediatric hematopoietic cell donors: ethical and clinical considerations. Recommendations from a working group of the Worldwide Network for Blood and Marrow Transplantation Association. *Biol Blood Marrow Transplant.* 2016;22:96–103.

3. *Huskey v Harrison*, Eq. No. 68666 (Mass 1957); *Foster v Harrison*, Eq. No. 68674 (Mass 1957); and *Masden v Harrison*, Eq. No. 68651 (Mass 1957).

4. Ross LF. *Children, Families and Health Care Decision Making.* Oxford UK: Oxford University Press, 1998, at p. 112.

5. Delmonico FL, Harmon WE. The use of a minor as a live kidney donor. *Am J Transplant.* 2002;2:333–336.

6. OPTN Data.

7. *Hart v Brown*, 29 Conn Super Ct 368, 289 A2d 386 (Conn Super Ct 1972).

8. Webb NJ, Fortune PM. Should children ever be living kidney donors? *Pediatr Transplant.* 2006;10:851–855.

9. Greenaway K. Baie-d'Urfé twin receives first successful kidney transplant in Canada. June 21, 2017. https://montrealgazette.com/news/local-news/west-island-gazette/baie-durfe-twin-receives-first-successful-kidney-transplant-in-canada

10. Delmonico and Harmon, "The use of a minor; Berney T, Genton L, Buhler LH, et al. Identical 13-year-old twins have donated small bowel: five-year follow-up after pediatric living related small bowel transplantation between two monozygotic twins. *Transplant Proc.* 2004;36(2):316–318; *Hart v Brown*, 29 Conn Super Ct 368, 289 A2d 386 (Conn Super Ct 1972); and Tilden SJ. Ethical and legal aspects of using an identical twin as a skin transplant donor for a severely burned minor. *Am J Law Med.* 2005;31:87–116.

11. This is discussed in Capitaine L, Thys K, Van Assche K, Sterckx S, Pennings G. Should minors be considered as potential living liver donors? *Liver Transpl.* 2013;19:649–655.

12. Wolstenholme GEW, O'Connor M, eds. *Ethics in Medical Progress: With Special Reference to Transplantation.* Boston, MA: Little, Brown and Company; 1966.

13. Wolstenholme and O'Connor, *Ethics in Medical Progress,* at p. 203.

14. Wolstenholme and O'Connor, *Ethics in Medical Progress,* at p. 198 and p. 203.

15. Lafranca JA, Spoon EQW, van de Wetering J, IJzermans JNM, Dor FJMF. Attitudes among transplant professionals regarding shifting paradigms in eligibility criteria for live kidney donation. PLoS One. 2017;12(7):e0181846. Published July 21, 2017. Accessed August 16, 2021. https://doi.org/10.1371/journal.pone.0181846

16. Delmonico F, Council of the Transplantation Society. A report of the Amsterdam Forum on the care of the live kidney donor: data and medical guidelines. *Transplantation.* 2005;79(6 suppl):S53–66.

17. Abecassis M, Adams M, Adams P, et al. Consensus statement on the live organ donor. *JAMA*. 2000;284: 2919–2926.
18. Ross LF, Thistlethwaite JR, Jr, Committee on Bioethics. Minors as living solid organ donors. *Pediatrics*. 2008;122:454–461, at p. 454.
19. Thys K, Van Assche K, Nobile H, et al. Could minors be living kidney donors? A systematic review of guidelines, position papers and reports. *Transpl Int*. 2013;26:949–960.
20. Lafranca et al, "Attitudes among transplant professionals."
21. Abecassis et al, "Consensus statement."
22. Ross et al, "Minors as living," at p. 457.
23. The National Commission for the Protection of Human Subjects of Biomedical and Behavioral Research. *The Belmont Report: Ethical Principles and Guidelines for the Protection of Human Subjects of Research*. Washington, DC: Government Printing Office, 1978. Hereinafter referred to as the *Belmont Report*.
24. *Belmont Report*.
25. See the 3 cases cited earlier: *Huskey v Harrison, Foster v Harrison*, and *Masden v Harrison*.
26. *Nathan v Farinelli*, Eq. No. 74–87 (Mass 1974).
27. See, for example, *In re Richardson*, 284 So2d 185 (La App 4th Cir) *writ denied*, 284 So2d 338 (La 1973); and *In re Pescinski*, 226 NW2d 180 (Wis 1975).
28. Diekema DS. Adolescent refusal of lifesaving treatment: are we asking the right questions? *Adolesc Med State Art Rev*. 2011;22(2):213–228.
29. See, for example, Grisso T, Vierling L. Minors' consent to treatment: a developmental perspective. *Prof Psychol*. 1978;9:412–427; Scherer DG, Reppucci ND. Adolescents' capacities to provide voluntary informed consent: the effects of parental influence and medical dilemmas. *Law Hum Behav*. 1988;12:123–141; and Weithorn LA, Campbell SB. The competency of children and adolescents to make informed treatment decisions. *Child Dev*. 1982;53:1589–1598.
30. Ross, *Children*, esp. chapter 3, "Constrained parental autonomy," at pp. 39–55.
31. American Academy of Pediatrics Committee on Bioethics, "Policy statement," at p. 454.
32. See, for example, Muzaale AD, Massie AB, Wang MC, et al. Risk of end-stage renal disease following live kidney donation. *JAMA*. 2014;311:579–586; Mjøen G, Hallan S, Hartmann A, et al. Long-term risks for kidney donors. *Kidney Int*. 2014;86:162–167; Lam NN, Lentine KL, Levey AS, Kasiske BL, Garg AX. Long-term medical risks to the living kidney donor. *Nat. Rev. Nephrol*. 2015;11:411–419; and Gaston RS, Kumar V, Matas AJ. Reassessing Medical Risk in Living Kidney Donors. *J Am Soc Nephrol*. 2015;26:1017–1019.
33. MacDonald D, Kukla AK, Ake S, et al. Medical outcomes of adolescent live kidney donors. *Pediatric Transplant*. 2014;18:336–341.
34. See, for example, Ibrahim HN, Akkina SK, Leister E, et al. Pregnancy outcomes after kidney donation. *Am J Transplant*. 2009;9:825–834; and Garg AX, Nevis IF, McArthur E, et al. Gestational hypertension and preeclampsia in living kidney donors. *N Engl J Med*. 2015;372:124–133.

35. American Academy of Pediatrics Committee on Bioethics, "Policy statement," at p. 455 (references omitted).

36. American Academy of Pediatrics Committee on Bioethics, "Policy statement," at p. 455 (references omitted).

37. Abecassis et al, "Consensus"; and American Academy of Pediatrics Committee on Bioethics, "Policy statement."

38. Wolstenholme and O'Connor, *Ethics in Medical Progress,* at p. 203.

39. Wolstenholme and O'Connor, *Ethics in Medical Progress,* at p. 198.

40. American Academy of Pediatrics Committee on Bioethics, "Policy statement," at p. 455.

41. Joseph JW, Thistlethwaite JR, Jr, Ross LF. An empirical investigation of physicians' attitudes towards intrasibling kidney donation by minor twins. *Transplantation.* 2008;85:1235–1239.

42. Wolstenholme and O'Connor, *Ethics in Medical Progress*; and American Academy of Pediatrics Committee on Bioethics, "Policy statement."

43. Muzaale AD, Massie AB, Al Ammary F, et al. Donor-recipient relationship and risk of ESKD in live kidney donors of varied racial groups. *Am J Kidney Dis.* 2020;75:333–341.

44. *Hart v Brown,* 29 Conn Super Ct 368, 289 A2d 386 (Conn Super Ct 1972).

45. See, for example, Spital A. Should children ever donate kidneys? Views of U.S. transplant centers. *Transplantation.* 1997;64(2):232–236; and Holm S. The child as organ and tissue donor: discussions in the Danish council of ethics. *Camb Q Healthc Ethics.* 2004;13(2):156–160.

46. For a discussion of Share 35, see Abraham EC, Wilson AC, Goebel J. Current kidney allocation rules and their impact on a pediatric transplant center. *Am J Transplant.* 2009;9:404–408. For a discussion of the impact of KAS, see OPTN. The New Kidney Allocation System (KAS) frequently asked questions. Updated 9-17-2014. To go into effect December 4, 2014. Last accessed August 16, 2021. https://optn.transplant.hrsa.gov/media/1235/kas_faqs.pdf

47. American Academy of Pediatrics Committee on Bioethics, "Policy statement."

48. Kasiske BL, Asrani SK, Dew MA, et al. The living donor collective: a scientific registry for living donors. *Am J Transplant.* 2017;17:3040–3048.

49. Sanders LM, Federico S, Klass P, Abrams MA, Drever B. Literacy and child health: a systematic review. *Arch Pediatr Adolesc Med.* 2009;163(2):131–140

50. Berkman ND, Sheridan SL, Donahue KE, Halpern DJ, Crotty K. Low health literacy and health outcomes: an updated systematic review. *Ann Intern Med.* 2011;155(2):97–107.

51. Winkelman TNA, Caldwell TM, Bertram B, Davis MM. Promoting health literacy for children and adolescents. *Pediatrics.* 2016;138(6):e20161937. https://doi.org/10.1542/peds.2016-1937

52. US Department of Health and Human Services, Advisory Committee on Organ Transplantation. Recommendations 1–18. Recommendation #2 available at: Date last reviewed June 2021. Date last accessed August 16, 2021. https://www.hrsa.gov/advisory-committees/organ-transplantation/recommendations/1-18;   Department of Health and Human Services part II. Centers for Medicare and Medicaid Services

42 DFR Parts 405, 482, 488, and 498. Medicare Program; Hospital Conditions of Participation: Requirements for approval and re-approval of transplant centers to perform organ transplants; Final Rule. *Fed Reg.* 2007(March 30, 2007);72:15198–15280. Of note, United Network for Organ Sharing (UNOS)/Organ Procurement and Transplantation Network (OPTN) modified its bylaws the same year. Appendix B, Section XIII, 2007. Updated in current UNOS/OPTN policy handbook in section 14.2 Independent Living Donor Advocate Requirements.

53. American Academy of Pediatrics Committee on Bioethics, "Policy statement," at p. 457.

54. American Academy of Pediatrics Committee on Bioethics, "Policy statement," at p. 458, (references omitted).

55. American Academy of Pediatrics Committee on Bioethics, "Policy statement," at p. 459.

56. American Academy of Pediatrics Committee on Bioethics, "Policy statement," at p. 457.

57. See, for example, Spital, "Should children"; Steinberg D. Kidney transplants from young children and the mentally retarded. *Theor Med.* 2004;25:229–241; Webb and Fortune, "Should children ever"; and Olbrisch ME, Levenson J, Newman JD. Children as living organ donors: current views and practice in the United States. *Curr Opin Organ Transplant.* 2010;15:241–244.

58. See, for example, Fost N. Children as renal donors. *N Engl J Med.* 1977;296:363–367; Lantos JD. Children as organ donors: An argument for involuntary altruism. In: Burgio GR, Lantos JD, eds. *Primum Non Nocere Today: A Symposium on Pediatric Bioethics.* New York: Elsevier; 1994:67–75.

59. See, for example, Delmonico F and the Council of the Transplantation Society, "Amsterdam Forum."

6

Prisoners as Living Organ Donors

6.1 Introduction

This chapter considers the special case in which a prisoner seeks to serve as a living donor and what lessons can be learned from human subjects protections for research participants given that both activities are done with the primary goal to benefit third parties. Human research subjects protections in the United States (US) are codified in the *Code of Federal Regulations* (45 CFR 46), and special protections are implemented when prisoners are recruited for research participation. Current Department of Justice Federal Bureau of Prisons policy allows prisoners to serve as living donors but only for first-degree relatives. In this chapter we describe what special considerations should be assessed for prisoners to ethically serve as potential living donors using a vulnerability approach adapted from the human research subjects protection literature.

6.2 The History of Prisoners as Living Donors

In a 1964 article on kidney transplantation in the *Journal of the American Medical Association*, Thomas Starzl, one of the pioneers of organ transplantation, described 12 kidney transplants that had been performed at the University of Colorado beginning in November 19662.[1] Two involved deceased donor kidneys while the other 10 involved living donor kidney grafts. The relationships between the living donors and recipients included 1 mother to child, 5 sibling pairs, 2 spouses, and 2 were unrelated: 1 was a volunteer who responded to an advertisement and the other was a prisoner (who 12 days postoperatively "disappeared from the ward and has not been seen since").[2] Later that year, Starzl and colleagues described 40 kidney transplants performed at the University of Colorado. Nine of the donors were prisoners.[3]

The Living Organ Donor as Patient. Lainie Friedman Ross and J. Richard Thistlethwaite, Jr, Oxford University Press.
© Oxford University Press 2022. DOI: 10.1093/oso/9780197618202.003.0006

The first symposium on ethics and transplantation was held in England in 1966, funded by the CIBA Foundation.[4] At that meeting, several participants challenged Starzl's practice of appealing for donors at state prisons. Starzl argued that fewer than 100 of the 4,000 inmates expressed any interest, supporting his position that they were free to refuse and were acting on their own volition. He also suggested that they were under less pressure than some people experience from their families. He emphasized that "the consent form contained two written stipulations: (1) no pay was involved and (2) no re-duction in the period of servitude was offered."[5] He also noted that many of the prisoners were nearing the completion of their sentence, supporting his position that they understood this action would not shorten their penal ob-ligation. However, by late 1966, Starzl stopped accepting prisoners as donors after "private and informal conversations with Professor David Daube," a British legal scholar who was an attendee at the CIBA-sponsored sympo-sium. Starzl stated:

> The latter discussant had convinced me that the use of penal volunteers, however equitably handled in a local situation would inevitably lead to abuse if accepted as a reasonable precedent and applied broadly.[6]

The interest in prisoners serving as living donors was also diminished as the medical community began to realize that conditions like hepatitis (and later on, human immunodeficiency virus (HIV)/acquired immune deficiency syndrome (AIDS)) were overrepresented in the prisoner population.[7]

In the intervening 50 years, prisoners have infrequently served as living donors, and in those cases, they have donated to family members.[8] But the participation of prisoners as living donors came to national attention in 2010 when Governor Haley Barbour of Mississippi offered indefinite suspensions of the life sentences of Jamie and Gladys Scott provided that Gladys donate a kidney to her sister Jaime who had end-stage renal disease (ESRD) within 1 year of their release (the follow-up will be discussed later in the chapter).[9]

In this chapter we examine the ethics of prisoners participating as living solid organ donors (liver or kidney). We compare the prisoner as living donor with the prisoner as participant in medical research, as both living donors and research participants agree to participate with the primary goal of benefiting third parties. We show how the concept of vulnerability used in research ethics can help us understand the challenges to voluntary con-sent faced by prisoners considering living donation. Finally, we argue that the offer of incentives such as sentence reduction to encourage living organ donation is unethical. We focus our discussion on the prisoner who seeks to donate directly to a family member, as current federal policy only allows prisoners to donate directedly to first-degree relatives.[10] We conclude this chapter by asking whether the current policy could be interpreted to allow a prisoner who is ABO-incompatible or crossmatch positive with a family member to participate in a paired exchange (which would mean that the prisoner donates to a stranger in exchange for another stranger donating to his or her intended recipient). To our knowledge this issue has not yet been discussed in the literature or challenged in the courts.

6.3 The Prisoner as Vulnerable Research Subject

In response to several egregious research studies, most notably the US Public Health Service Syphilis Study at Tuskegee,[11] the National Commission for the Protection of Biomedical and Behavioral Research (hereinafter referred to as the National Commission) was established in July 1974 under the National Research Act (Public Law 93-348).[12] The National Commission was specifically charged to develop federal human subjects protections for biomedical and behavioral research: prisoners were considered 1 vulnerable group that needed additional protections.[13] The resulting guidelines for the protection of human subjects were codified in 45 CFR 46, Subpart A: the Common Rule, which applies to all research participants, and additional protections were codified in the various subsections: Subpart B: Pregnant Women, Human Fetuses, and Neonates; Subpart C: Prisoners; and Subpart D: Children.[14]

In the decades prior to the promulgation of human subjects protection regulations by the National Commission, prisoners participated in research in large numbers. During World War II, prisoners were used "to develop treatment for infectious diseases that afflicted our armed forces" and continued to participate after the war due to the rapid expansion of biomedical research and the governmental policies for drug testing.[15]

The charge given to the National Commission was timely. Investigative reports from the 1960s and 1970s described widespread abuse in medical research conducted in prisons.[16] The National Commission's Report, *Research Involving Prisoners*, published in 1976, questioned whether incarceration truly allowed for free choice in deciding whether to participate in research: "the availability of a population living in conditions of social and economic deprivation makes it possible for researchers to bring to these populations types of research which persons better situated would ordinarily refuse."[17] The National Commission concluded that, given the vulnerabilities of the prisoners, they should only participate in research that offers direct benefit to the prisoners as individuals or to prisoners as a group. The research should also focus on health problems that are serious for or within the prison population. The result was the closing down of much prison-based medical research.

During the decades prior to the National Commission's reports and the federal regulations that were developed from them, research subjects were typically paid. This was also true of the prisoner research subjects. The National Commission noted that prisoners were willing to participate for very small financial incentives because alternative opportunities to earn money in the prison were few and meager. To avoid "coercion or undue influence," Subpart C restricted the use of incentives in research involving prisoners:

> §46.305 (a)(2) Any possible advantages accruing to the prisoner through his or her participation in the research, when compared to the general living conditions, medical care, quality of food, amenities and opportunity for earnings in the prison, are not of such a magnitude that his or her ability to weigh the risks of the research against the value of such advantages in the limited choice environment of the prison is impaired; and . . .
>
> §46.305 (a)(6) Adequate assurance exists that parole boards will not take into account a prisoner's participation in the research in making decisions regarding parole, and each prisoner is clearly informed in advance that participation in the research will have no effect on his or her parole.[18]

That is, the federal regulations were designed to protect the vulnerable prisoners from participating in research against their better judgment by removing 2 disparate sources of "undue influence" that could interfere with their ability to give an informed and voluntary consent—large financial incentives and sentence reduction.

Another means to protect prisoners enumerated in the *Federal Regulations* was to require institutional review boards—committees that oversee human subjects protections—to include a prisoner, or a prisoner representative with appropriate background and experience when reviewing a research project involving the recruitment and participation of prisoners.[19]

6.4 Incentivizing Prisoners to Serve as Living Donors

The prisoners whom Starzl recruited as living donors were unique both because they were incarcerated and because they were living donors with no genetic nor emotional relationship to the recipient. In fact, at that time, most centers would not have accepted law-abiding citizens who volunteered to donate to strangers,[20] although this attitude changed over the decades.[21] Today, US prisoners are not permitted to donate to strangers, but they can and do donate to family members on a case-by-case basis.[22]

More recently, however, there have been some proposals to incentivize prisoners to serve as nondirected donors or Good Samaritan donors by offering a reduction in prison term in exchange for organ or tissue donation. In 1998, Missouri state representative Chuck Graham proposed a bill that offered "a life for a life."[23] The bill targeted death row inmates and offered them a reprieve from execution to a sentence of life without parole if they donated a kidney for transplantation. In 2007, South Carolina state senator Ralph Anderson introduced Senate Bill 480 (SB 480) which offered to reduce a prisoner's sentence by 180 days for a kidney.[24] Neither bill passed.

Even had the proposals passed in the US, they would not have been implementable without modifications to the National Organ Transplantation Act (NOTA) of 1984, which specifically prohibits "any person to knowingly acquire, receive, or otherwise transfer any human organ for valuable consideration for use in human transplantation if the transfer affects interstate commerce."[25] The phrase "valuable consideration" can be understood to prohibit payment as well as any other form of benefit like reduction of prison sentence. As Emily Lee, a legal scholar, explains, "Liberty, unlike monetary compensation, is not quantifiable, but it is still undeniably valuable."[26]

Thus, it came as a surprise when, in late 2010, Mississippi Governor Haley Barbour released Jamie and Gladys Scott who had served 16 years of their life sentences for armed robbery convictions on the condition of organ donation by Gladys to Jamie. Jamie Scott had ESRD and her release is what is known as a humanitarian or medical release. Her sister Gladys had offered to donate a kidney, which led to the Governor offering her a conditional release. She was given 1 year to donate a kidney to her sister, or she could be sent back to prison.

Although the illegality of this conditional release seems obvious, Jamila Jefferson-Jones explains that this is not how the Mississippi governor understood the situation:

The Governor's spokesperson denied that the exchange may have been illegal and instead pointed to Gladys's petition to the parole board in which she indicated her willingness to donate. Gladys Scott even publicly claimed that it was her idea to donate her kidney to Jamie and that she would have done so willingly, even without the promise of freedom. This Article argues that one may therefore surmise that both Gladys and the Governor thought that the potential issue of valuable consideration (to the extent that they were aware of the issue) was meaningless because Gladys actually wanted to give a kidney to Jamie.[27]

Jefferson-Jones goes on to explain that they were wrong in their interpretation and the deal was a violation of NOTA, whether or not Gladys volunteered.[28]

Denouement: After their release, it was determined that Jamie needed to lose weight to be eligible for an organ and Gladys needed to lose weight to be eligible to donate. In January 2014, Jaime remained on dialysis.[29] Despite breaking this condition of parole, there were no attempts to re-incarcerate the sisters. In 2019, having lost the weight necessary, Jaime was the recipient of a deceased donor kidney transplant. The sisters continue to seek a pardon or to have their sentence commuted.[30]

6.5 Is It Ethical to Allow Prisoners to Serve as Living Donors? A Vulnerability Analysis

Although the courts have specifically stated that there is no legal right for a prisoner to be a living donor,[31] Aviva Goldberg and Joel Frader have argued persuasively that respect for persons would require that prisoners, as members of humanity, be allowed to donate to help a loved one if they can give a voluntary and informed consent.[32]

Whether a potential donor can give a voluntary and informed consent is not a concern unique to prisoners and was recognized early on. At the 1966 CIBA Foundation symposium entitled *Ethics in Medical Progress: With Special Reference to Transplantation*, some transplant professionals described incorporating a psychological evaluation into the living donor work-up to ensure voluntariness and adequate information.[33] Over 3 decades later, in the year 2000, an international committee of transplant personnel proposed the idea of an independent donor advocate.[34] These independent donor advocates are now referred to as living donor advocates (LDAs) or, when it involves 2 or more persons, living donor advocate teams (LDATs). The team approach acknowledges that all the skills needed to provide the appropriate medical and psychosocial care of a living donor may not reside in 1 individual and instead involves a team to evaluate, educate, and advocate for the living donor.[35]

When the donor is a prisoner there are additional vulnerabilities that may interfere with a free and voluntary consent process. The LDAT serves to help empower the potential donor to understand the risks, benefits, and alternatives before deciding whether to donate. However, most LDATs are unlikely to have the expertise to determine a potential donor's ability to understand risks and benefits in the setting of incarceration where the individual's autonomy is compromised and daily life activities and well-being are controlled by others. The training and experience of the LDAT enables them to detect and address the nuanced differences among potential living donors and their individual personal and social circumstances, but is unlikely to give them adequate insight into the additional vulnerabilities incarceration is likely to impose and how these vulnerabilities affect decision-making for individual prisoners. We propose the mandatory inclusion on the LDAT of a social worker or psychologist who works or has worked with prisoners when a prisoner is being considered as a living donor. We will call this person a prisoner liaison (PL). The PL will have a better understanding of the constraints of prison life and its impact on decision-making and can help determine whether the prisoner's consent is informed and voluntary.

A vulnerability analysis can help us understand the additional challenges and concerns that are faced by the prisoner who is contemplating serving as a living donor. We use the modified vulnerability taxonomy enumerated in Table 3.3 and describe how these incarceration-related vulnerabilities can be addressed by including a PL as a member of an LDAT when the potential living donor is a prisoner.

Capacitational: Consider the first vulnerability trait: "Do prisoners as potential living donors have the capacity to deliberate about and decide whether or not to participate as a living donor?" J. Michael Millis and Mary Simmerling argue that most prisoners have the decisional capacity to serve as living donors because otherwise they would not have been allowed to stand trial.[36] They also argue for symmetry because prisoners are empowered to consent to be a solid organ recipient.

Millis and Simmerling may be a bit too quick in making their capacity assessment. First, capacity is not all-or-none, but decision-specific.[37] This means that just because one can voluntarily consent to receive a kidney does not mean that one can voluntarily consent to donate a kidney. There is a lower threshold for consenting to receive a life-saving treatment than for consenting to undergo a surgery that offers no clinical benefit to the patient but only to a third party.[38] Second, the data about prisoners are skewed to those of lower educational attainment. In 1997, approximately 41% of inmates in US State and Federal prisons and local jails and 31% of probationers had not completed high school or its equivalent. In comparison, 18% of the general population age 18 or older had not finished the 12th grade.[39] In 2002, Mark Cunningham and Mark Vigen reviewed 13 clinical studies of death row inmates conducted over the past 35 years and found that they were frequently intellectually limited and academically deficient.[40] While low educational attainment or low IQ is not an absolute contraindication to donation, it does raise red flags regarding the candidate donor's ability to understand the risks of the procedure as well as their right to renege.[41]

Mental illness may also impair an individual's ability to make an informed decision, and mental illness is common among prisoners. In a 2002 analysis of 62 surveys of prisoners from 12 countries, Seena Fazel and colleagues found:

> 3.7% of men (95% CI [Confidence Interval] 3.3–4.1) had psychotic illnesses, 10% (9–11) major depression, and 65% (61–68) a personality disorder, including 47% (46–48) with antisocial personality disorder. 4.0% of women (3.2–5.1) had psychotic illnesses, 12% (11–14) major depression, and 42% (38–45) a personality disorder, including 21% (19–23) with antisocial personality disorder.[42]

A review of studies from 16 US states found wide heterogeneity between studies although the range of prevalence estimates for particular disorders was much higher than found in community samples.[43]

Drug and alcohol problems are also common. Fazel and colleagues analyzed 13 studies and found that:

> estimates of prevalence for alcohol abuse and dependence in male prisoners ranged from 18 to 30% and 10 to 24% in female prisoners. The prevalence estimates of drug abuse and dependence varied from 10 to 48% in male prisoners and 30 to 60% in female prisoners.[44]

Again, these are only risk factors, but they do suggest that a thorough capacity assessment is necessary when incarcerated individuals are being evaluated for living donation. This is not to deny that many smart, sober, mentally well individuals also have difficulty understanding risks, especially in the high-stakes health care arena such as transplantation, but only to emphasize the need for a robust LDAT including a PL who helps the potential donor think through the issues, and the risks, benefits and alternatives.

Juridic: "Is the potential living donor liable to the authority of others who may have an independent interest in that donation?" One problem with prisoners serving as living donors is that they are liable to the authority of prison officials who have legal authority over them, even if the prison officials are not particularly invested in organ transplantation. No data exist, but one could imagine that an advertising campaign to promote Good Samaritan donation would be supported by some prison authorities who believe that prisoners "owe" it to the rest of society or even think that the prisoner is of little social value and, therefore, should be used to do some "good" for others. The task for the health care team is "to devise a consent procedure that will adequately insulate the prisoner from the hierarchical system to which he or she is subject."[45] Some question whether prisoners can ever give a truly voluntary consent given "the inherently coercive nature of prison."[46] Most LDATs will not have a true grasp of the constraints of prison life and its impact on decision-making. This insight may be achieved with the addition of a PL to the team. In addition, even though prisoners may be told that a reward is not permitted and that information about donation cannot be included in a parole hearing, some expectation of reward for good behavior may remain (eg, earlier parole, better work assignment). An LDAT that includes a PL should only permit the donation to go forward if they are convinced that the prisoner is not motivated by an expectation of external reward.

Deferential: "Is the potential living donor given to patterns of deferential behavior that may mask an underlying unwillingness to participate?" While juridic and deferential vulnerabilities certainly overlap and are often present together, juridic vulnerability entails a relationship in which 1 person has formal authority or power over the other whereas deferential vulnerability involves subjective responses (from respect to fear to insecurity) by the individual to certain others.[47] Although becoming a living donor is elective, the prisoner may feel some degree of familial pressure. Family ties are often of great importance for prisoners. Family members are the most likely individuals to visit a prisoner and are the most important source of support when released.[48] There may be deferential vulnerability because prisoners may feel some degree of dependence on their family that is often their prime external contact. Thus, when a prisoner is informed that a family member needs an organ transplant, the prisoner may offer to be the donor either out of fear that not donating may lead to alienation or out of hope to do something positive. Many prisoners provided financial support to their families before incarceration; they may have also offered physical and emotional support. Incarceration takes away these abilities to give back and, as such, the idea of donation may become a way to "give back."[49] In other scenarios, the prisoner may be asked to serve as the donor either because he is more "expendable" than other family members or because other family members cannot afford to take the time off for the work-up and recuperation. The British Transplantation Society recently promulgated guidelines in which they asserted that the prisoner must be a "last resort";[50] but that is not a requirement of US guidelines, which only require that the donor be a first-degree relative.[51] Again, the LDAT, supplemented with a PL, should work with the prisoner to ensure that the donation is truly what he wants to do, to reassure the prisoner that third parties (both prison staff and family) need not be told the reasons for exclusion if he elects not to proceed, and to ensure that the prisoner understands what, if anything, is and is not being offered in return.

Social: "Does the potential living donor belong to a group whose rights and interests have been socially disvalued?" Prisoners are socially disvalued.[52] While they retain many of their constitutional rights, there are restrictions on their rights and interests including limitations on their rights to privacy and to freedom of movement. Prisoners have the right to "adequate" health care, although options and access may be limited due to the need for security.[53] The PL's role in the LDAT is to evaluate the threats that incarceration poses to donor voluntariness, to ensure that the prisoners have privacy in medical decision-making regarding donation, and to ensure that prisoners who are prospective living donors receive evaluation and treatment comparable to that provided to prospective non-prisoner donors.

Medical: "Has the potential living donor been selected, in part, because of the presence of a serious health-related condition in the intended recipient for which there are only less satisfactory alternative remedies?" For example, there may be external pressures if the intended recipient is doing poorly with dialysis, or even if just unhappy with the burdensomeness of therapy. External pressures may be exacerbated if the intended recipient is sensitized to other family members who were tested for compatibility for living donation. It is critical that the LDAT supplemented with a PL ensure that the prisoner understands that there may be other options for the candidate recipient. There are different modes of dialysis (eg, peritoneal as well as hemodialysis). In addition, there is the possibility of desensitization protocols that would make it feasible for another family member to donate either directly or in a donor exchange program. And yet, even if the other alternatives are less effective, the prisoner must understand that he or she may still choose not to donate without repercussions from the penal system and without disclosure of the reason to the candidate recipient and family.

Situational: "Is the potential living donor in a situation in which medical exigency prevents the education and deliberation needed to decide whether to participate as a living donor?" Consider, for example, a patient who presents in acute liver failure (ALF) and the physicians fear that a deceased donor will not become available in time. They ask about potential living donor volunteers. This scenario creates both a medical and a situational vulnerability for any potential living donor, whether a prisoner or a civilian. The medical vulnerability is that there is a very high likelihood that a deceased donor organ will not become available in time. To avoid the risk of recipient death, the physicians may encourage parallel work-ups of willing family members. ALF creates a situational vulnerability for all potential living donors because they have to undergo a complete medical and psychosocial work-up in a very short period of time without much time for reflection about the risks and benefits.

We believe a compressed work-up is inadequate for evaluating a prisoner given the numerous additional vulnerabilities incarceration can bring about. It is also strategically problematic because of the complexities of getting the requisite resources (eg, getting permission from appropriate prison authorities, hiring of guards, arranging transport) to undergo the work-up in such a limited time frame. When time is so limited (situational vulnerability), it is difficult to ensure that even a nonincarcerated competent adult has adequate time to make an informed decision, and transplant teams should restrict donation to those who are not at increased vulnerability.

Allocational: "Is the potential living donor lacking in subjectively important social goods that will be provided as a consequence of participation as a donor?" Incarceration threatens many social goods because prisoners lose most opportunities to control their own environment and must follow externally imposed constraints on activities and relationships. Prisoners may want to donate for personal, emotional, or spiritual redemption, or because they believe it will improve their self-esteem and self-respect or improve their relationships with the recipient and the wider family. While there are data that show these benefits accrue to some donors,[54] there are no guarantees that any particular donor will gain these benefits. These intangible benefits may be harder to secure for a prisoner given that, after donation, the prisoner will return to the isolation and hierarchy of the prison environment where redemption may seem illusory. It is critical that the LDAT and PL both help the prisoner understand what can and cannot be promised or guaranteed as a result of donation.

Infrastructural: "Does the political, organizational, economic, and social context of the setting possess the integrity and resources needed to manage living donation?" This vulnerability includes both whether potential living donors who are incarcerated have adequate access to the resources necessary to get optimal medical and psychological evaluation at the transplant hospital and whether potential prisoner donors can get adequate evaluation and counseling by an LDAT that includes a PL. As important is whether there will be adequate access to resources necessary in the setting of incarceration for recovery from the donor procedure (access to adequate pain medication, skilled specialty nurses and physicians, and recovery-appropriate physical activities) and assured access for long-term transplant donor-specific follow-up care. Given the limitations of health care access in most prisons,[55] the answer may well be no.

While all prisoners have access to (some) health care while in prison, given the increasing awareness of the long-term health implications of living donation, especially kidney donation,[56] adequate health care is needed after release. Given that health insurance is often employment-based in the US, these donors are at high risk for lack of health care access after release. The poor health literacy of the prison population is a further barrier to appropriate long-term follow up and compliance with healthy behaviors necessary for persons with a single kidney.[57] One should hesitate to promote greater numbers of prisoners serving as living donors unless these infrastructural vulnerabilities can be addressed.

6.6 How Do Incentives Impact the Vulnerability Analysis?

One difference between research participation and living donation is the permissibility of tangible incentives. In the research world, some incentives are permitted, provided they do not exert "undue influence" such that the potential participant feels as if he or she cannot refuse the offer.[58] There are even greater restrictions on what can be offered to prisoners because of the actual circumstances in which they live (infrastructural vulnerability). In contrast, incentives are prohibited in organ donation for both prisoners and the general population. Freedom is the overarching allocational good that prisoners lack, and the possibility of a reduction in sentence time is an offer that can be categorized as exerting "undue influence": it is so tempting that donors may be unable or unwilling to truly consider the actual donation risks. As such, the offer interferes with the prisoner's ability to give a truly informed consent. This incentive may also exacerbate the juridic vulnerability of the prisoner who may be unable to critically evaluate or refuse an offer made by those in positions of power. As such, it is appropriately prohibited by the US Department of Justice (DOJ).[59]

6.7 Restricting Prisoners to Donations to First-Degree Relatives

Transplant programs may be reluctant to accept prisoners as living donors, even if the prisoner is a first-degree family member. Prisoners are at increased risk of being infected with HIV and/or hepatitis and transmitting infection(s) unintentionally with the donor organ.[60] The increased risk status must be disclosed to potential recipients even if the potential prisoner donor screens negative for these infections.[61] There is a period of time during which the newly infected may not test positive. An individual may also become infected between the time of testing and the time of donation.[62] Improvements in viral testing have reduced but not eliminated this window of risk. While donors are told to refrain from high-risk activities in the time between evaluation and donation, compliance cannot be assured in any case, but especially with prisoners because they are at greater risk of engaging in high-risk activities involuntarily.

The PL can help strategize with the prisoner regarding risk reduction. While the LDAT may be best situated to discuss the risks of infection transmission by organ transplantation and its frequency, the PL is best situated to evaluate and discuss these risks in the context of incarceration in general and in the context of the individual prisoner's life within the prison. One proposed solution is to put prisoners in "medical isolation" between evaluation and donation, which may unfortunately translate into solitary confinement.[63] Solitary confinement may cause serious psychological harm and may not be in a prisoner's best interests. The PL must evaluate the potential ill effects that solitary confinement might cause the prisoner and such a strategy should not be imposed without the potential donor's understanding and informed consent.[64] Even if the potential donor agrees to voluntary medical isolation, the PL must ensure that the prisoner understands that he or she has the right to withdraw from voluntary solitary confinement if the burdens become too great. The PL must also ensure that the prison staff understands the voluntary nature of this specific confinement.

Even if a potential prisoner donor can successfully overcome the vulnerability threats enumerated, the practicalities may be too overwhelming for the prison system to permit the donation. There is also the issue of who will pay for the additional resources needed, such as guards for inpatient care pre- and postsurgery, for transporting the prisoner to and from the transplant clinic, and for overseeing prisoners during appointments both before and after the donor surgery admission. The DOJ program statement on patient care explicitly states that it does not cover these expenses:

> Hospitalizations or fees involved will not be at the Government's expense including all costs associated with guarding the inmate at off-site facilities. This includes the US Marshals Service.[65]

If the costs are not covered by the recipient's insurance, they may have to be paid for privately or the donation process cannot go forward.

To be eligible to donate to a loved one, the prisoner should be ABO-compatible, or the candidate will need to undergo a desensitization protocol. While civilians who are ABO-incompatible can also elect to participate in a living donor paired exchange, this might not be possible with a prisoner donor because the DOJ currently only permits donation to first-degree relatives. Logistical issues justify excluding them from being considered for paired exchanges and domino chains. First, it would seem unlikely that a donor-recipient pair would agree to an exchange with a prisoner donor-recipient pair given the increased risk of hepatitis and HIV infections in the prison population. Second, security issues raised by prisoner donation could lead to serious delays and unexpected cancellations due to infrastructural vulnerabilities beyond the prisoner's control that would discourage allocation modelers from including them in chains or exchanges. Third, the costs of these security issues would be the responsibility of the prisoner or his family, which may interfere with the coordination of the multiple surgeries.

Prisoners should be the donors of last resort due to the juridical, deferential, social and infrastructural vulnerabilities that incarceration creates and that threaten the voluntariness of their consent. We believe it is fair to exclude them from paired exchanges and domino chains.

6.8 Conclusion

A vulnerability analysis helps illuminate potential threats to the prisoner's decision-making process. To overcome these threats, the prisoner requires access to an LDAT that includes a PL as well as access to appropriate education and resources. It will be critical that the prisoner understand the risks, benefits, and alternatives to living kidney donation for him- or herself and for the potential recipient. An LDAT which includes a PL can attempt to provide the resources to overcome the vulnerabilities that may interfere with the prisoner's comprehension. These resources can help the prisoner examine his or her own motivation and willingness, as well as the added psychological and physical burdens that incarceration may create for the potential donor. If either the PL or any other member of the LDAT believes the donor is not acting freely and knowledgeably, the donation should be prohibited.

In sum, we agree with Goldberg and Frader that prisoners should not be uniformly prohibited from serving as living donors out of respect for their humanity (personhood).[66] However, modifying current federal regulations to permit sentence reduction or other tangible benefits related to incarceration status would exert "undue influence" and is ethically impermissible. Incarceration imposes specific additional psychological and logistical vulnerabilities that may make organ donation an inappropriate course of action for many incarcerated individuals and justifies restricting their donation to first-degree relatives.

Notes

1. Starzl TE, Marchioro TL, Brittain RS, Holmes JH, Waddell WR. Problems in renal homotransplantation. *JAMA.* 1964;187:734–740.
2. Starzl et al, "Problems."

3. Marchioro TL, Brittain RS, Hermann G, Jolmes J, Waddell WR, Starzl TE. Use of living donors for renal homotransplantation. *Arch Surg*. 1964;88:711–720.
4. Wolstenholme GEW, O'Connor M, eds. *Ethics in Medical Progress: With Special Reference to Transplantation*. Boston, MA: Little, Brown and Company; 1966, at pp. vii–viii.
5. Wolstenhome and O'Connor, *Ethics in Medical Progress*, at p. 75.
6. Wolstenhome and O'Connor, *Ethics in Medical Progress*, at pp. 76–77.
7. See, for example, Krotoski WA. Hepatitis in prisoner blood donors. *N Engl J Med*. 1972;286:149; and Hammett TM, Harmon MP, Rhodes W. The burden of infectious disease among inmates of releases from US correctional facilities. *Am J Public Health*. 2002;92:1789–1794.
8. Indiana University Center for Bioethics. Organ Donation by Death Row Inmates. https://medicine.iu.edu/research-centers/bioethics/reference-center/death-row-organ-donation; and Miller J. A life for an afterlife: assessing the potential redemption of capital inmates' requests to posthumously donate organs under the Religious Land Use and Institutionalized Persons Act. *Rutgers J L and Religion*. 2011;13(part 1):87–137.
9. Williams T. Jailed sisters are released for kidney transplant. *The New York Times*. January 7, 2011. August 18, 2021.https://www.nytimes.com/2011/01/08/us/08sisters.html
10. See US Department of Justice (DOJ), Federal Bureau of Prisons. Program Statement: Patient Care. Section 38: Organ Donation by Inmates: 45. June 3, 2014. August 18, 2021 for both the US and the British. http://www.bop.gov/policy/progstat/6031_004.pdf. Of note, in April 2015, the British Transplantation Society published guidelines that allow prisoners to serve as a living kidney or living liver donor to either a family member or a stranger after an intensive case review, although it does acknowledge that practical and logistical issues may be too overwhelming. See Working Party of the British Transplant Society. *UK Guidelines for Living Organ Donation from Prisoners*. Draft posted on December 2015. https://bts.org.uk/wp-content/uploads/2016/09/04_BTS_Donation_Prisoners-1.pdf
11. Jones J. *Bad Blood: The Tuskegee Syphilis Experiment*. New York, NY: Free Press; 1981.
12. National Research Act, Pub L No. 93–348 (1974).
13. The National Commission for the Protection of Human Subjects of Biomedical and Behavioral Research. *The Belmont Report: Ethical Principles and Guidelines for the Protection of Human Subjects of Research*. Washington, DC: Government Printing Office; 1978. http://www.hhs.gov/ohrp/humansubjects/guidance/belmont.html
14. Department of Health and Human Services. Code of Federal Regulations (CFR) Title 45 Public Welfare Part 46. Final Regulations Amending Basic HHS Policy for the Protection of Human Research Subjects. *Fed Regist*. 1981;46:8366–8391. Most recently revised *Fed Regist*. 2017;82:7259–7273. Last accessed August 18, 2021. https://www.ecfr.gov/cgi-bin/retrieveECFR?gp=&SID=83cd09e1c0f5c6937cd9d7513160fc3f&pitd=20180719&n=pt45.1.46&r=PART&ty=HTML. Hereinafter referred to as 45 CFR 46.
15. National Commission for the Protection of Biomedical and Behavioral Research. *Report and Recommendations: Research Involving Prisoners*. DHEW Publication

No. (OS) 76–131. Washington, DC: National Commission for the Protection of Biomedical and Behavioral Research; 1976, at p. 1.

16. See, for example, Kondo KK, Johnson ME, Ironside EF, Brems C, Eldridge GD. HIV/AIDS research in correctional settings: perspectives on training needs from researchers and IRB members. *AIDS Educ Prev.* 2014;26:565–576; and Hatfield F. Prison research: the view from inside. *Hastings Cent Rep.* 1977;7(1):11–12.

17. National Commission, *Research Involving Prisoners*, at pp. 7–8.

18. 45 CFR 46 at §46.305 (a) (2) and (a) (6).

19. 45 CFR 46 at §46.304 (b).

20. Sadler HH, Davison L, Carroll C, Kountz SL. The living, genetically unrelated, kidney donor. *Semin Psych.* 1971;3:86–101; and Simmons RG, Klein SD, Simmons RL. *Gift of Life: The Social and Psychological Impact of Organ Transplantation.* New York, NY: John Wiley and Sons; 1977.

21. Spital A. Unconventional living kidney donors—attitudes and use among transplant centers. *Transplantation.* 1989;48:243–248; Spital A. Unrelated living kidney donors: an update of attitudes and use among US transplant centers. *Transplantation.* 1994;57:1722–1726; and Spital A. Evolution of attitudes at US transplant centers toward kidney donation by friends and altruistic strangers. *Transplantation.* 2000;69:1728–1731.

22. For US policy prohibiting prisoners from donating to strangers, see Federal Bureau of Prisons, "Program Statement." For examples of prisoners serving as living donors to family members, see Indiana University Center for Bioethics, "Organ Donation" and Miller, "A life."

23. Hinkle W. Giving until it hurts: prisoners are not the answer to the national organ shortage. *Indiana Law Rev.* 2002;35(2):593–619, at p. 609.

24. Visconti JL. Exchanging a kidney for freedom: the illegality of conditioning prison releases on organ donations. *New Engl J Crim and Civil Confinement.* 2012;38(1):199–217, at p. 211.

25. National Organ Transplantation Act (NOTA), Pub L No. 98–507. Approved October 19, 1984, at 42 USC § 274e.

26. Lee EC. Trading kidneys for prison time: when two contradictory legal traditions intersect, which one has the right of way. *Univ San Francisco Law Rev.* 2009;43(3):507–556, at p. 549.

27. Jefferson-Jones J. The exchange of inmate organs for liberty: diminishing the "yuck factor" in the bioethics repugnance debate. *J Gender Race Justice.* 2013;16(105):105–137, at p. 115 (footnotes omitted).

28. Jefferson-Jones, "The exchange," at p. 115.

29. Second Chances Lead to Hope for Scott Sisters. Michles and Booth Accident and Injury Lawyers Website. Published January 17, 2014, Accessed August 18, 2019. https://www.michlesbooth.com/blog/2014/january/second-chances-lead-to-hope-for-scott-sisters/

30. Gater H. Scott sisters, who got life for armed robbery, continue to ask Gov. Bryant for release. *Mississippi Clarion Ledger.* July 29, 2019. Last accessed August 18, 2021. https://www.statesmanjournal.com/story/news/2019/07/29/

scott- sisters- continue- ask- gov- bryant- pardon- commutation- armed-robbery-haley-barbour-kidney-donation/1856618001/

31. See, for example, *Lee v Quarterman*, No. C-07-476, 2008 WL 3926118 at *2 (SD Tex 2008); and *Campbell v Wainwright*, 416 F2d 949, 950 (5th Cir 1969).

32. Goldberg AM, Frader J. Prisoners as living organ donors: the case of the Scott sisters. *Am J Bioeth*. 2011;11(10):15–16.

33. Wolstenhome and O'Connor, *Ethics in Medical Progress*, at pp. 14–15 and 66.

34. Department of Health and Human Services Advisory Committee on Organ Transplantation Recommendations. Meeting archives: Full Consensus Recommendations, Recommendations 1–18. November 2002. Accessed August 18, 2021. https://www.hrsa.gov/advisory-committees/organ-transplantation/recommendations/1-18

35. See, for example, Rudow DL, Brown RS, Jr. Role of the independent donor advocacy team in ethical decision making. *Prog Transplant*. 2005;15:298–302; and Rudow DL. The living donor advocate: a team approach to educate, evaluate, and manage donors across the continuum. *Prog Transplant*. 2009;19:64–70; and Hays RE, LaPointe Rudow D, Dew MA, Taler SJ, Spicer H, Mandelbrot DA. The independent living donor advocate: a guidance document from the American Society of Transplantation's Living Donor Community of Practice. *Am J Transplant*. 2015;15:518–525.

36. Millis MA, Simmerling M. Prisoners as organ donors: is it worth the effort? Is it ethical? *Transplant Proc*. 2009;41:23–24.

37. Appelbaum PS, Grisso T. Assessing patients' capacities to consent to treatment. *N Engl J Med*. 1988;319:1635–1638.

38. Appelbaum and Grisso, "Assessing."

39. Harlow CW. Bureau of Justice Statistics Special Report: Education and Correctional Populations. Revised April 15, 2003. Last accessed August 18, 2021. http://www.bjs.gov/content/pub/pdf/ecp.pdf

40. Cunningham MD, Vigen MP. Death row inmate characteristics, adjustment, and confinement: a critical review of the literature. *Behav Sci Law*. 2002;20(1–2):191–210, at pp. 191–192.

41. Dew MA, Jacobs CL, Jowsey SG, et al. Guidelines for the psychosocial evaluation of living unrelated kidney donors in the United States. *Am J Transplant*. 2007;7:1047–1054.

42. Fazel S, Danesh J. Serious mental disorder in 23,000 prisoners: a systematic review of 62 surveys. *Lancet*. 2002;359:545–550.

43. Prins SJ. Prevalence of mental illnesses in US state prisons: a systematic review. *Psychiatr Serv*. 2014;65:862–872.

44. Fazel S, Bairns P, Doll H. Substance abuse and dependence in prisoners: a systematic review. *Addiction*. 2006;101:181–191.

45. Kipnis K. Vulnerability in Research Subjects: A Bioethical Taxonomy. In: The National Bioethics Advisory Commission. *Ethical and Policy Issues in Research Involving Human Participants. Volume II: Commissioned Papers and Staff Analysis*. Bethesda, MD: National Bioethics Advisory Commission; 2001:G1–13, at p. G8.

46. Patton L-HM. Note: a call for common sense: organ donation and the executed prisoner. *Virginia J Soc Policy Law.* 1996;3:387–434, at p. 418.

47. Kipnis, "Vulnerability," at pp. G-7 and G-8.

48. See, for example, La Vigne NH, Naser RL, Brooks LE, Castro JL. Examining the effect of incarceration and in-prison family contact on prisoners' family relationships. *J Contemp Crim Justice.* 2005;21(4):314–335; Hairston CF. Family ties during imprisonment: important to whom and for what? *J Sociol and Social Welfare.* 2015;18(1):87–104; and Minnesota Department of Corrections. The effects of prison visitation on offender recidivism. November 2011. Last accessed August 18, 2021. https://mn.gov/doc/assets/11-11MNPrisonVisitationStudy_tcm1089-272781.pdf

49. Travis J, McBride EC, Solomon AL. Families left behind: the hidden costs of incarceration and reentry. October 2003; revised June 2005. Accessed August 18, 2021. http://www.urban.org/sites/default/files/alfresco/ publication-pdfs/310882-Families-Left-Behind.PDF

50. British Transplant Society, *UK Guidelines*.

51. Federal Bureau of Prisons, "Program Statement."

52. Kipnis K. Social justice and correctional health services. In: Kleing J, ed. *Prisoners' Rights*. Burlington VT: Ashgate Publishing Co; 2014:203–214.

53. Do inmates have rights? If so, what are they? HG.org Legal Resources. Last accessed August 18, 2021. https://www.hg.org/legal-articles/do-inmates-have-rights-if-so- what-are-they-31517#:~:text=Inmates%20generally%20lose%20 their%20right,include%20 any%20form%20of%20contraband

54. Tong A, Chapman JR, Wong G, Kanellis J, McCarthy G, Craig JC. The motivations and experiences of living kidney donors: a thematic synthesis. *Am J Kidney Dis.* 2012;60:15–26; and Clemens KK, Thiessen-Philbrook H, Parikh CR, et al. for the Donor Nephrectomy Outcomes Research (DONOR). Psychosocial health of living kidney donors: a systematic review. *Am J Transplant.* 2006;6:2965–2977.

55. See, for example, Wilper AP, Woolhandler S, Boyd JW, et al. The health and health care of US prisoners: results of a nationwide survey. *Am J Public Health.* 2009;99:666–672; and Benbow S, Hall J, Heard K, Donelle L. Conducting research with criminalized women in an incarcerated setting: the researcher's perspective. *Canad J Nurs Res.* 2013;45:80–91.

56. Mjøen G, Hallan S, Hartmann A, et al. Long-term risks for kidney donors. *Kidney Int.* 2014;86:162–167; and Muzaale AD, Massie AB, Wang MC, et al. Risk of end-stage renal disease following live kidney donation. *JAMA.* 2014;311:579–586.

57. Hadden KB, Puglisi L, Prince L, et al. Health literacy among a formerly incarcerated population using data from the transitions clinic network. *Urban Health.* 2018;95(4):547–555.

58. See, for example, Grady C. Money for research participation: does in jeopardize informed consent? *Am J Bioeth.* 2001;1(2):40–44; and Grant RW, Sugarman J. Ethics in human subjects research: do incentives matter? *J Med Phil.* 2004;29:717–738.

59. Federal Bureau of Prisons, "Program Statement."

60. Seem DL, Lee I, Umscheid CA, and Kuehnert MJ. PHS Guideline for Reducing Human Immunodeficiency Virus, Hepatitis B Virus, and Hepatitis C Virus Transmission Through Organ Transplantation. *Public Health Rep.* 2013;128(4):247–343.

61. Organ Procurement and Transplantation Network (OPTN) policies. Table 15–1: Requirements for Donors with Risk Identified Pre-Transplant. Last updated effective Date: 6/17/2021; last accessed 8/18/2021. https://optn.transplant.hrsa.gov/media/1200/optn_policies.pdf

62. Seem et al, "PHS Guidelines."

63. See, for example, Millis and Simmerling, "Prisoners"; and Satel S. A kidney for a kidney. *Slate*. April 15, 2013. Last accessed August 18, 2021. http://www.slate.com/articles/health_and_science/medical_ examiner/2013/04/let_prisoners_donate_organs_it_ could_be_fair_ethical_and_just.html

64. Kaba F, Lewis A, Glowa-Kollisch S, et al. Solitary confinement and risk of self-harm among jail inmates. *Am J Public Health*. 2014;104:442–447; and Anonymous. The Istanbul Statement on the Use and Effects of Solitary Confinement. Adopted December 9, 2007. Last accessed August 18, 2021. https://irct.org/assets/uploads/Opinion.pdf

65. Federal Bureau of Prisons, "Program Statement."

66. Goldberg and Frader, "Prisoners."

PART 3
EXPANDING LIVING DONOR TRANSPLANTATION

7

The Good Samaritan or
Non-Directed Donor

Case 7-1: This is a case from our institution that we
previously discussed in the medical literature. We reprint
the case itself verbatim.

. . . [A] 40-year-old man with no significant medical history approached our
institution about the possibility of serving as a kidney donor. In the medical work-up, the individual was found to have a family history of hypertension, to be moderately obese (40% over ideal body weight), and to have
high normal- to stage-2 systolic hypertension (with blood pressure readings
ranging from a low of 138/78 to a high of 163/89). A 24-hour ambulatory
blood-pressure study revealed a mean blood pressure within the normal
range of 128/82 but with 18% of daytime readings greater than 140/90.[1]

Although the nephrologist noted that the potential donor's profile was
not perfect, the profile would have been deemed "acceptable" if the man
were the usual emotionally related donor at our institution and would be
considered to fall within published clinical practice guidelines. In a clinical patient review conference, the nephrologist and transplant surgeons
agreed that, if this donor were the recipient's brother, they would inform
the donor of the intermittent blood pressure elevations, counsel him on
diet and exercise, and stress the need for medical follow-up. They would
explain to him that he had a significant possibility of developing hypertension that needed medical treatment in the next 2 decades; and, furthermore, that if hypertension did develop, it could potentially have a
deleterious effect on his own renal function. However, they agreed that
they would not discourage him from donating and would proceed with
the transplant if he remained willing. However, given these same medical
facts, all members of the transplant team were uncomfortable in assisting
this individual to donate a kidney to a person to whom he had no previously established emotional relationship.

The Living Organ Donor as Patient. Lainie Friedman Ross and J. Richard Thistlethwaite, Jr, Oxford University Press.
© Oxford University Press 2022. DOI: 10.1093/oso/9780197618202.003.0007

Case Report 7-2: This is a case described by Reginald Gohh and colleagues from Brown and Harvard Universities that we reprint verbatim.

A 50-year-old white woman (the volunteer) contacted our transplant center offering to donate one of her kidneys to any eligible person on our cadaver transplant list. When asked about her motivation, she stated that she was an ordained Buddhist monk and as part of her faith, placed a high value on helping mankind to the best of her ability. . . . Notably, she had made a similar request to a transplant center closer to her home, but had been turned down. . . .

[The volunteer] was interviewed by the transplant co-ordinator, social worker, transplant nephrologist, and transplant surgeon. She was found to be sincere in her request and her judgement and insight were considered to be sound. She had discussed her intention with her husband who was supportive of her decision. . . . She had no history of psychiatric illness nor did she have current psychological problems.

The patient placed only two conditions prior to donating. She requested that the donation be entirely anonymous in nature without public media consideration and the recipient be a person who is not associated with a killing vocation of any type (eg, hunter, fisherman, military person). Although she preferred that the recipient be of an ethnic or racial minority [she had done research and understood that they were more disadvantaged], this was not a major consideration in her mind.[2]

7.1 History

From the outset of kidney transplantation, some living donors were "Good Samaritan" donors—that is, individuals who donated a kidney without a specific recipient in mind. By definition, then, they did not have a genetic or an emotional relationship with the prospective candidates. Historically, Good Samaritan donors were individuals who either were solicited or responded to media requests or requests directly from transplant programs. For example, Thomas Starzl recruited prisoners in the 1960s,[3] and in 1971, H. Harrison Sadler and colleagues reported on 9 living kidney donors who had no relationship to the recipient but rather had responded to media requests.[4] However, non-genetically related donors fell out of favor quickly because the results were no better than deceased donor grafts.[5]

About 3 decades later, on September 7, 1999, Joyce Roush (now Joyce Roush Mason) made headlines as the first person in recent history to donate a kidney to a stranger.[6] At about the same time, the University of Minnesota announced "that a 50-year-old woman had also given a kidney to a stranger but that both she and the recipient had requested anonymity."[7] The concept of the "nondirected donor" (also known as a "Good Samaritan donor" or a "Stranger donor" or an "Altruistic donor"[8]) gained in both popularity and acceptability in the transplant community with the 2000 publication of "Nondirected Donation of Kidneys from Living Donors" by Arthur Matas and colleagues at the University of Minnesota in the *New England Journal of Medicine*.[9]

As we saw in chapter 2, Aaron Spital had empirical data to show that transplant centers were not keen on non-genetically related donors in the 1980s.[10] The public expressed greater and earlier support than transplant professionals, with support greatest for spouses, then friends, then acquaintances, and lastly strangers.[11] These attitudes were buoyed by a report in 1995 by Paul Terasaki and colleagues that kidney transplants between spouses were as effective as kidney transplants between HLA-mismatched genetic relatives.[12] In this chapter, we will examine controversies raised by Good Samaritan donors, focusing on whether it is ethical using the living donor ethics framework we developed in chapter 3. We will also examine the ethics of the donor and recipient selection processes.

7.2 Is It Ethical?

Let us examine how the living donor ethics framework can evaluate the living donor who is neither genetically nor emotionally related to the recipient, but is rather a stranger.

7.2.1 The Principle of Respect for Persons

The principle of respect for persons focuses on the living donor acting autonomously and giving an informed consent, free of undue pressure. To some extent, one could argue that a Good Samaritan donor like the one in case 7-1 is less vulnerable than a related donor because there can be no external pressure from a recipient or recipient family who do not know the potential donor. In fact, recipients are often not aware that they may have been matched with a potential Good Samaritan donor until late in the process. This is not to say that Good Samaritan donors do not feel self-induced internal pressure once they have started the work-up or that they may feel some degree of external pressure if they have heard about a particular individual with ESRD through the media.[13] It is also the case that if the Good Samaritan donor contacts a potential recipient or his or her family in response to a media appeal, for example, then the candidate and his or her family may put some pressure on the donor. In this chapter we focus on the (at least initially) anonymous Good Samaritan donor.

Consider the potential donor in case 7-1 from the University of Chicago transplant center. He had a thorough psychological evaluation to ensure that his motivations were appropriate in that he had no expectation of financial reward or the establishment of a social relationship with the recipient or recipient's family. The evaluation by the living donor advocate team (LDAT) also ensured that he did not have unrealistic expectations about what his or her donation would do (including an understanding that the kidney transplant could fail and/or that the recipient could choose not to have any relationship with him). Psychological pathology was ruled out and his consent was deemed voluntarily and informed, but the LDAT requested an ethics consult because of their discomfort with the degree of risk that the donation would cause this "not-so-healthy" donor. We will discuss this below.

Case 7-2 also expresses the autonomous wishes of a potential donor who in this case is a Buddhist monk and has a lifelong history of good deeds. In her case she was medically healthy, but she had requested 2 stipulations to her donation based on her religious values: (1) that the recipient not be associated with "killing occupations"; and (2) her preference for a minority given her understanding that they had longer wait times and were therefore "worst off" and in most need of her gift. The ethics of these stipulations will be discussed in the section on recipient selection in §7.2.3.

7.2.2 Beneficence

In the context of living donation, beneficence looks at the benefit and potential harms to the potential donor and the potential recipients as individuals and jointly. Consider, first, the benefits. The benefit to the living donor is psychological. The recipient benefits from both a longer life expectancy and lower expected morbidity. Some have argued that Good Samaritan donors, particularly those who donate non-directedly (ie, they do not know their recipients and never do learn the recipient's identity) gain less potential psychological benefit because they do not get the benefit of knowing their recipients and sharing in their improved quality of life.[14] Others disagree, stating that the benefits may be different, but one cannot presume the quantity or quality of the benefit is greater or less.[15] The empirical data from both the United States and around the world find that both directed and non-directed living donors describe positive psychological outcomes, improved self-esteem, and do not regret donation.[16]

Donor benefits must be weighed against the risks of living donation, which are nontrivial: there are both short-term perioperative risks as well as long-term risks that were not appreciated until the last decade when a number of retrospective studies found increased risk of kidney disease, pregnancy complications, and cardiovascular disease.[17] But these risks exist whether or not the living donor is emotionally related to the recipient.

The benefits to the recipients are the potential for longer life expectancy and better quality of life from a living donor transplant compared with a deceased donor transplant or remaining on dialysis.[18] The major risks to the recipients are the early risks of transmitted infections and cancers from the donor graft, and the later risks of secondary cancers and infections from the immunosuppression. All donors go through an extensive work-up but there are no guarantees. This is the case, however, for both genetically and non-genetically living related kidney transplants. Given the risks of the alternative therapies (deceased donor transplantation has similar risks with overall lower graft longevity, and dialysis has both greater morbidity and mortality), the benefits of living donor transplant for recipients usually outweigh the risks.[19]

7.2.3 Justice and the Fair Selection of Donors

The principle of justice focuses on the fair selection of donors. Case 7-1 raises the question of whether it is fair to hold non-directed donors to different standards than directed donors. As noted above, the transplant team conceded that if the donor were donating to his sibling, they would explain to him his risks and benefits, but ultimately they would respect his informed decision. However, they were uncomfortable in assisting him to donate to a stranger.

In their original article, Arthur Matas and colleagues did not propose different medical criteria for emotionally related versus Good Samaritan donors.[20] The use of the same medical criteria for kidney donations from Good Samaritan and emotionally related donors has been affirmed by numerous transplant guidelines.[21] However, Matas and colleagues did require different psychosocial evaluations. While emotionally related donors were routinely evaluated for both clinical and psychosocial issues in their own local communities, Matas and colleagues required Good Samaritan donors to have the psychosocial evaluation performed at the University of Minnesota "to ensure a detailed discussion of the operative risks as well as the reasons for the offer" and to include "a detailed psychosocial evaluation."[22]

Guidelines have been developed to address the psychosocial evaluation for Good Samaritan donors.[23] Similar to the psychosocial evaluation for emotionally related donors, these guidelines recommended that the psychosocial evaluation of the Good Samaritan donor be conducted by an independent living donor advocate (LDA) or LDAT and it should be followed by a "cooling off period" to give the prospective donor a chance to renege.[24] When the donor was a Good Samaritan, they also recommended "an additional interview or telephone conversation that included both the prospective donor and his or her significant other."[25]

Leonieke Kranenburg and colleagues in the Netherlands also describe stricter psychological criteria, in part because they are not sure if these donors are truly equivalent to "conventional living kidney donors" or just that they "have insufficient data available yet that describe the differences between the conventional and the Samaritan donation experience."[26] In a systematic review of the psychological evaluation of Good Samaritan kidney donors, Kranenburg and colleagues found 5 articles that met their criteria, and although samples were small, they concluded that "[a]t present, data seem to be accumulating that support the view that Samaritan donation leads to satisfactory outcomes in terms of the psychological health of these donors."[27]

Initially, Matas and colleagues also treated Good Samaritan and emotionally related donors differently because they restricted Good Samaritan donors to living kidney donation whereas emotionally related donors could donate a kidney or liver lobe. Matas et al explained their practice:

> As we gain more experience with transplanting parts of other organs from living donors, it is likely that the risks of donation will decrease. We will

then need to reconsider our policy of restricting nondirected donation to kidney transplantation.[28]

Now that Good Samaritan donors are widely accepted and the results are excellent, some centers are allowing individuals to serve as Good Samaritan living liver donors, although some restrict Good Samaritan living liver donors to left lateral lobe donations (which is a safer procedure than a full lobe hepatectomy, but usually can only provide adequate liver mass for a young pediatric candidate).[29] Moreover, in their follow-up report in 2004, Matas and colleagues noted that they had increased the age of Good Samaritan donors from 18 years to 21 years of age—although emotionally related donors were still allowed to donate at age 18 years.[30] Thus, despite their claim, Matas et al had different clinical and psychosocial criteria for emotionally related donors compared with Good Samaritan donors.

We believe that one can morally justify more stringent clinical and psychosocial criteria for Good Samaritan donors compared to emotionally related donors. Kane and colleagues, coming from a feminist ethics of care tradition, argue similarly:

> The further one moves out of immediate relationships, the more cautious must be the selection of donors. In this "sliding scale" approach, more rigorous screening of stranger donors would be required for their own protection and to ensure that their motivation was not to fulfill some psychological need.[31]

This is not to say that all Good Samaritan donations should be prohibited, nor that emotionally related donors should be allowed to donate regardless of the health or psychosocial risks. The position is that intimates (family) should be allowed to accept slightly more risk.[32] We base our argument on the fact that individuals experience different expectations and obligations when they stand in relationship with others.[33] We have argued elsewhere that family relationships create a prima facie obligation to donate (the duty may be overridden depending on the degree of risk, and to a lesser extent on the probability of successful engraftment).[34] We argue that the moral basis for this obligation is intimacy. Nancy Jecker clearly articulates this position:

> the closer and more personal a relationship is, the stronger the claims it can make ethically on our allegiance. This is not to say that persons can

legitimately exploit those with whom they are most intimate. Rather, it establishes that family members are governed by stronger ethical responsibilities than strangers, and we expect them to serve each other's welfare to a greater extent.[35]

Jeffrey Kahn objects to the notion that family members may have a moral duty, suggesting that this would lead to imposing a duty of heroism—which is self-contradictory since heroism is, by definition, supererogatory.[36] We disagree. Rather, we argue that intrafamilial donations are not purely altruistic (supererogatory), but entail some degree of moral obligation, even if these obligations are defeasible. As we explained in the manuscript in which this case was originally presented:

> To say that family members have a degree of moral obligation to serve as organ donors needs to be clarified. The expectation to do more for a family member is based on the principle that relations of intimacy generate moral obligations within families. Intimacy implies the sharing of common interests and needs. Insofar as donating an organ meets the needs of one who is intimate, there can be a moral obligation for intrafamilial donation, even if it entails some risk to the donor. Similarly, such a moral obligation can also exist outside a familial relationship in which a preexisting emotional bond is clearly established between donor and recipient, and the donor is well situated to help the recipient fulfill a specific need.[37]
>
> The moral obligation in these cases is not absolute but prima facie and, thus, may be contingent on several factors. These factors include, but are not limited to, the degree of intimacy between the donor and the recipient, the presence of other conflicting obligations the donor may have, the risk of donation, and the likelihood of success of the transplant. Any of these factors can diminish, or even override, the duty to donate.

In another manuscript on this topic, we suggested that the difference in expectations is more clearly seen in the case of non-donation.

> It is the case of non-donation that clarifies precisely the moral distinction between altruistic versus intimate donors. Few would blame an anonymous individual who considered and then decided not to donate to a stranger. But family members who decide not to donate to their siblings, parents, or children are viewed with contempt. This is because of the moral obligations

we expect of those who stand in intimate relations with others. An altru-istic donor has no obligation to donate. The decision to donate goes beyond the obligatory and permissible to the supererogatory, and a decision not to donate does not invite or warrant moral criticism because there is no moral basis on which to criticize not performing an act that would have been beyond the call of duty. In contrast, the family member who is a po-tential donor has a prima facie obligation to donate because of the nature of relationships within the family. A decision to donate is morally praise-worthy, though partly obligatory, and that is why a decision not to donate may be morally blameworthy—because the individual fails to discharge a duty. Yet, in both anonymous and familial donations, many of the reasons for not donating would be the same.[38]

The basis for the moral obligation then derives from intimacy. This means that:

nonintimate family members do not have an obligation to donate an organ to others in the same family. Because of the common scenario of divorce and the less common scenario of adoption, siblings and half-siblings reared apart would have no more moral obligation to donate than a stranger would, despite a known biological connection. Donations between any and all of these individuals would be altruistic [supererogatory].[39]

Aaron Spital agrees that intimates should be permitted to accept greater risk than strangers.[40] However, he rejects our argument that this is due to a moral duty. Rather he bases his position on the fact that emotionally related donors "are likely to derive more benefit than strangers from helping each other."[41] Kahn disagrees, arguing that we cannot judge how much benefit either party may derive from donating because both "stand to realize sub-stantial benefits, albeit of different varieties, and it is difficult to understand why one sort of benefit is of greater value than the other, particularly when they are both of such subjective nature."[42] Kahn takes the position that since it is not clear whether emotionally related donors derive greater benefit, we cannot justify holding Good Samaritan donors to stricter standards.

While we agree with Kahn that one cannot assume that emotionally re-lated donors derive greater benefits, we disagree with Kahn because there are other reasons that justify the different standards. One such reason as discussed above is intimacy. Another reason is that living donation requires the participation of the transplant team who are moral agents in their own right. In an earlier manuscript, one of us (LFR) wrote:

> While the risks to emotionally related donors and altruistic donors are the same, they may not be perceived as such by the surgeons or by the community at large. The media might characterize the death of a sibling as a result of being an organ donor as a valiant, but tragic attempt to save the life of a loved one. However, the media might castigate an institution for unethical practices if an individual died while donating to a stranger. Media coverage can influence public opinion regarding donation both positively and negatively and the influence can go beyond the specific issue at hand. Following negative publicity surrounding a non-heart beating donor program in Cleveland, cadaveric donations in northeast Ohio experienced a short-term decrease. Transplant personnel may decide that the threat of bad publicity from the tangible risk of death to living donors justifies restrictions on who can serve as a donor and which organs they may donate.[43]

In case 7-1, the surgeons perceived the risk to the Chicago donor was too great because he had no relationship to the recipient. We have argued that it is morally justifiable to hold Good Samaritan living donors to stricter criteria.

7.2.4 Vulnerabilities

As we explored in chapter 3, all donors are vulnerable. Let us consider whether there are vulnerabilities that are unique to Good Samaritan donors.

In general, one would think that Good Samaritan donors would not be at risk for incapacitational, juridic, deferential, medical, or situational vulnerability as there is no potential candidate or family pushing the individual to donate. The Minnesota experience was that no donor felt pressure to donate.[44] David Serur and colleagues examined whether "solicited" Good Samaritan donors (donors who answered ads or attended donor drives) were coerced, and they found that "community solicitation of NDDs [nondirected donors] . . . [did not] confer a subtle coercion. . . ."[45]

To determine whether Good Samaritan living donors are socially or allocationally vulnerable, it is useful to examine who are the Good Samaritan living donors. Using the UNOS/OPTN website, Komal Kumar et al noted that most Good Samaritan donors are White (93%), over half (50.3%) had a college degree or post-college education, and 85.7% had insurance. This is not a group that is usually considered to be lacking social goods.[46] The only demographic that suggests any social or allocational vulnerability is that the majority of Good Samaritan donors are female (~57%), but this is comparable to the percentage of women who are directed donors (~60%).[47] In sum, the demographics do not suggest serious social or allocational vulnerability.

Finally, Good Samaritan donors often have less infrastructural vulnerability than other donors as they are more likely to have health insurance and a higher educational level that empowers them to have greater access to health care.[48]

The 20-year experience with Good Samaritan donation does show that some of these donors experience some negative outcomes—some of which were not anticipated at the onset. For example, many Good Samaritan donors find that they must explain their decision to family, friends, and even medical personnel who question it.[49] Some will be disappointed if their recipient does not want any contact even after the recommended non-contact period. They may also face some financial burden and some physical and mental health problems.[50] The LDAT should ensure that Good Samaritan donors are aware of these potential events and help the potential donor preemptively address them.

There are exceptional cases where Good Samaritan donors may have serious vulnerabilities. Consider, for example, the case of kidney donations by members of the Jesus Christians, a cult founded by David McKay in 1982 in Australia that practices communal living, voluntary work, and activism. Members were encouraged to disavow their families and friends and sell books by their founder.[51] In 2002, McKay offered to be an altruistic living unrelated kidney donor. According to the Mayo physicians who later wrote up this case, "He did, however, identify (using the Internet) a potential recipient and requested that his kidney be directed to that recipient."[52] The transplant took place at the Mayo clinic in 2003. Mueller and colleagues explain that "Subsequently, our transplant center was contacted by the religious community and informed that 6 of its members desired coming to our institution to donate kidneys to 6 potential recipients (identified using the Internet)."[53] In this case, concern was expressed whether the religious community members were acting voluntarily. The members were beholden to McKay who claimed that "his interpretation of New Testament scripture. . . calls believers to be 'living sacrifices.'"[54] According to some accounts, over half of the group of 30 members have been living kidney donors.[55]

From a vulnerability perspective, one must ask whether the followers were deferentially if not juridically vulnerable given their leader's own donation and his call to his followers. In addition, the Jesus Christians may have felt some degree of social or allocational vulnerability, because to join the community they had to relinquish all their possessions and external relationships. The Mayo transplant group elected not to permit additional members of this cult from donating because of these vulnerabilities and the institution's inability to ensure that these vulnerabilities were being adequately addressed. They published their experience to warn other transplant programs and to protect other cult members, but still some members have found ways to donate.[56]

7.2.5 Special Relationships Create Special Obligations

The LDAT stands in a special relationship with the potential living donor. The LDAT must ensure that the donor give an informed and voluntary consent. The LDAT also has moral agency and must believe that the risks are justified.[57]

In case 7-1, the living donor's transplant team (which included one of us, JRT) acknowledged that the donor was informed and gave voluntary consent, but members of the LDAT were concerned about the amount of risk that the potential donor was willing to take for a stranger. The team elected to explain their reluctance of exposing a Good Samaritan donor to that degree of risk. The potential donor appeared quite disappointed. The team did leave open the possibility of reconsidering his candidacy in 6–12 months if he undertook lifestyle changes (diet and exercise) that resulted in improved blood pressure control. They also acknowledged to the donor that other transplant programs might not be as stringent and that he could look elsewhere.[58]

7.3 Recipient Selection

Initially, there were no systematic algorithms to determine who should receive a Good Samaritan donor kidney. In the early 1960s, Starzl stated that among his first 12 transplants, 1 was in response to a media appeal by a patient's spouse and 1 was a prisoner. Starzl does not explain how he selected the latter's recipient or whether the recipient was aware that the donor was a prisoner.[59] As transplant outcomes improved, allocation policies and practices have become more salient. In the more modern period, Matas and colleagues formally described their selection process:

> We decided that the recipient of a nondirected kidney would be chosen from the pool of patients on the waiting list for a cadaveric transplant and that we would rank the potential recipients according to the same point system used to allocate cadaveric kidneys. This system takes into account the extent of HLA matching between donor and recipient and the length of time the recipient has been on the waiting list.
>
> To maximize the chance of success, we decided to limit the pool of recipients to patients on the waiting list at our institution who were candidates for a first or second transplant and who had no history of non-compliance with a medical regimen.[60]

Thus, within the boundaries of HLA matching and waiting time, the Minnesota recipient algorithm was designed to cherry pick recipients who were expected to maximize the utility of the Good Samaritan kidney grafts. While this selection process makes sense from an efficiency perspective, it is unfair because it may bypass someone worse off and in more urgent need of the transplant. Strategizing to ensure a good outcome for the Good Samaritan implies that the recipient outcome is of greater importance for living donors than for deceased donors (and their families). This not only harms those individuals on the waitlist who are "worst off,"[61] but also risks diminishing public trust in the fairness of the transplant system.[62]

Alternatively, the Good Samaritan can choose her own recipient (for example, by responding directly to a media appeal). While Starzl described such a case in 1966,[63] the 21st century has seen an expansion of media appeals, from billboards to broadcast media to social media,[64] and even websites dedicated to matching donors and recipients.[65] The disadvantages of this approach are threefold: (1) the patient or family making the appeal may not be telling the truth about the candidate's health status; (2) the histocompatibility matching may not be ideal; and (3) the approach favors those with resources who can make a more appealing website/pitch to potential donors. Nevertheless, the Uniform Anatomical Gift Act permits directed donations of both living and deceased donor grafts.[66]

Case 7-2 proposes a third option. In this case, the potential Good Samaritan donor does not necessarily want to pick a candidate, but instead, a class of candidates (or at least a class of non-candidates). Again, other scenarios have been described in the literature. For example, in 1994, a family requested that the decedent's organs be allocated to a White person given the decedent's membership in the Klu Klux Klan.[67] Negative public outcry led Florida to ban directed donation according to group membership.[68] In case 7-2, a Buddhist monk requested that her kidney be allocated to someone who was not "associated with a killing vocation of any type (eg, hunter, fisherman, military person)."[69] Anticipating potential negative reactions, Gohh and colleagues acknowledged that "the donor for reasons related to her own moral beliefs, imparted some restriction on her gift," but they noted that "she did not exclude a group of persons based on sex, creed or colour," which they stated "would have been deemed unacceptable by our institution."[70] Others, however, might find the monk's restrictions discriminatory, particularly the fact that she excluded all military personnel. To avoid tacit endorsement of discriminatory preferences, Matas and colleagues prohibited any selection based on particular characteristics, whether gender, race, religion and age.[71] In contrast, the surgeons at Johns Hopkins University intentionally selected a child to be the recipient of the Good Samaritan kidney donated by Joyce Roush Mason.[72]

Should recipients be allowed to request that their kidney be allocated to a member of a particular social group? Public preferences in the United States are divided. Aaron Spital sought to determine public attitude about directed donations by strangers. Spital performed 2 surveys, each involving more than 1000 participants. In the first survey, he found that respondents were more willing for Good Samaritans to select a specific recipient (47% yes or probably yes) than a specific type of recipient (36% yes or probably yes), although neither achieved support of a majority of the respondents.[73] When asked about specific groups in the second survey (engaging different survey respondents), 74% were willing for strangers to be permitted to request a child candidate, but less than half would allow a Good Samaritan to choose someone of a specific religion (30%), a specific racial group (28%), or a person who advertised in the media (43%).[74] Thus, giving priority to some groups was more socially acceptable than others, although even children, the most socially acceptable group, had a significant number of respondents who objected. Spital's data also showed that transplant programs that refuse to honor such a request may not significantly reduce the number of Good

Samaritan donor organs available: 93% of individuals who wanted to select a candidate would donate (or probably donate) even if they could not choose a specific group to which their kidney would be allocated.[75]

During the early years of this debate, one of us (LFR) argued in favor of allowing Good Samaritans to choose a class of recipients:

> The decision to serve as a nondirected living donor is a charitable act. And while we have an imperfect duty to act charitably, no particular charity can demand that they have a right to our donation. Although recipients of charities prefer unrestricted gifts, they also accept restricted gifts. As such, I can donate to the general endowment of my alma mater or I can donate directly to the university's softball team. Why then, should I not be able to choose who will be the recipient of the gift of my kidney?
>
> This is not to say that a transplant surgeon should not be disturbed if an individual insisted on donating to a white person because he thought others were inferior. In fact, the transplant surgeon could refuse to do the surgery. Institutions have been known to refuse restricted gifts when the terms have been unacceptable. But, what if an individual insisted on donating to a black person because she knew that blacks had a much longer waiting time? The donor herself may be white or black, and her decision may reflect a desire to respond to this particular community's need.
>
> Kahn's position to refuse all directed donations is the safe one. The question of whether it is morally permissible for an individual to choose to donate only to a particular type of stranger raises many moral questions: How do we judge what are good and not so good reasons to direct a gift toward one group or away from another? Would this be permissible for all organ donations, or just for living donations? It also raises an important policy question about what impact such a policy would have on organ donation rates generally.
>
> Donating a kidney to a stranger is altruistic. Selecting the type of recipient may raise some eyebrows. There are moral arguments to support a policy that permits, and other arguments to support a policy that prohibits, selecting a class of recipients. Since those on the waiting list are most harmed by a policy that excludes donors who seek to donate restrictively, the appropriate policy may not be for the transplant community to draft a policy unilaterally, but rather, to engage those on the waiting list in a discussion about what policy they would believe is fair.[76]

We believe that transplant centers must be transparent about what group traits are permissible. Children are an easy example.

The potential donor in case 7-2, however, wanted to donate an individual in the "nonkilling professions." She also had a preference for an ethnic minority as she understood they were "worse off" in terms of waiting time for a kidney transplant. The transplant program had 3 options: (1) refuse her gift unless she agrees to donate without stipulations; (2) accede to her request; or (3) recommend that she locate a specific candidate.

The first option can be seen as taking the high road but at high cost given that her classifications did not violate any civil rights and comes from true religious tenets. However, it is clearly within a transplant program's prerogative to state that, as moral agents, they will refuse all stipulations. The third option puts the onus of finding a candidate of a particular trait (eg, a minor child) on the prospective Good Samaritan. This protects the transplant program from being accused of bias. Locating a candidate should not be difficult in today's world of ubiquitous access to social media and the internet (although it would have been more difficult when the actual case was described in 2001). But even in 2001, the potential Good Samaritan donor could have solicited a candidate through more traditional media including posting an ad in a Church bulletin, an alumni magazine, or looking for such ads in a variety of sites that match her own values.[77]

Requiring the Good Samaritan donor to find her own recipient when the donor wants a recipient who meets specific criteria has the disadvantage in that it tends to favor those recipient-candidates who are media savvy or more capable of writing a compelling story,[78] and not necessarily those in greatest need (eg, lacking dialysis access) or those who have waited the longest. It also has the disadvantage of forcing the donor to create a preference for a particular candidate when another candidate of the same social group may be in greater need or be a better match (with a better likelihood of success). Thus, requiring the Good Samaritan to find an amenable candidate may fail to maximize utility and may fail to achieve fairness. For example, if a Good Samaritan of blood type O randomly selects a child-recipient of blood type A, this disadvantages those candidates of blood type O who can only get an organ of blood type O and often have some of the longest waiting times because of ABO-incompatibility. As David Steinberg concludes: "A fair balance of equity and utility cannot be achieved when altruistic strangers allocate their donated organs in response to patients' publicly issues emotional pleas."[79] But such is the case for conventional living donors as well who allocate their donated organs in response to a plea from a family member or acquaintance. While it does not treat all candidates as equal, it is morally permissible given that the Good Samaritan kidney is a private good and is not held to the same allocation criteria.

The second option, then, to accede to her wishes and thereby allocate the kidney to the next candidate on the waitlist who meets the donor's requirements, would be more efficient than option 3, and it is within the bounds of fairness that can be set for living donors who donate a private good as long as the traits are not offensive (eg, a demand that a kidney only be allocated to a White candidate) to the public at large.

7.4 Implementing a Good Samaritan Kidney Donor Program

In the first 6 years of their Good Samaritan kidney program, the Minnesota program has only performed 22 Good Samaritan donations despite 360 requests for information.[80] During the initial 30 months of their program operations, Martin Jendrisak and colleagues at Washington University in St Louis received 731 donor inquiries, of which 131 individuals called back after review of mailed information materials. Forty-seven candidates initiated and 19 completed the evaluation process. Seven underwent donation, including 6 kidneys and 1 liver segment, and 5 were actively pending donation at the time the article was published.[81] In other words, identifying Good Samaritan donors is a time-consuming and inefficient process and will not produce the large numbers needed to make a significant impact on the waitlist.

Creativity however is never to be underestimated. One way to make the Good Samaritan donation more "productive" would be to consent the individual to consider catalyzing a kidney domino chain.[82] While this is discussed in detail in the next chapter, it does raise 1 equity question that we address here.

7.5 The Good Samaritan Catalyzes a Domino Chain

In 2006, Robert Montgomery and colleagues proposed the allocation of a kidney from a Good Samaritan donor to catalyze a domino chain.[83] As we mentioned in chapter 2 a chain involves allocating a kidney from a good

Samaritan donor to a candidate with an incompatible living donor who then donates her kidney to another candidate with an incompatible donor who "pays it forward"—that is, the donor donates to a candidate after her intended recipient has received an organ (see Figure 7.1).

Catalyzing a chain maximizes the utility of Good Samaritan kidneys. The Good Samaritan kidney benefits not just 1 recipient but often several candidates (and their families). It does have the risk of creating additional pressure on the potential Good Samaritan to go ahead with the donation even if she becomes ambivalent about proceeding.

However, catalyzing a chain has similar justice concerns raised by case 7-2 because it does require that the Good Samaritan donor donate to a candidate who has a particular trait—a willing but incompatible living donor. Candidates who have an incompatible living donor are not among the worst off because they have the option of being listed on the deceased donor waitlist similar to other prospective recipients who do not have appropriate living donors and the additional option of participating in a kidney paired exchange that those without any available living donor do not have.

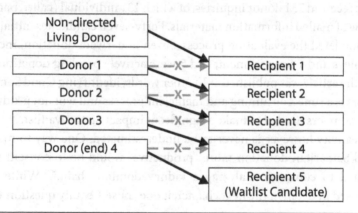

Dashed gray arrows with an X: Histo*incompatible* donations that *cannot* occur.
Solid black arrows: Histocompatible donations that occur.

Figure 7.1 Domino Chain Catalyzed by a Non-Directed Living Donor
A domino chain involving multiple donor-recipient pairs is catalyzed by a non-directed or Good Samaritan donor. In this domino chain, all of the donors are incompatible with their paired recipients, but they are able to donate to other recipients. The domino chain ends with the end donor donating to a candidate on the deceased donor waitlist who does not have a paired living donor.

Thus, like option 3, catalyzing a chain entails that the donor be allowed to donate to a group. Whereas the donor in case 7-2 wanted to donate to a person who was not a member of a killing profession, the Good Samaritan donor who catalyzes a chain wants to donate to a person who has an incompatible living donor (or more realistically, is encouraged to donate to a candidate who has an incompatible living donor) to make it possible for more candidates to receive transplants through domino chains.[84] While neither of these groups are inherently among the worst off, we believe it is still permissible for a potential living donor to make that choice because it is a private good which can be allocated based on donor preference provided that the preference is within the realm of reasonable moral boundaries.

7.6 Conclusion

How did the cases with which we began this chapter resolve? As explained previously, the University of Chicago transplant team explained their reluctance to the potential donor in case 7-1 and he was rejected at that time, with the transplant team stating that he could be reconsidered if he undertook lifestyle changes and improved his health. Nine months later, the donor returned, having become a regular at a gym and having lost 15 lbs. His 24-hour blood pressure measurements without medication were now within normal limits without significant periods of hypertension. He was found to be medically and psychologically sound and was approved to be a living donor. He also stated that he was committed to keep up his new habits to protect his remaining kidney.[85]

In case 7-2, the transplant team decided to go forward with the donation despite their misgivings regarding her stipulations. They stated that there were certain stipulations that they would not have accepted: "she did not exclude a group of persons based on sex, creed or colour ... [which] would have been deemed unacceptable by our institution."[86] Such a decision is supported by David Steinberg, who proposes that "altruistic strangers attend a mandated education program that encourages their adherence to allocation guidelines, yet ultimately preserves their freedom of choice."[87] We agree with Steinberg's analysis. It is imperative, however, that the transplant community be transparent about what stipulations are permissible.

In sum, Good Samaritan donors can choose to donate to (1) an individual on the deceased donor waitlist of the center to which she presents (preferably the top candidate on the waitlist for whom her kidney is an acceptable match); (2) a specific individual identified by a media appeal; or (3) an individual member of a particular group, provided that the classification is determined to be nondiscriminatory and acceptable to the wider community. Children, for example, represent a group that the public supports being selected to receive a Good Samaritan donor organ.[88] Catalyzing chains (that is, donating to those who have a histo-incompatible but willing living donor) is another such group. We discuss this in greater detail in the next chapter.

Notes

1. Ross LF, Glannon W, Josephson MA, Thistlethwaite JR, Jr. Should all living donors be treated equally? *Transplantation*. 2002;74:418–421, at p. 418 (references omitted).
2. Gohh RY, Morrissey PE, Madras PN, Monaco AP. Controversies in organ donation: the altruistic living donor. *Nephrol Dial Transplant*. 2001;16:619–621, at pp. 619–620.
3. Wolstenholme GEW, O'Connor M, eds. *Ethics in Medical Progress: With Special Reference to Transplantation*. Boston, MA: Little, Brown and Company; 1966, citing Starzl at pp. 74–77.
4. Sadler HH, Davison L, Carroll C, and Kountz SL. The living genetically unrelated kidney donor. *Semin Psychiatry*. 1971;3:86–101.
5. Murray JE, Barnes BA, Atkinson J. Fifth report of The Human Kidney Transplant Registry. *Transplantation*. 1967;5(4):752–774. See also, Wolstenholme and O'Connor, *Ethics in Medical*, citing Schreiner at p. 68.
6. Grady D. The new organ donors are living strangers. *The New York Times*. September 20, 1999. Accessed August 18, 2021. https://www.nytimes.com/1999/09/20/us/the-new-organ-donors-are-living-strangers.html
7. Grady, "The new organ donors."
8. There is confusion and controversy about how to describe individuals who donate outside of a biological or long-standing emotional relationship. The Ethical, Legal and Psychosocial Aspects of Organ Transplantation (ELPAT) committee of the European Society of Transplantation attempted a standardization in 2011. See Dor FJMF, Massey EK, Frunza M, et al. New classification of ELPAT for living organ donation. *Transplantation*. 2011;91(9):935–938. In this book, we use Good Samaritan donation to refer to all donations outside of traditional biological and emotional relationships. Some of these can also be referred to as nondirected donors, which means that the donor is not involved in the selection of the recipient. Donors who respond to a specific media request to help a particular person would be donating directedly even if still identified as a Good Samaritan.
9. Matas AJ, Garvey CA, Jacobs CL, Kahn JP. Nondirected donation of kidneys from living donors. *N Engl J Med*. 2000;343:433–436. Many different terms are used to

describe these donors. While Matas used the phrase "non-directed donors," in our own work we have used "Good Samaritan" and nondirected donors interchangeably, although we now attempt to be more precise and refer to all such donors as Good Samaritan donors, referring to them as nondirected donors only if the donor has no role in the selection of the recipient and does not know and will not know the recipient's identity.

10. Spital A. Unconventional living kidney Donors—attitudes and use among transplant centers. *Transplantation*. 1989;48:243–248.

11. See Spital, "Unconventional"; Spital A. Unrelated living kidney donors: an update of attitudes and use among US transplant centers. *Transplantation*. 1994;57:1722–1726; and Spital A. Evolution of attitudes at US transplant centers toward kidney donation by friends and altruistic strangers. *Transplantation*. 2000;69:1728–1731.

12. Terasaki PI, Cecka JM, Gjertson DW, Takemoto S. High survival rates of kidney transplants from spousal and living unrelated donors. *N Engl J Med*. 1995;333:333–336.

13. See, Serur D, Bretzlaff G, Christos P, Desrosiers F, Charlton M. Solicited kidney donors: are they coerced? *Nephrology*. 2015;20:952–955. Serur and colleagues found that nondirected donors did as well psychologically as directed donors.

14. See, for example, Spital A. Justification of living-organ donation requires benefit for the donor that balances the risk: commentary on Ross et al, *Transplantation*. 2002;74:423–424; and UNOS Ethics Committee. Ethics of organ transplantation from living donors. *Transplant Proc*. 1992;24:2236–2237.

15. See, for example, Khan J, Matas AJ. What's special about the ethics of living donors? Reply to Ross et al, *Transplantation*. 2002;74:421–422.

16. 4:1110–1116; Clemens KK, Thiessen-Philbrook H, Parikh CR, et al. Psychosocial health of living kidney donors: a systematic review. *Am J Transplant*. 2006;6:2965–2977; Massey EK, Kranenburg LW, Zuidema WC, et al. Encouraging psychological outcomes after altruistic donation to a stranger. *Am J Transplant*. 2010;10:1445–1452; Rodrigue JR, Schutzer ME, Paek M, Morrissey P. Altruistic kidney donation to a stranger: psychosocial and functional outcomes at two US transplant centers. *Transplantation*. 2011;91:772–78; Timmerman L, Zuidema WC, Erdman RA, et al. Psychologic functioning of unspecified anonymous living kidney donors before and after donation. *Transplantation*. 2013;95(11):1369–1374; Maple H, Chilcot J, Burnapp L, et al. Motivations, outcomes, and characteristics of unspecified (nondirected altruistic) kidney donors in the United Kingdom. *Transplantation*. 2014;98:1182–1189; Clarke A, Mitchell A, Abraham C. Understanding donation experiences of unspecified (altruistic) kidney donors. *Br J Health Psychol*. 2014;19(2):393–408; and Jacobs C, Berglund DM, Wisemans JF, et al. Long-term psychosocial outcomes after nondirected donation: a single-center experience. *Am J Transplant*. 2019;19:1498–1506.

17. See, for example, Garg AX, Prasad GV, Thiessen-Philbrook HR, et al. Cardiovascular disease and hypertension risk in living kidney donors: an analysis of health administrative data in Ontario, Canada. *Transplantation*. 2008;86:399–406; Ibrahim HN, Foley R, Tan L, et al. Long-term consequences of kidney donation. *N Engl J Med*. 2009;360:459–469; Muzaale AD, Massie AB, Wainwright J, McBride MA, Wang M, Segev DL. Long-term risk of ESRD attributable to live kidney donation: matching with

healthy non-donors. *Am J Transplant.* 2013;13(suppl 5):204–205; Mjoen G, Hallan S, Hartmann A, et al. Long-term risks for kidney donors. *Kidney Int.* 2014;86:162–167; Reese PP, Bloom RD, Feldman HI, et al. Mortality and cardiovascular disease among older live kidney donors. *Am J Transplant.* 2014;14(8):1853–1861; Maggiore U, Budde K, Heemann U, et al. Long-term risks of kidney living donation: review and position paper by the ERA-EDTA DESCARTES working group. *Nephrol Dial Transplant.* 2017;32:216–223; and O'Keefe LM, Ramond A, Oliver-Williams C, et al. Mid- and long-term health risks in living kidney donors: a systematic review and meta-analysis. *Ann Intern Med.* 2018;168:276–284.

18. See, for example, Tonelli M, Wiebe N, Knoll G, et al. Systematic review: kidney transplantation compared with dialysis in clinically relevant outcomes. *Am J Transplant.* 2011; 11(10): 2093–2109; and Lentine KL, Kasiske BL, Levey AS, et al. KDIGO Clinical Practice Guideline on the Evaluation and Care of Living Kidney Donors. *Transplantation.* 2017;101(8S suppl 1):S1–S109.

19. See Tonelli et al, "Systematic review"; and Lentine et al, "KDIGO."

20. Matas et al, "Nondirected."

21. Abecassis M, Adams P, Adams M, et al. The live donor consensus conference. *JAMA.* 2000;284:2919–2926; and Adams PL, Cohen DJ, Danovitch GM, et al. The nondirected live-kidney donor: ethical considerations and practice guidelines: A National Conference Report. *Transplantation.* 2002;74:582–590.

22. Matas et al, "Nondirected."

23. Adams et al, "The nondirected live-kidney"; and Dew MA, Jacobs CL, Jowsey SG, et al. Guidelines for the psychosocial evaluation of living unrelated kidney donors in the United States: meeting report. *Am J Transplant.* 2007;7:1047–1054.

24. Dew et al, "Guidelines," at p. 1051.

25. Dew et al, "Guidelines," at p. 1051.

26. Kranenburg L, Zuidema W, Erdman R, Weimar W, Passchier J, Busschbach J. The psychological evaluation of Samaritan kidney donors: a systematic review. *Psychol Med.* 2008;38:177–185, at p. 183.

27. Kranenburg et al, "The psychological," at p. 183.

28. Matas et al, "Nondirected," at p. 436.

29. Otte JB. Good Samaritan liver donor in pediatric transplantation. *Pediatr Transplant.* 2009;13:155–159; and Reichman TW, Fox A, Adcock L, et al. Anonymous living liver donation: donor profiles and outcomes. *Am J Transplant.* 2010;10:2099–2104; and Raza MH, Aziz H, Kaur N, et al. Global experience and perspectives on anonymous nondirected live donation in living donor liver transplantation. *Clin Transplant.* 2020;34(4):e13836.

30. Jacobs CL, Roman D, Garvey C, Kahn J, Matas AJ. Twenty-two nondirected kidney donors: an update on a single center's experience. *Am J Transplant.* 2004;4:1110–1116.

31. Kane F, Clement G, Kane M. Live kidney donations and the ethics of care. *J Med Humanit.* 2008;29:173–188, at p. 183.

32. Glannon W, Ross LF. Do genetic relationships create moral obligations in organ transplantation? *Cambr Q Healthc Ethics.* 2002;11(2):153–159.

33. Glannon and Ross, "Do genetic relationships," at p. 155.

34. Glannon and Ross, "Do genetic relationships"; and Ross LF, Glannon W, Josephson MA, Thistlethwaite JR. Should all living donors be treated equally? *Transplantation.* 2002;74:418–421.

35. Jecker N. Conceiving a child to save a child: reproduction and filial ethics. *J Clin Ethics.* 1990;1:99–103, at p. 102.

36. Kahn J. Commentary: making the most of strangers' altruism. *J Law Med Ethics.* 2002;30:446–447, at p. 447

37. Ross et al, "Should all donors," at p. 419.

38. Glannon and Ross, "Do genetic relationships," at pp. 155–156.

39. Glannon and Ross, "Do genetic relationships," at p. 157.

40. Spital, "Justification."

41. Spital, "Justification," at p. 423 (reference omitted).

42. Kahn, "Commentary," at p. 447.

43. Ross LF. Solid organ donations between strangers. *J Law Med Ethics.* 2002;30:440–445, at p. 442 (references omitted).

44. Jacobs et al, "Twenty-two."

45. Serur et al, "Solicited kidney donors," at p. 954. While Serur refers to these individuals as nondirected donors, we would identify them as Good Samaritan donors because their donation is directed.

46. Kumar K, Holscher CM, Luo X, et al. Persistent regional and racial disparities in non-directed living kidney donation. *Clin Transplant.* 2017;31(12):10.1111/ctr.13135.

47. Organ Procurement and Transplantation Network. (OPTN). National Database. Accessed August 18, 2021. https://optn.transplant.hrsa.gov/data/view-data-reports/national-data/

48. Kumar et al, "Persistent regional."

49. Clarke et al, "Understanding"; Jacobs et al, "Long-term psychosocial"; and Balliet W, Kazley AS, Johnson E, et al. The non-directed living kidney donor: why donate to strangers? *J Ren Care.* 2019;45:102–110.

50. See, for example, Rodrigue et al, "Altruistic kidney"; Massey et al, "Encouraging"; and Sharif A. Unspecified kidney donation: a review of principles, practice and potential. *Transplantation.* 2013;95:1425–1430

51. For a description of the Jesus Christians cult founded by David McKay, and its relations to nondirected kidney donation, see the archive of related articles at The Cult Education Institute website. Last accessed August 18, 2021. https://culteducation.com/group/1001-the-jesus-christians.html

52. Mueller PS, Case EJ, Hook CC. Responding to offers of altruistic living unrelated kidney donation by group associations: an ethical analysis. *Transplant Rev.* 2008;22:200–205, at p. 201.

53. See Mueller et al, "Responding," at p. 201.

54. See Mueller et al, "Responding," at p. 201.

55. Meckler L. For religious group, true charity begins on operating table: sect's kidney donations pose dilemma for doctors; a member's mom objects. *The Wall Street Journal.* December 13, 2007. Last accessed August 18, 2021. https://www.wsj.com/articles/SB119747536833823793

56. Godfrey A. "secret" surgery to donate healthy organ: a man has donated a healthy kidney in a "secret" operation after his first attempt was thwarted. *News.Com.Au.* March 17, 2009. Last accessed August 18, 2021. https://www.news.com.au/national/ secret-surgery-to-donate-healthy-organ/news-story/f3f8e8af57f4e137c3d62acd155 b7218?sv=fda11601ca2bb5e1e2a5143f1c721a00

57. Elliott C. Doing harm: living organ donors, clinical research and *The Tenth Man. J Med Ethics.* 1995;21:91–96, at 95.

58. Ross et al, "Should all donors."

59. In an article entitled "Problems in Renal Transplantation," Starzl and colleagues wrote:

> In two cases living donors were obtained from rather unusual sources. A 42-year-old male volunteered a kidney to a 50-year-old man with polycystic renal disease as the result of a newspaper appeal by the patient's wife. A second kidney was donated by a convict from the Colorado State Prison.

> Starzl TE, Marchiori TL, Brittain RS, Homes JH, Waddell WR. Problems in renal homotransplantation. *JAMA.* 1964;187:734–740, at p. 734.

60. Matas et al, "Nondirected," at p. 433.

61. The equity argument in support of prioritizing those who are worst off is based on the arguments of John Rawls' in *A Theory of Justice.* Cambridge, MA: Harvard University Press; 1971.

62. On December 9–10, 2020, the National Academy of Medicine launched a project entitled "A Fairer and More Equitable, Cost-Effective, and Transparent System of Donor Organ Procurement, Allocation and Distribution." The short description reads:

> Challenges exist in ensuring deceased donor organs are allocated to individuals on the transplant recipient waitlist in a fair, equitable, cost-effective and transparent manner. In response to the Consolidated Appropriations Act, 2020, the National Academies of Sciences, Engineering, and Medicine will establish an ad hoc committee to conduct a study to examine the economic (costs), ethical, policy, regulatory, and operational issues relevant to organ allocation policy decisions involving deceased donor organs.

> As of August 4, 2021, 9 meeting have occurred with at least 2 more scheduled. More information is available on the National Academies website https://www. nationalacademies.org/our-work/a-fairer-and-more-equitable-cost-effective-and-transparent-system-of-donor-organ-procurement-allocation-and-distribution

63. Starzl et al, "Problems."

64. One of us (LFR) discussed this elsewhere and provided many references. See Veatch RM, Ross LF. Chapter 15: The Media's Impact on Transplants and Directed Donation. In: *Transplantation Ethics.* 2nd ed. Washington, DC: Georgetown University Press; 2015:251–267

65. See, for example, the website Matching Donors. Publication date 2004. Last revised August 18, 2021 Last accessed August 18, 2021. https://matchingdonors.com/life/

66. National Conference of Commissioners on Uniform State Laws. Revised Uniform Anatomal Gift Act (2006). (Last revised or Amended in 2009). On the web at: uaga_ final_aug09.pdf (donornetworkwest.org). Last accessed August 18, 2021.

67. Testerman J. Should donors say who gets organs? *Tampa Bay Times*. Oct. 6, 2005. August 18, 2021. https://www.tampabay.com/archive/1994/01/09/should-donors-say-who-gets-organs/

68. 1998 Florida Code Title XLII—Estates and Trusts, Chapter 732 Probate Code: Intestate Succession and Wills, Part X—Anatomical Gifts (ss. 732. 910-732.922).

   The amendment reads:

   > However, the Legislature declares that the public policy of this state prohibits restrictions on the possible recipients of an anatomical gift on the basis of race, color, religion, sex, national origin, age, physical handicap, health status, marital status, or economic status, and such restrictions are hereby declared void and unenforceable.

   https://www.flsenate.gov/Laws/Statutes/1998/Chapter732/PART_X. The quote is Chapter 732, Section 913. It was published July/August 1998. Last accessed August 18, 2021.

69. Gohh et al., "Controversies," at pp. 619–620.

70. Gohh et al., "Controversies," at p. 621. Last accessed August 18, 2021.

71. Matas et al., "Nondirected," at p. 436.

72. We believe that there is an ethical argument to support the Hopkin's policy based on the work of Rawls, *A Theory of Justice*. Rawls, one of the most important political theorists of the 20th century, argued for an egalitarian conception of justice known as "justice as fairness." In this conception of justice, inequities are permitted only if they benefit those who are worst off. Since children in end-stage renal disease have had a shorter healthy life than their adult counterparts, they are among the worst off. Today, Johns Hopkins often allocates Good Samaritan kidneys to catalyze chains. This policy is justified on the grounds of maximizing the benefit of the Good Samaritan donor. We argue in chapter 8 that such a practice can be ethical provided that the living donor advocate team educates and empowers donors to consider their donation options and the donor freely chooses to catalyze a chain. We do discuss in section 6 of this chapter (chapter 7) one ethical issue that this raises. See text corresponding to references 82–88.

73. Spital A. Should people who donate a kidney to a stranger be permitted to choose their recipients? Views of the United States public. *Transplantation*. 2003;76(8):1252–1256, at p. 1254.

74. Spital, "Choose their recipients," at p. 1254.

75. Spital, "Choose their recipients."

76. Ross LF. All donations should not be treated equally: a response to Jeffrey Kahn's commentary. *J Law Med Ethics*. 2002;30(3):448–451, at p. 449 (references omitted).

77. See, for example, Brennan P. Public solicitation of organs on the internet: ethical and policy issues. *J Emerg Nurs*. 2006; 32(2):191–193; Hanto DW. Ethical challenges posed by the solicitation of deceased and living organ donors. *N Engl J Med*. 2007;356(10):1062–1066; and Verghese PS, Garvey CA, Mauer MS, Matas AJ. Media appeals by pediatric patients for living donors and the impact on a transplant center. *Transplantation*. 2011;91(6):593–596.

78. Ross LF. Media appeals for directed altruistic living liver donations. *Perspect Biol Med.* 2002;45:329–337.

79. Steinberg D. The allocation of organs donated by altruistic strangers. *Ann Intern Med.* 2006;145(3):197–203, at p. 201.

80. Jacobs et al, "Twenty-two."

81. Jendrisak MD, Hong B, Shenoy S, et al. Altruistic living donors: evaluation for nondirected kidney or liver donation. *Am J Transplant.* 2006;6(1):115–120.

82. Burnapp L, Assche KV, Lennerling A, et al. Raising awareness of unspecified living kidney donation: an ELPAT* (Ethical, Legal and Psychosocial Aspects of Transplantation) view. *Clin Kidney J.* 2020;13(2):159–165.

83. Montgomery RA, Gentry SE, Marks WH, et al. Domino paired kidney donation: a strategy to make best use of live non-directed donation. *Lancet.* 2006;368(9533): 419–421.

84. See, for example, Burnapp et al, "Raising awareness" or Sharif, "Unspecified," p. 1427. Sharif states, "In countries such as the United States and the Netherlands, unspecified donors have been successfully diverted toward kidney paired donation frameworks to maximize the number of transplantations."

85. Ross, "Should all donors."

86. Gohh et al., "Controversies," at p. 621.

87. Steinberg, "The allocation," at p. 201.

88. Spital, "Choose their recipients."

8

Kidney Paired Exchanges and Variants

Case 8-1: This description is copied verbatim from Jeffrey
Veale and Garet Hil.[1]
On October 3, 2000 the first recorded US paired exchange occurred at
Rhode Island Hospital. The pairs consisted of 2 offspring, each of whom
wanted to donate to their corresponding mother but had blood type
incompatibilities (reciprocal A/B and B/A). This historic exchange was
performed in sequence by Dr. Paul Morrissey and Dr. Anthony Monaco
with minimal media attention.

Case 8-2: Advance donor program.
Mr. Howard Broadman is a 64-year-old retired judge. His grandson,
Quinn, was born with 1 kidney and it does not function well. On the
University of California at Los Angeles (UCLA) Newsroom website, Mr.
Broadman explains:
   I know Quinn will eventually need a transplant, but by the time he's
ready, I'll be too old to give him one of my kidneys. So I approached UCLA
and asked, "Why don't I give a kidney to someone who needs it now, then
get a voucher for my grandson to use when *he* needs a transplant in the future?" And that's just what we did.[2]

8.1 Introduction

In a 1997 article published in the *New England Journal of Medicine*, the
authors (LFR and JRT) and colleagues at the University of Chicago explored
the ethics (and legality) of a kidney paired exchange (KPE) program between 2 recipients who were ABO-incompatible or crossmatch positive with
their intended donors.[3] In an exchange program, recipient 1 is ABO-incompatible (or crossmatch positive) with Donor 1 but is ABO-compatible (or

The Living Organ Donor as Patient. Lainie Friedman Ross and J. Richard Thistlethwaite, Jr, Oxford University Press.
© Oxford University Press 2022. DOI: 10.1093/oso/9780197618202.003.0008

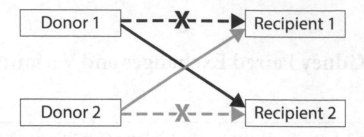

Dashed arrows with an X: Histo*incompatible* donations that *cannot* occur.
Solid arrows: Histocompatible donations that occur.

Figure 8.1 Paired Exchange of Organs Between Two Living Donor-Recipient Pairs Due to ABO- or HLA-incompatibility, Donor 1 cannot donate to Recipient 1, and Donor 2 cannot donate to Recipient 2, but Donor 1 can donate to Recipient 2, and Donor 2 can donate to Recipient 1. This is referred to as a kidney paired exchange.

crossmatch negative) with Donor 2. Recipient 2 is ABO-incompatible (or crossmatch positive) with Donor 2 but is ABO-compatible (or crossmatch negative) with Donor 1. Thus Donor 1 does not give to her intended recipient (recipient 1) but to Recipient 2 and Donor 2 does not give her kidney to her intended recipient (Recipient 2) but to Recipient 1 in a paired exchange (see Figure 8.1).

Although the idea had been proposed in the literature by Felix Rapaport in 1986,[4] the first exchange did not occur in the United States (US) until 2000 (see case 8-1), although a few had occurred in the 1990s in South Korea.[5] The first 3-way swap in the US occurred at Johns Hopkins in August 2003 (see Figure 8.2).[6] Initially, donors had to travel to their paired exchange recipient's institution, but within a few years it became more common to transport the organs rather than the donors, which allowed for exchanges to include programs at greater distance.[7]

Approximately one-third of all potential living donors in the United States (US) are either ABO-incompatible or crossmatch positive with their intended recipients.[8] The most common ABO-incompatibility involves a potential recipient of blood type O. Whereas donors of blood type O (O-donor) are universal donors and can donate to candidates of all blood types, recipient candidates of blood type O (O-candidates) can only receive organs from O-donors. As such, donor-recipient pairs with an O-donor rarely need to

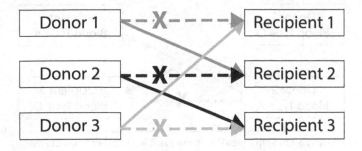

Dashed arrows with an X: Histo*incompatible* donations that *cannot* occur.
Solid arrows: Histocompatible donations that occur.

Figure 8.2 Exchange of Organs Between Multiple Living Donor-Recipient Pairs
The original kidney paired exchange was envisioned to involve 2 incompatible
donor-recipient pairs. Exchanges can, however, involve any number of pairs
although the logistics become more complicated. Several practice changes
have made it possible to include a larger number of donor-recipient pairs in
exchanges. First, transplant programs became willing to do the procedures
asynchronously. Second, once good results were shown from flying the kidneys
rather than the kidney donors, algorithms that included donor-recipient pairs
from a wider geographic area became more acceptable which allowed for more
matches.

participate in an exchange. Rather, the most common blood type incompatibility in donor-recipient pairs seeking to participate in a paired exchange is a
donor of blood type A or B with a paired recipient of blood type O. The lack
of incompatible donor-recipient pairs with O-donors makes finding matches
for O-candidates difficult. This resulted in the slow uptake of KPE at the level
of individual transplant programs. Multi-center registries were created to increase the chances of finding matches.[9] In July 2007, the National Kidney
Registry (NKR) was founded,[10] and the United Network of Organ Sharing
(UNOS) began its registry in 2010.[11]

However, what if an O-donor were willing to participate in an exchange
even if she could donate directly in order to help 2 recipients rather than just
her own compatible recipient? This type of exchange involves a compatible
donor-recipient pair in which the donor electively participates in the exchange (see Figure 8.3). We say electively because Donor 1 could donate directly to recipient 1. Donor 2, however, cannot donate directly to Recipient
2 and without a trade, Recipient 2 will not get a kidney. If Donor 1 agrees

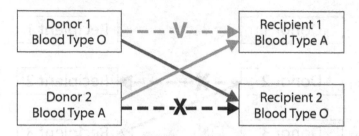

Figure 8.3 Altruistically Unbalanced Living Paired Kidney Exchange
The exchange involves a compatible Donor-Recipient Pair 1 who elect to participate in a paired exchange with an incompatible Donor-Recipient Pair 2. It is unbalanced because Donor 1 can donate directly but voluntarily elects not to, in order to help realize 2 living donor kidney transplants.

to participate in an exchange, then both recipients can get compatible living donor kidneys. The ethical challenge is how to inform Donor-Recipient pair 1 about this option and determine if they are interested in participating without causing undue pressure. We refer to this as an unbalanced exchange because donor-recipient pair 1 does not need to participate in the exchange. We discuss the ethical issues Section 8.5 Compatible Pairs.

Another variation on KPE involves an ABO-incompatible or ABO cross-match positive pair exchanging with the deceased donor waitlist (see Figures 8.4 and 8.5). In a list-paired exchange, the living donor donates to a candidate on the waitlist in exchange for her intended recipient getting special priority for the next ABO-identical crossmatch negative deceased donor kidney.[12]

In 2006, Robert Montgomery and colleagues first proposed a shift from donor-recipient pairs participating in a KPE to donor-recipient pairs participating in a domino chain catalyzed by a non-directed donor (see Figure 8.6).[13] Recall in the last chapter that Arthur Matas and colleagues allocated non-directed living donor grafts to candidates on the University of Minnesota's waitlist. What Montgomery proposed was to match this non-directed donor to a candidate (Recipient 1) who has an incompatible living donor (Donor 1) and Donor 1 would now donate to another recipient (Recipient 2) of an incompatible living donor-recipient pair and the domino effect would continue until no additional incompatible donor-pair recipients could be matched. The last paired donor would donate to a candidate on the

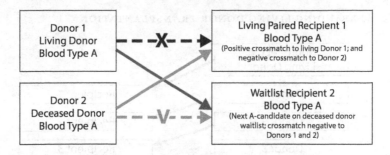

Dashed black arrow with an X: His*toincompatible* donation that *cannot* occur.
Dashed grey arrow with a V: Histocompatible but candidate declines deceased
donor kidney in order to receive a living paired exchange kidney.
Solid grey and black arrows: Histocompatible donations that occur.

Figure 8.4 List Paired Kidney Exchange (Between ABO-Compatible Crossmatch Positive) Living and Deceased Donors

The exchange involves a living donor (Donor 1) who is HLA-incompatible with her recipient (Recipient 1). Donor 1 elects to donate to a waitlist candidate (Recipient 2) who is concurrently being offered a deceased donor kidney (Donor 2). Recipient 1 is compatible with the Donor 2. Recipient 2 elects to accept the living donor graft from Donor 1 rather than the deceased donor kidney from Donor 2 because living donor grafts tend to have better graft survival. In the exchange, Recipient 1 is transplanted with the kidney from Donor 2.

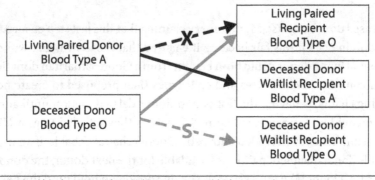

Dashed black arrow with an X: His*toincompatible* donation that *cannot* occur.
Dashed grey arrow with an S: Histocompatible donation that would have
occurred if exchange did *not* happen.
Solid grey and black arrows: Histocompatible donations that occur.

Figure 8.5 List Paired Kidney Exchange Between Living and Deceased (ABO-Incompatible) Donors

The exchange involves a living donor (Donor1) who is ABO-incompatible with her recipient (Recipient 1). Donor 1 (blood type A) elects to donate to a waitlist candidate of blood type A (Recipient 2) in order to get a deceased donor O-kidney that matches her recipient (Donor 2). This means that the waitlist candidate who benefits from this list paired exchange (Recipient 2) differs from the waitlist candidate of blood type O (Recipient 3) who would have benefited had the exchange not occurred.

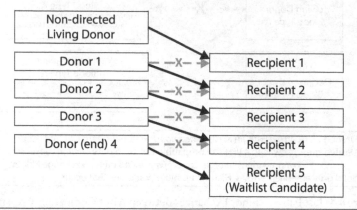

Dashed gray arrows with an X: Histo*incompatible* donations that *cannot* occur.
Solid black arrows: Histocompatible donations that occur.

Figure 8.6 Domino Chain Catalyzed by a Non-directed Living Donor
A domino chain involving multiple donor-recipient pairs is catalyzed by a non-directed or Good Samaritan donor. In this domino chain, all of the donors are incompatible with their paired recipients, but they are able to donate to other recipients. The domino chain ends with the end donor donating to a candidate on the deceased donor waitlist who does not have a paired living donor.

deceased donor waitlist. Montgomery claimed that this last step ensured that the domino chain was fair because it ensured that those with and without a potential living donor could both benefit from a Good Samaritan donation.[14]

In contrast, Michael Rees and colleagues then proposed to create never-ending chains by having the last paired donor delay donation until another chain could be formed (see Figure 8.7) which they referred to as a NEAD (Nonsimultaneous Extended Altruistic Donor) chain.[15] That is, if an incompatible donor-recipient pair is not available for the next donor, the donor (in this case, Donor N) would serve as a bridge donor, on hold until the next appropriate and willing incompatible donor-recipient pairs were found. When the next incompatible donor-recipient pairs were located, the bridge donor would then begin this new chain. The ethics and practicalities of NEAD will be discussed below.

The NKR was the first organization to successfully coordinate multiple exchanges and chains involving many centers nationwide. Its goal is to maximize the number of transplants performed. In 2008, NKR facilitated 21 transplants and the number has increased annually with 399 transplants performed in 2016 and 760 transplants performed in 2019.[16] The NKR

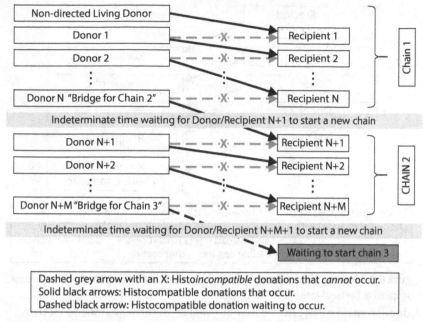

Figure 8.7 Nonsimultaneous Extended Altruistic Donor (NEAD) Domino Chain
A domino chain involving multiple donor-recipient pairs is catalyzed by a non-directed or Good Samaritan donor. In this domino chain, all of the donors are incompatible with their paired recipients, but they are able and willing to donate to other recipients. There is no candidate ready for Donor N, who becomes a "bridge donor"—a donor waiting to resume the chain. Once additional donor-recipient pairs are located, Donor N donates to the next recipient (N + 1) and the chain continues. This may entail a wait of weeks to months (nonsimultaneous). There is no candidate to whom donor N + M can donate, so she becomes a "bridge donor" as well. These chains are never-ending because end donors do not donate to the waitlist (see Figure 8.6) but instead wait for another donor-recipient pair.

quickly learned that (1) maximizing efficiency is not achieved by creating the longest chains possible because sometimes hard-to-match candidates can only match to a shorter chain, but this allows for the transplantation of a candidate who may otherwise never get transplanted, which allows his donor who may otherwise never donate to do so and thus catalyze yet another transplant; (2) long chains may require bridging, and the longer a donor waits after her intended recipient is transplanted, the more likely she is to opt out; and (3) the larger the number of donor-recipient pairs enrolled,

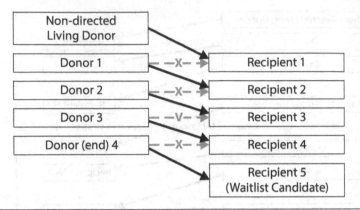

Figure 8.8 Domino Chain Catalyzed by a Non-directed Living Donor Including a
Compatible Living Donor-Recipient Pair
A domino chain catalyzed by a non-directed or Good Samaritan donor that
includes a compatible pair—a pair in which Donor 3 could donate directly to
her recipient (Recipient 3) but instead elects to participate in a chain to promote
additional kidney transplants. The compatible donor-recipient pair may
participate for purely altruistically reasons, to get a younger or better matched
graft, or for a combination of reasons.

the more chains can be generated by match runs, leading to more transplants
being performed.[17] To maximize the number of pairs enrolling in chains
and exchanges, some transplant centers began to list compatible pairs into
the NKR (see Figure 8.8). The ethics of including compatible pairs in paired
exchanges and chains are also discussed Section 8.3 Domino Chains.

A final alternative is to start a chain with an advance donor program
(ADP) donor—an ADP donor is an individual who donates in the present in
order that a loved one can access a kidney in the future (see case 8-2).

Our focus in this chapter is on the ethics of KPE and chains and their novel
variants. There are also legal issues. When we first conceived of the idea of the
KPE, we sought legal counsel from our own institution regarding whether
exchanging kidneys would be considered exchanges of "valuable consideration," which was prohibited by the National Organ Transplant Act of 1984.[18]
We were told we could proceed even though it was not until the Charlie
W. Norwood Living Organ Donation Act was passed in 2007 that the legal

issue was fully clarified.[19] However, the Norwood Act only clarified paired exchanges for immunologically incompatible exchanges and did not address the participation of compatible donor-recipient pairs nor kidney chains, although many transplant programs may assume that these variations are covered.[20]

In this chapter, then, we examine the ethical controversies raised by KPE and chains and their novel variants. We begin by examining whether KPE is ethical using our living donor ethics framework, which is based on 5 principles: respect for persons, beneficence, justice, vulnerabilities, and special relationships creating special obligations. We will then consider unique issues raised by the variants: (1) chains catalyzed by a non-directed donor, (2) chains catalyzed by an ADP donor, (3) the inclusion of compatible donor-recipient pairs in paired exchanges or domino chains, and (4) list-paired exchanges or domino chains.

8.2 Are Exchanges Between Two ABO-Incompatible Donor-Recipient Pairs Ethical?

8.2.1 Respect for Persons

In our living donor ethics framework, the first principle is respect for persons, which focuses on the autonomous individual being able to provide an informed and voluntary consent, free from undue coercion. This is 1 of the key concerns raised by KPE and its variants. Historically ABO-incompatibility served to exclude a potential donor. While many individuals may have been disappointed that they could not help their potential intended recipient, others may have been relieved.[21] With paired exchanges, whether a potential donor is ABO-incompatible or crossmatch positive with an intended recipient is less important. Since there is a strong possibility that there is another candidate with whom she matches, she can donate to this other candidate, whose paired donor can then donate to her intended recipient. Thus, paired exchanges and chains eliminate donor-recipient ABO and crossmatch incompatibility as medical excuses that were traditionally available to the hesitant donor.[22]

One way to try to limit the potential for undue pressure of the reluctant donor is to address the possibility for KPE early in the educational process. The Consensus Conference on Kidney Paired Donation, held on March

29–30, 2012, in Herndon, VA, involved 73 diverse stakeholders, and concluded that:

> All potential living donors should be informed about KPD [kidney paired donation] early in the educational process, prior to compatibility testing. This allows sufficient time for the potential donor to consider donation preferences, discuss options with their family and the donor evaluation team, and attenuate feelings of pressure or coercion if KPD is presented after incompatibility is determined.[23]

Educating prospective donors before compatibility testing is performed allows donors to decide if they are willing to be recontacted if they are not able to donate directly to their intended recipient. If they are not willing, and a donor is incompatible with her intended recipient, this stops the transplant center from recontacting her (and the added pressure this may cause). Recipients are not authorized to learn why the process has ended from the transplant center. They are only told the potential donor is ineligible.[24]

A second way to reduce the pressure is to have separate health care teams for the donor and candidate. The introduction of the independent donor advocate in 2007[25] requires all living donor transplant programs to have separate sets of health care providers for the recipient candidate and the donor, whose team consists of the living donor advocate (LDA), a transplant surgeon, a nephrologist, and other health care professionals as needed. This living donor advocate team (LDAT) focuses on the donor's well-being and explores the donor's voluntariness and understanding in a private confidential way. The LDAT also provides donors with many opportunities to opt out, the reasons for which are to be kept confidential because donors are patients and have the right to privacy regarding their health information.[26] If the potential donor decides it is not in her best interests to donate, members of the transplant team caring directly for the potential recipient should just inform the potential recipient that his potential donor has been excluded.[27] No further explanation is needed and, indeed, it would be a breach of patient confidentiality for the recipient's transplant team to say anything more. In contrast, if a potential donor herself wanted to explain her reluctance to her intended recipient, there is no prohibition to her doing so.

To ensure that donors have the right to opt out, we suggested in our original KPE article that donors must be offered the opportunity to opt out of the exchange up until the moment the surgery takes place. To both ensure that recipients get their kidney and permit the donors to renege at any time, we proposed that the procedures be done simultaneously.[28] With the move from 2 donor-recipient paired exchanges, to multi-donor recipient paired exchanges, and then to domino chains of larger and larger sizes and matches involving donor-recipient pairs across the country, simultaneous procedures became unfeasible, and transplants have been performed asynchronously. Experience, however, shows that synchronicity is less important than we had hypothesized, as few donors opt out.[29]

And yet, even with a right to opt out, participation in an exchange or chain may create additional pressures on donors who no longer have just one can- didate dependent upon their decision, but other donor-recipient pair(s) as well. Thus, it is critical that donors undergo extensive counseling to ensure that their participation is voluntary and that they are not experiencing exces- sive external pressure. While the data are limited, at least 1 study has found that exchange donors do not feel greater pressure than other donors.[30]

Another ethical concern is what additional information, if any, is needed by incompatible donor-recipient pairs in order to ensure that the donors and recipients in an exchange are informed about their options and that their participation is voluntary. Clearly, donors and recipients need to be ed- ucated about the risks, benefits, and alternatives of participating in a KPE. Some kidneys are acutely rejected and some recipients experience early graft loss (this is more common in deceased donor organ transplantation but can occur even in living donor transplantation). It is critical that both donor-re- cipient pairs understand that there is no guarantee that a transplant will be successful, whether donated directly or through in an exchange.[31] Both the donor and the recipient in each pair must agree to the participation in the paired exchange.

8.2.2 Beneficence

This principle requires an evaluation of the risks, benefits, and alternatives from the perspective of the donor, of the recipient, and of the donor-recipient jointly.

In many ways, the physical risks and benefits for exchange donors and recipients are the same as they would be for any living donor and recipient. Do the psychosocial risks and benefits change? There is a small older literature that does show that some recipients and other laypersons are (or think they would be) cognitively and emotionally affected by the origin of the donated organ.[32] But there are only limited data about whether exchange donation (versus direct donation) has any impact on long-term donor psychological benefit or regret. In 2014 Serur et al published data comparing 44 exchange/chain donors with 44 directed donors. They found that "the chain donors and traditional donors have similar positive psychological outcomes."[33] They also found no difference in coercion measures.[34] The only difference was that direct donors felt that their recipients were more indebted to them.[35]

The benefit for the recipient is a living donor kidney. The risk for the recipient is that the donor is unknown. A clinical difference is that the exchange recipients are not first-degree biological relatives, which translates into slightly lower 1- and 5-year graft survival because of both HLA and minor histocompatibility factors. However, as we saw in chapter 4, there is already a shift away from genetically related relatives, particularly in the White community, where less than half of living donors are first-degree relatives, but more likely to be spouses, other emotionally related extended family members, or friends.[36] Given current immunosuppression regimens, graft and patient outcomes from nonrelated living donors do almost as well as genetically related living donor grafts (with few exceptions like identical twins and other zero-antigen mismatched donor-recipient pairs).[37] Whether the source of the non-genetically related living kidney graft (emotionally related donor versus exchange donor versus non-directed donor) has any effect on recipient compliance has not yet been studied.

Another concern is not knowing who your donor or recipient is, the type of person he or she may be, their actual health status and health behaviors, and their familial or environmental risks, which may have some impact on kidney graft longevity. Although the exchange donors and recipients all go through similar extensive work-ups, the exchange donor may have unidentified transmissible health risks (infectious or cancer). This is also true of directed donors. Still, the concern is real and limits participation in KPE. In 2006, Amy Waterman et al found that 36% of donors would not consider participation in a living donor KPE,[38] whereas James Rodrigue et al reported in 2015 that 63.5% of donors would not consider participation.[39] Although both studies are limited in their geography (Waterman in St. Louis and Florida and Rodrigue in Boston) and used different questionnaires, both studies found that the main reasons not to participate in a KPE or domino chain were lack of trust by both donors and recipients that the intended recipient would get as good a kidney as the one being donated.[40] Steinberg points out that this may be illusory. We often don't know the nuanced health status of our own emotionally or genetically related donors, and our emotionally and genetically related donors do not have to reveal all personal health information to their recipients: "Donors who feel pressure to help a relative or friend may be 'less than fully truthful' and hide unhealthy habits or addictions."[41]

While the risk:benefit of exchanges and chains is generally perceived as positive for incompatible donor-recipient pairs who participate, there are alternatives. First, candidates can stay on dialysis and/or wait for a deceased donor organ. Second, candidates can undergo desensitization and get transplanted with the kidney of his intended donor. However, desensitization protocols work best for recipient candidates who have low-strength donor specific antibodies (DSA), but even then they are expensive, performed at only a few centers, and have, on average, shorter graft survival. Recipients who undergo desensitization still require a greater level of immunosuppression than recipients who have no DSA, and greater levels of immunosuppression increase the risks of infection and malignancy.[42]

It may be better not to view desensitization and KPE as competing options but as synergistic. Candidates who are highly sensitized to their own donor—that is, have high-strength donor specific antigens (DSA)—may have low-strength DSA to another donor on a paired exchange and domino chain registry. Imagine the situation where Recipient 1 has high DSA to Donor 1 but only low DSA to Donor 2, and Recipient 2 has high DSA to Donor 2 but no DSA to Donor 1 (see Figure 8.9). While each recipient-candidate could attempt desensitization to receive a direct donation from their paired donor, desensitization protocols work best for recipient-candidates who have low DSA. Recipient 1 has a better chance of a successful transplant if desensitized to Donor 2 rather than his own paired donor (Donor 1). Recipient 2 can receive a kidney from Donor 1 without any need for desensitization. A paired exchange after desensitization of Recipient 1 will result in better outcomes for both recipients (at least statistically).[43]

8.2.3 Justice

The principle of justice focuses on the fairness of the donor selection process (and, in this case, in the donor-recipient selection process). A candidate may have more than 1 potential living donor. Participation in an exchange or chain is usually only considered if no direct donation is possible (compatible

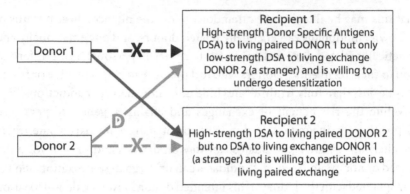

Dashed black and grey arrows with an X: Histo*incompatible* donations that *cannot* occur.
Solid black arrow: Histocompatible donation that occurs.
Solid grey arrow with a D: After desensitization of recipient, histocompatible donation occurs.

Figure 8.9   Living Donor Paired Exchange After Desensitization of Recipient 1
This paired exchange involves 2 donor-recipient pairs in which each recipient
has high donor specific antigen (DSA) to their respective donors. While each
recipient-candidate could attempt desensitization to receive a direct donation
from their paired donor, desensitization protocols work best for recipient-
candidates who have low DSA. Recipient 1 has low DSA to Donor 2 and high
DSA to Donor 1 such that desensitization of Recipient 1 has a better chance
of a positive outcome with a transplant from Donor 2 rather than from Donor
1. Recipient 2 has no DSA to Donor 1 and can be transplanted with a kidney
from Donor 1 without any desensitization. A paired exchange is beneficial to
Recipient 1 because it is unlikely that desensitization could adequately reduce
his DSA to Donor 1 to produce a successful direct transplant. Likewise it is
unlikely that desensitization could adequately reduce the high DSA of Recipient
2 to Donor 2. Recipient 2 would greatly benefit from a paired exchange because
transplants where the recipient has no DSA have better overall outcomes than
transplants where the recipient initially has DSA to their donor, even after
undergoing desensitization. Thus, a paired exchange would achieve the best
possible outcomes for both recipients.

pairs will be discussed in section 5). If a candidate has more than 1 incompatible donor, 2 questions arise: (1) which potential incompatible donor will
participate in the exchange or chain, and (2) who makes that decision?

Donors of blood type O are the easiest to match in a paired exchange
or domino chain registry. But if transplant teams tell the candidate to
proceed to exchange or chain with their donor of blood type O, this may

cause undue pressure because this may be a more reluctant donor who was only glad to have a positive crossmatch. Thus, to reduce pressure, all donors and candidates should be educated about ABO and compatibility testing and what options exist if they are healthy enough to be a donor but are not able to donate directly to their emotionally related candidate. All donors should be asked upfront, even before ABO and histocompatibility testing (identification of both HLA type and anti-HLA antibodies) for direct donation, whether they would be willing to be considered for a paired exchange or domino chain if a direct donation is not feasible.[44] The LDAT should assess the degree of willingness and only recontact those interested in recontact and should not recontact simply because a donor has a more desirable blood type. Upon recontact, the donor must be given additional opportunities to decline participation before any attempt to include the donor-recipient pair in a match run (a computer algorithm designed to identify individuals to participate in paired exchanges or domino-chains).

8.2.4 Vulnerabilities

Donors who agree to be evaluated to participate in KPE or domino chains face many of the same potential vulnerabilities faced by those who donate directly to their known intended recipient, and these vulnerabilities should be addressed with the LDAT. Potential KPE or domino chain donors are at risk for additional juridic and deferential vulnerabilities which may be difficult to discern because it is often not transparent how an intrafamilial donor is selected to be the designated donor.[45] Although we believe the donor should self-select (ie, volunteer), we would be naïve to think this is always the case. The deferential concern is compounded by the fact that paired chains and domino exchanges take away the medical excuse, removing what is seen as a "legitimate medical reason not to donate" because the emotionally or biologically related donors no longer needs to be compatible with their intended recipients.[46] The LDAT should extensively explore the willingness and engagement of living donors who are considering exchange donation to ensure that the decision reflects the donor's reflective decision. The LDAT also needs to explore motivation to minimize donors opting out late in the process, which could compromise multiple donors and candidates who are downstream of the donor in a domino chain.

Savvy families in which several potential donors have all been excluded from direct donation may pressure potential donors of blood type O to participate in a domino chain because they will be easier to match. Therefore, being a potential O-donor increases one's medical vulnerability. Even if the potential donor expressed initial willingness to participate in a paired exchange or domino chain, they must be given other opportunities to decline after recontact to ensure genuine voluntariness.

Potential paired exchange and domino chain donors may also face infrastructural vulnerability in that exchanges and domino chains complicate attempts to ensure privacy and confidentiality, and it becomes even more logistically complicated when the number of donor-recipient pairs in the paired exchange or domino chain increases. In 2012, the *New York Times* published the photos and names of 59 of the 60 individuals involved in a 30-kidney chain.[47] In general, in the US, transplant centers try to maintain strict privacy between donor-recipient pairs prior to the transplants, and then only to disclose if all parties agree. Different programs have different policies regarding a required period of "silence."[48] Some programs have different rules, including the prohibition of contact.[49] For example, in the Netherlands, Marry de Klerk and colleagues conducted a pilot study involving 14 donor-recipient pairs who were eligible to participate in a paired exchange program that was just being developed, and all stated they would prefer anonymity.[50] Based on these data, when the program was implemented, the decision was made to maintain anonymity permanently.[51] However, data from the first 24 donor-recipient pairs who actually participated in exchanges in the Netherlands found that 21% (5/24) donors and 17% (4/24) recipients would have preferred to have been able to meet.[52] A recent study in the Netherlands found that while many donors and recipients continue to support anonymity, they do not feel a stringent no-contact anonymous policy is always necessary.[53] These data suggest that the policy may need to be re-evaluated.

If several donors and recipients are all recovering in 1 hospital as is the case in single-center exchanges and chains, unwanted or premature identity disclosure between the pairs is more likely to occur. In 1986, Rapaport suggested that the exchanges should take place at different institutions.[54] Today, that may be inadequate given greater connectivity through the internet and social media. Families also need to be educated and counseled about the right to privacy of domino-chain and paired-exchange participants. The stress caused by unwanted disclosure may be particularly acute if 1 donor has complications or 1 kidney fails. More data are necessary regarding the clinical, psychological, and emotional follow-up of the parties involved in exchanges in which identities have and have not been revealed to determine if, when, and whether privacy and confidentiality policies need to be more or less stringent.

8.2.5 Special Relationships Create Special Obligations

Exchanges and chains differ from directed donation because the donor-recipient pairs are strangers. It is important to maintain privacy preoperatively to prevent any additional pressure. Currently most programs in the US allow donors and recipients to meet post-transplant after a specified period if all parties agree. This allows the donors and recipients time to recuperate and to reflect upon the pros and cons of establishing a relationship. Some donor-recipient pairs may not want to meet, especially if an adverse event occurs. The LDAT must ensure that privacy is maintained and respected.

Overall, then, an evaluation of KPE using our living donor ethics framework appears to show broad similarity in benefits and concerns for donors and recipients involved in directed donation and donors and recipients involved in paired exchanges and domino chains. Donors may face some greater risks of deferential and infrastructural vulnerabilities which must be adequately addressed with the aid of an LDAT before the surgeries are scheduled.

In the next sections we consider ethical issues raised by some of the exchange variants and domino chains.

8.3 Domino Chains

Recall in chapter 7 that we suggested offering Good Samaritan donors 3 options: (1) to donate to the next person on their chosen center's deceased donor waitlist; (2) to donate to a particular person whom they select from personal contacts or media appeals; or (3) to donate to an individual who is a member of a group that society agrees should be given priority. While children were initially such a group, today the focus is on donating to a candidate who has an incompatible donor in order to catalyze a domino chain which benefits not 1 person, but several persons.

From a utilitarian perspective, non-directed donors should be encouraged to catalyze domino chains because this maximizes the number of transplants performed. If anything, the altruistic non-directed donor ought to be pleased if her donation leads to more than 1 transplant being performed. But if the non-directed donor elects to donate to a particular person or to the top of the waitlist, their preference should be respected.

Chains can be open (never ending). The last donor in an open-ended chain becomes a "bridge" donor—a donor whose recipient has already received a kidney, but her donation is on hold until another eligible donor-recipient pair is located. One disadvantage of bridge donation is that there will be some donors who, when contacted weeks or months later, may not be willing (or able) to donate. Although the data show that the number of donors who opt out is small,[55] it does happen and is more likely to happen the longer the delay.[56] There are a variety of reasons for opting out, including the donor becoming ineligible during the waiting period or the timing not working for the donor due to other life circumstances. This has led some to argue to close the chain after a certain number of donor-recipient pairs or a certain period of time has elapsed for the bridge donor.[57]

Open-ended domino chains raise a justice concern because they benefit those who are already advantaged (those with a potential living donor, albeit an incompatible living donor) over those who do not have a potential living donor. If the chain is not closed by allocating the last paired kidney donor to a waitlist candidate, all those without a potential living donor are denied the benefits of the non-directed donor. This is inconsistent with a Rawlsian notion of justice, in which inequities are permitted only if they benefit those who are worst off, and those without a potential living donor are worse off than those with a living donor.[58] In the original non-directed donor protocol described by Matas, the Good Samaritan kidney was allocated to a patient near or at the top of the waitlist at the University of Minnesota.[59] If a Good Samaritan is now encouraged to donate to a chain rather than to the next candidate on the waitlist, those on the waitlist who don't have a living donor are disadvantaged because they are no longer eligible for kidneys donated by these Good Samaritans. It would be fairer from a justice perspective if the chain is closed by a candidate who is at the top of the deceased donor waitlist where the Good Samaritan donor donated.[60]

Another justice issue involves the algorithm used for identifying exchanges and chains. It is not the case that there is only 1 algorithm for a registry at any 1 time, but rather there may be several potential chains that can be catalyzed from a particular non-directed donor. In fact, in an article published in 2015, NKR stated that only 1 in 4.6 match offers resulted in a transplant:

> Of the 3,180 match offers issued, 2,228 (70%) were accepted, 454 (14%) were rejected, and there was no center response for 498 (16%) match offers. To expedite the matching process, match offers were often withdrawn by the registry before the deadline because another center had already rejected one of the offers within the chain. In these situations, centers may not have responded yet to their match offers, accounting for most of the 498 nonresponders. Among the 2,228 accepted match offers, only 1,335 (42% of total offers, 59% of accepted offers) actually advanced to the next stage because 893 offers that were accepted did not proceed because they were part of chains that fell through. The NKR facilitated 690 kidney transplants within this period. Therefore, one in 4.6 match offers resulted in a transplant.[61]

The reasons why match runs do not materialize are varied. For example, 1 candidate may have already received a deceased donor transplant; a donor may have become ineligible; or the planned match is refused by a potential chain participant if the participant (donor and/or recipient) does not perceive the offer to be satisfactory.[62]

We believe chain algorithms should attempt to include highly sensitized candidates, even if it means a shorter chain length. This is both fair (because the very highly sensitized are worst off because they otherwise might not ever find a match) and maximizes utility (the number of kidney transplants performed). While it may seem counter-intuitive for a system that seeks to maximize the number of transplants performed to perform shorter chains to accommodate the highly sensitized, it actually increases the number of transplants in the long run (because the paired donor of the highly sensitive recipient might otherwise never participate). Still, even with these attempts to give priority to highly sensitized candidates, highly sensitized candidates do accumulate on the waitlist.[63]

8.4 Advance Donor Program Donor

The origin of the concept of an Advance Donor Program (ADP) was detailed by one of us (LFR) in an article with James Rodrigue and Bob Veatch:

In 2014, Howard Broadman conceived of the idea of an "advanced donation" (Hawryluk 2016). Broadman's grandson was born with a congenital
kidney abnormality and was expected to need a kidney transplant by young
adulthood. Broadman, who was 64 years old when his 4-year-old grandson
was diagnosed, realized he might be too old to donate when his grandson
might need a kidney, and proposed donating now in exchange for providing
his grandson with a kidney voucher to be utilized when he needed it. The
National Kidney Registry, (NKR), a private not-for-profit organization was
created in 2007 to facilitate exchanges, developed the Advanced Donation
Program (ADP) to allow individuals to donate a kidney in exchange for a
voucher for one of up to 5 specified individuals who might require a kidney
transplant in the future. Broadman is not the only one to donate under this
system. In 2007, Garet Hil, the founder of NKR, was unable to donate to his
daughter due to a positive crossmatch. His experience finding her a kidney
was the inspiration behind his creation of NKR. Although a cousin who
was a match eventually donated to Hil's daughter, Hil has donated one of his
kidneys to provide a voucher for his daughter in case his daughter needs a
second transplant in the future.[64]

In these cases, the ADP donor elects to donate now while he is still young
enough and healthy enough to meet the living donor inclusion criteria although his intended recipient (Broadman's grandson (detailed in case 8-2
at the start of this chapter) and Hil's daughter in these 2 cases), may not
need one for years or decades, if ever. Their future recipients are known
as voucher holders. The ADP donor-recipient pair is a donor-recipient
pair stretched out over a long time frame. ADP programs raise unique
ethical issues for 3 principles in our framework: beneficence, justice, and
vulnerabilities.

8.4.1 Beneficence

The risk:benefit calculation for an ADP donor is unique because, while the
risks of donation are the same for the ADP donors as for other living donors,
the clinical benefits to their intended recipients may or may not accrue during
their lifetime, depending on when the voucher holder develops ESRD. But
either way, the ADP donor may judge that the peace of mind he experiences
for providing an insurance policy for his intended recipient is a tangible

immediate benefit that justifies the donation. However, it is critical that ADP donors realize that they may never get a payback for their donated kidney because (1) their intended recipient may not need a kidney and (2) the doctors can't guarantee a kidney will be found when their loved one needs it.[65]

8.4.2 Justice

NKR's policy is to offer chain-ending organs to the candidate ranked highest on the deceased donor waitlist from the site where the chain catalyst (usually a Good Samaritan donor but also possibly an ADP donor) donated unless a priority candidate (eg, a voucher holder or a donor in the NKR system who has since developed ESRD themselves). In June 2021, Jeffrey Veale and colleagues reported that there have been 250 voucher donors and 6 vouchers had been redeemed.[66] It is fair to give the voucher holder priority to end a chain because the present value of an ADP donor catalyzing a chain that is closed by a waitlist candidate outweighs this future payback of ending a chain with a voucher holder. If the voucher holder never needs a kidney, this is an additional bonus for waitlist candidates.

8.4.3 Vulnerabilities

On the face of it, neither Broadman nor Hil seem to have any additional vulnerabilities. Broadman may have felt a bit socially vulnerable due to his age. He wanted to donate now because he understood that he might not be eligible to be a living donor when his grandson would need the kidney. Hil may have felt the same. Although both have been proactive about helping a young family member, whether the voucher system that they created will be honored in the future cannot be guaranteed, a fact that both are well aware of (infrastructural vulnerability), and a fact that must be explained clearly to others who may express interest in becoming an ADP.

Overall, we concluded that "the concept of ADP is ethical in principle, but there are many logistical issues that will require further evaluation to avoid confusion, conflict, and complaints of lack of transparency."[67] We also emphasized the need for transparency and public participation in the development and implementation of policies and practices to promote and preserve public trust.[68]

8.5 Compatible Donors

Donor-recipient pairs with O-donors whose intended recipient is not sensitized to the donor's HLA antigens do not need to participate in KPE because O-donors are universal donors. The question is, however, whether it can be ethical for transplant teams to ask compatible donor-recipient pairs, especially those with O-donors, to participate in paired exchanges (see Figure 8.3) or domino chains (see Figure 8.8) even though they could donate directly to their intended recipient. We named this exchange an altruistically unbalanced exchange because 1 donor-recipient pair can donate directly (compatible pair) and does not need to participate in an exchange.[69] By agreeing to participate in an exchange, the donor who can donate directly fosters the opportunity for both her intended recipient and her exchange or chain recipient to get a living donor kidney transplant. One of us (LFR) called this donor "doubly altruistic" because the donor was not only being altruistic by agreeing to serve as a living donor, but also was now agreeing to donate to a stranger rather than to her intended emotionally related recipient to promote 2 transplants rather than 1.[70] The exchange is unbalanced because 1 recipient can receive a transplant whether or not the donor-recipient pair participates in an exchange. The same analysis holds when compatible pairs participate in domino chains.

Gentry and colleagues found that the participation of compatible donor-recipient pairs would nearly double the match rate for incompatible pairs regardless of whether the program was a single-center program or a national program.[71] Interviews of 19 Canadian providers found most were quite positive about including compatible pairs in kidney exchanges and chains, although they expressed some concern it would lead to long delays for the compatible pairs.[72]

Compatible pairs, themselves, have been less enthusiastic. In the Dutch national KPE program, only one-third of the donors and recipients were willing to consider participation.[73] Ratner et al surveyed donors and their compatible recipients and found that they were ambivalent about participating in paired exchanges and domino chains, but expressed greater willingness if the paired exchange or domino chain provided an advantage to the recipient (eg, a younger donor kidney).[74] A major concern expressed by both donors and recipients was the delay caused by the logistics of arranging for paired exchanges or domino chains, even if the delay was relatively short.[75] Time sensitivity is particularly acute for those who are seeking to donate preemptively before their intended recipient needs to begin dialysis. And even if all the logistics are worked out quickly, there may be last-minute circumstances that lead to further delays (eg, an intercurrent illness or the decision by 1 pair not to pursue a paired exchange or domino chain). David Steinberg mentions other logistical challenges that may reduce compatible pair participation:

> There may be a delay in time to transplantation; because there are two or more transplants, there may be limits in scheduling flexibility and raised hopes dashed because of last minute circumstances of one of the pairs. There may also be additional testing, interviews and clinic visits, and further scrutiny for donor suitability if other institutions are involved. Surgeries may be performed at separate hospitals, and the donors and recipients might find themselves in unfamiliar clinical settings.[76]

To examine the ethics of proposing that compatible pairs participate in an exchange or chain, we will again use our living donor ethics framework.

8.5.1 Respect for Persons

A major ethical challenge is how a member of the transplant team morally can ask a compatible donor (Donor 1) to donate to a stranger (Recipient 2) in such a way that Donor 1 does not agree to participate in the exchange against her better judgment.[77] This is why we recommend that KPE be raised even before compatibility testing is done, so that donor- recipient pairs can think about this option while it is only a theoretical possibility, not an actual choice. Being presented with the option of compatible pair participation in a KPE or domino chain after a donor has found out that she can donate directly adds a stressful element of choice and confusion. The request by the transplant team for a donor-recipient pair to participate in an unbalanced exchange is not a neutral act but creates some degree of undue influence or pressure on the donor-recipient pair who may accede in order to please the transplant program where they are registered even if they perceive the exchange to be contrary to their best interests. As such, the offer threatens the voluntariness of the donation. Survey data support our concern. Ratner and colleagues found that 38% of potential recipients and 46% of potential donors stated that the opportunity to participate as a compatible paired would put pressure on them to participate.[78] The concern of undue pressure by the transplant team's request for compatible pairs to participate in an exchange is further exacerbated because opting out also becomes more burdensome if the compatible donor now feels responsible for helping 2 (or more) individuals.

A main reason a compatible pair may not want to participate is that coordinating paired exchanges and domino chains can take time. As such, if a compatible donor-recipient pair is willing to participate, they should determine a priori how long they would be willing to delay.

A second reason compatible pairs may not want to participate is due to mistrust. This may be amplified if some compatible pair participants have poor outcomes. As one of us (LFR) wrote elsewhere:

> The ethical propriety of the request is most likely to be raised when an adverse event occurs. If an individual (Donor 1) is donating to his brother (Recipient 1) and the kidney develops a blood clot, both are harmed in that they suffer a setback to their goals. Imagine, however, that Donor 1 donates to a stranger (Recipient 2), but the kidney his brother is supposed to receive from donor 2 develops a blood clot. Although in both cases, Donor 1 and Recipient 1 are harmed, they might claim in the second case that they also were wronged—treated unjustly—because they did not need to participate in the exchange, but felt compelled to do so because of the request, and the compulsion invalidated their consent.[79]

A third reason that compatible pairs may not want to participate is due to privacy concerns. Although identity sharing is only supposed to occur if all parties agree, unintentional disclosures occur especially if multiple pairs are at the same hospital or the media decides it is a human interest story worth investigating.

To overcome these concerns, John Gill and colleagues from Canada have suggested that compatible exchange kidney donors should be informed that if their intended recipient were to experience early or acute graft failure, that their intended recipient would be given high priority on the deceased donor waitlist for a deceased donor kidney.[80] While this may promote more compatible pairs to participate, we do not believe it is fair. A small number of recipients of living kidney donor grafts do experience acute or early graft failure.[81] This is a known risk that must be discussed in the consent process although it is important to note that this can occur whether the graft is from a biologically or emotionally related donor or from a stranger. When a living donor graft given directly fails, the recipients are not given high priority for a deceased donor organ. Thus, Gill and colleague's proposal unfairly promotes the compatible exchange recipient to the front of the line, an inducement to increase the participation of compatible pairs that cannot be ethically justified. To our knowledge, no program has implemented this proposal.

8.5.2   Beneficence

What are the benefits and risks of compatible pairs participating in paired exchanges or domino chains? As we discussed previously, in many ways, the benefits and harms raised by a paired exchange are the same as the benefits and harms raised by a direct donation. Participation provides the additional benefit for the compatible donor who can now help 2 candidates in end-stage renal disease rather than 1. While some potential donors may be thrilled about this opportunity, others may be ambivalent. Participation in a paired exchange or domino chain introduces additional clinical risk for the compatible donor-recipient pair because there is no guarantee that the quality of the exchange kidney is as good or better than her own.

Some compatible donors may expect their intended recipient to get some additional benefit—whether a kidney from a younger donor or in some other way a better quality kidney. However, even if this is incorporated into the algorithm, there are no guarantee that the outcome is actually better. (Whether it is fair to "trade-up" will be discussed in the following sections on vulnerability and on special relationships creating special obligations).

The psychological risks and benefits of the participation of compatible pairs in paired exchanges or domino chains have not been adequately studied. There is the possibility that direct donation offers a greater psychological benefit to the donor and/or recipient and that recipient compliance with post-transplantation treatment may be better when recipients face their donors on a regular basis. There is also the psychological risk felt by some donors and recipients who now feel responsible for the well-being of either the paired exchange recipient or of the domino chain recipient.

In some cases, it may be the compatible paired recipient who is more positive about participation in an unbalanced paired exchange or domino chain and may put pressure on their intended donors to participate in exchanges or chains even though they could be a direct recipient. Why might a recipient prefer receiving a kidney from a stranger? Marie-Chantal Fortin hypothesizes that donation can "alter the relationships in the sense that recipients might find it easier to manage their indebtedness to an anonymous stranger than to a known donor."[82] Other compatible paired recipients may be ambivalent or even reluctant, but feel pressured to go along with their intended donors. They may fear an additional time delay as well as the risks to which an unknown donor graft exposes them.

8.5.3   Vulnerabilities

Compatible pairs may agree to participate in exchanges or chains due to juridic or deferential vulnerability, in this case due to the tendency of patients to accede to the requests of their physicians, even if they would prefer to do otherwise. Dominick Frosch and colleagues conducted 6 focus groups with 48 people in the San Francisco Bay Area. They found that

> even relatively affluent and well-educated patients feel compelled to conform to socially sanctioned roles and defer to physicians during clinical consultations; that physicians can be authoritarian; and that the fear of being categorized as "difficult" prevents patients from participating more fully in their own health care.[83]

Although the doctor-patient relationship and obstacles to shared decision-making were the subject of these focus groups, the concern can be easily extrapolated to the situation in which the transplant team is encouraging a compatible pair to participate in an unbalanced exchange. Frosch and colleagues explore the fear that participants feel when disagreeing with their provider and the potential for retribution:

> If I were to do that I would think . . . is the guy going to be pissed at me for not doing what he wanted? . . . Is it going to come out in some other way that's going to lower the quality of my treatment? . . . Will he do what I want but . . . resent it and therefore not quite be as good . . . or in some way . . . [be] detrimental to my quality of care. . . .[84]

Frosch and colleagues "argue that physicians may not be aware of a need to create a safe environment for open communication to facilitate shared decision-making."[85] More specifically in the transplant arena, the LDAT needs to realize the perceived juridic vulnerability of compatible donors to requests by their providers and empower the donors to refuse to participate in exchanges that are not necessary for their intended recipient.[86]

Requests for the participation of compatible pairs in exchanges or chains are not focused on the compatible pair's best interest. The transplant team may be focused on the maximal number of transplants (to help the greatest number) rather than to maximally benefit any particular donor-recipient pair. It may be perceived as coercive and may cause psychological burden. While directed kidney donors feel personally responsible for their kidney's function in their intended recipient, now these donors may experience stress and responsibility for 2 recipients—their intended recipient and their exchange recipient.[87]

Emma Clark and colleagues surveyed US kidney transplant programs and found that 32% of programs would encourage compatible pairs with blood type O-donors to participate in paired exchanges and domino chains without reservation and another 21% would encourage compatible pairs with blood type O-donors if the intended recipient could obtain a "better" organ.[88] Madison Cuffy and colleagues suggest incentivizing compatible pairs to participate by ensuring that they receive benefit in the form of "a better quality kidney or a better matched kidney" which they termed "risk mitigation."[89] They cited Sommer Gentry and colleagues at Johns Hopkins who considered a 10-year reduction in kidney donor age as an acceptable benefit.[90] Of note, the Hopkins group showed that designing an algorithm with this risk mitigation strategy does not substantially reduce match rates.[91]

Is it ethical to incentivize compatible donors by suggesting that the exchange will yield a better kidney than their own for their intended recipient? We believe it plays on their medical vulnerability. While some living kidney donor grafts are better than others, often these statistical differences do not have significant clinical implications. As such, the suggestion of an improved graft may be somewhat disingenuous. The transplant team must be transparent about their conflict of interest, which breach the special obligations owed to the living donor. We explore this in the following section.

8.5.4 Special Relationships Create Special Obligations

In 1998 and 2000, one of us (LFR), with colleague Steve Woodle, objected to compatible-incompatible live donor kidney exchanges because of the potential for coercion the donor may experience as the result of "psychological pressure" to "participate in the exchange to maximize the number of organs available."[92] We further noted that "most donors agree to donate because a loved one is ill" and asking them to accept a "more generalized concept of altruism" may be construed as coercive.[93] While Woodle has reversed his position for utilitarian reasons (it will increase the number of possible pairs and exchanges),[94] we remain ethically concerned about such participation unless stringent restrictions are followed, which ensure that the LDAT's primary fiduciary obligation is directed at the compatible donor. While some compatible donors may be glad to learn about the opportunity to participate in a paired exchange or domino exchange, others will not be and it is critical that they not feel pressure to participate. The LDAT's fiduciary obligation to the compatible donor must prevail over the transplant center's desire to increase the number of transplants overall.[95]

Our objection to encouraging compatible pair participation is a minority opinion that highlights our concern that the transplant community does not always treat the living donor as a full patient in her own right. At a minimum, we propose that programs willing to consider the participation of compatible pairs must ensure that 3 criteria are met. First, risks are minimized by explaining the option clearly and thoroughly in as neutral a way as possible before ABO testing and compatibility matching are done. This way, donors can choose whether or not paired exchanges or domino chains are options they would be willing to consider—both in the situation in which they are incompatible (where paired exchanges and domino chains may be their only option other than the potential recipient waiting on the deceased donor waitlist) and where they are compatible with their intended recipient (thus making paired exchanges and domino chains elective and altruistic).

It is less coercive for living donors to consider these options behind a (Rawlsian) veil of ignorance to minimize the pressure that may be felt if a transplant team were to propose an unbalanced exchange after a donor-recipient pair had learned that they were compatible to proceed with direct donation.[96] At that point, a transplant team's proposing participation in an unbalanced paired exchange or domino chain could be harder to refuse and even appear as a manipulative situation. Of course, the recipient would also have to consent in order for the compatible donor-recipient pair to participate in an exchange—either member of the pair can say no and/or change his or her mind. Both the donor and recipient must be given numerous opportunities to refuse because the decision impacts them both as individuals and as a compatible pair.

Second, to reinforce the voluntary nature of compatible pair participation in paired exchanges and domino chains, transplant programs would need to develop procedures to minimize the psychological pressure that donors and their intended recipients may feel to help their providers. For example, transplant programs could require the compatible pair and not the transplant team to re-initiate a discussion of this option after testing is completed. By taking a passive approach, the LDAT attempts to minimize perceived coercion or undue pressure that asking a compatible pair to participate in an unbalanced exchange might cause.

Third, the amount of time that the compatible pair would be willing to delay transplantation in order for the transplant program to coordinate a paired exchange or domino chain should be agreed upon in advance. Given the supererogatory nature of the compatible pair's participation, it should be short (eg, less than 1 month) to avoid an unnecessary delay in which the compatible candidate's health may worsen unnecessarily.

Whether these safeguards are adequate to protect the compatible pair from undue pressure will depend on whether all vulnerabilities can be adequately addressed and compatible donor-recipient pairs can consent freely. We are doubtful, especially about whether transplant team members can truly avoid unintentional pressure because just the act of asking the donor of a compatible pair to participate in an unbalanced chain makes her vulnerable. It implies that she should see her kidneys as a quasi-public good that ought to be allocated to benefit the program rather than herself.

8.6 Exchange Variations: List-Paired Exchanges

Another variation on living paired exchanges are list-paired exchanges (which we initially described in the literature as indirect paired exchanges[97]). This variant (see Figures 8.4 and 8.5) was raised by Robert Sells in the UK in response to our original *New England Journal of Medicine* paper.[98] It involved a relative of a recipient who came from overseas and was then found to be incompatible.

Despite our objections to Sells' proposal, the first list-paired exchanges took place in UNOS region 1 (New England) in the early 2000s.[99] In this protocol, the living donor donated to the waitlist first, and then his or her intended recipient got first choice for the next available ABO-identical deceased organ donor. The intended recipient could (and did) "cherry pick," that is, he or she waited for an ideal kidney to become available. Because the paired recipient is allowed to skip to the front of the queue, a variance from UNOS was required because deceased donor grafts are otherwise allocated according to a strict formula. Region 1 received a variance before they began these exchanges.[100] We did not support the variance because list-paired exchanges disadvantage O-waitlist candidates who do not have a potential incompatible living donor. Today this variance is no longer in effect, although the idea has been recently revived as a means to initiate chains (using a deceased donor rather than a Good Samaritan living donor).[101]

Why are incompatible donor-recipient pairs willing to participate in a list-paired exchange? If the only concern were to get the best kidney, a candidate would prefer a living donor graft. However, some donor-recipient pairs may reject living donor paired exchanges due to concerns around privacy and requests to meet or to avoid other potential obligations to the other pair, real or perceived.

Now in Figure 8.4, the waitlist candidate (recipient 2) is being offered a choice between a living donor kidney versus a deceased donor kidney. The living donor graft is almost always a better graft because living kidney grafts have a longer expected graft survival. However, it is unlikely to be the case that the candidate who would be on top of the match-run for the deceased donor kidney is the same as the candidate who would be on top of the match-run for the living donor kidney due to histocompatibility variation. This means that most list-paired exchanges look more like Figure 8.5 than Figure 8.4. This raises a host of policy issues that would need to be resolved before a list-paired policy could be implemented.

Most candidates who might seek a list-paired exchange would do so because they are of blood type O and their living donor is not. Donor-recipient pairs with O-recipients are unlikely to find a reciprocal living donor-recipient exchange pair.[102] Remember why this is so: the paired donor would need to be of blood type O, but O-donors are universal donors and can donate to their intended recipients who have blood types A, B, or AB.

In a list-paired exchange, the list-paired exchange candidate would get priority for deceased donor kidney of blood type O over the highest ranked person of blood type O on the waitlist, prolonging the wait of the highest ranked individual on the O blood type deceased donor waitlist as well as all other O blood type deceased donor candidates. A deceased donor waitlist candidate of another blood type (A, B, or AB), however, does benefit by getting a living donor kidney in exchange.

The potential harm to waitlist O-candidates was raised by Ross and Woodle before these exchanges were given a variance to proceed from UNOS.[103] The data from Region 1 confirmed our fears. In the first 17 transplants performed, only 1 donor was of blood type O (who had a positive crossmatch with his intended O-recipient) and 16 of the 17 list-paired recipients were of blood type O.[104] Francis Delmonico et al realized that this would lead to an increased wait for those on the waitlist with blood type O who did not have a willing living donor. However, they argued that the harm would be temporary:

the small initial disadvantage to the O-list disappears completely once an exchange program in any given area has been in place for a period equaling the waiting time threshold for unsensitized O-patients in that area.[105]

With a colleague, Stefanos Zenios, one of us (LFR) argued that this is false:

If the pool of transplant candidates is divided into two groups, one group with higher priority and another group with lower (or standard) priority, then the average waiting time for the patients in the standard group will be higher than their average waiting time in a system where no patients enjoy higher priority. This effect is not transient, it persists over time, and can only be mitigated if the supply of organs in the system with priorities is sufficiently higher than in the second system with no priorities (which it will never be). Furthermore, the long-term harm will only get worse as the standard waitlist grows at a faster rate than the supply of kidneys (both living and deceased donor).[106]

Thus, even though the number of organs is increased by the list-paired exchange program, it is increased at the expense of those who are already worst off. O-candidates already have a longer than average wait time, and these exchanges will further disadvantage those who are already worse off. Rawlsian justice permits inequities provided that it benefits those who are already worst off.[107] Thus, list-paired exchanges are inconsistent with a Rawlsian theory of justice by being unfair to those individuals who are already waiting for a deceased blood type O donor kidney.

Bob Veatch, however, argued that inequalities that do not benefit the worst off can be ethical if the least well-off consent to waive the requirements of

Rawlsian justice.[108] That is, Veatch argued that disparities are ethically permissible if those who will be disadvantaged are willing to suffer setbacks for the greater good (to increase the overall number of available organs, even though it means that they will have to wait longer).

To determine if blood type O waitlist candidates would consent to an incremental increase in waiting time, we asked a student, Paul Ackerman (now a neurosurgeon) to interview patients on dialysis about their attitude about list-paired exchanges.[109] While 100% supported ABO-compatible list-paired exchanges, only 57% supported ABO-incompatible list-paired exchanges (p<.001).[110] Half of the respondents of blood type O supported these exchanges even though it would increase their wait.[111] While we were surprised by the degree of altruism shown by those of blood type O, the interests of the nearly half who stated that they would not want to wait any additional time cannot be ignored. Without their support, justice demands that ABO-incompatible list-paired exchanges should not be performed. In contrast, we argued that ABO-compatible list-paired exchanges may be permissible. These were supported by all interviewed dialysis participants, who recognized that they presented no disadvantage to any group of waitlist individuals.[112]

A second issue also arose in the pilot study by Delmonico and colleagues: of the list-paired recipients, 2 had acute graft failure due to renal vein thrombosis. Because they had not planned for this adverse event, both list-paired recipients were given priority for a second deceased donor kidney.[113] Although the original replacement was approved by the UNOS Kidney Pancreas Committee, the Renal Transplant Oversight Committee of Region 1 "subsequently agreed that any future exchange could only offer the opportunity for a single cadaver renal transplantation with this special allocation priority."[114] We agree: if list-paired exchanges are permitted, the living donor-recipient pair must be informed of the risk of acute or early graft failure, the fact that the exchange is a gamble and the organ will not be replaced out of turn, with the recipient of a failed transplanted kidney having to enter the deceased donor waitlist with no accumulated waiting time.

8.7 Conclusion

The original KPE variant between 2 ABO-incompatible donor-recipient pairs (see Figure 8.1) is ethically sound but will only yield a small increase in the number of living donors. Exchange variants such as list-paired exchanges could modestly increase the number of transplants, but they raise ethical issues that should lead to restrictions if not prohibitions on their performance. The participation of compatible pairs in paired exchanges or domino chains could increase the number of transplants performed, but they should not be incentivized, and it is not clear whether one can even ask donors without creating undue pressure. ADPs could also increase the number of transplants but raise many logistical concerns. Domino chains catalyzed by a Good Samaritan donor can significantly increase the number of living donor kidney transplants. We believe that domino chains are ethically permissible provided that the end kidney is allocated to a deceased donor waitlist candidate.

Notes

1. Veale J, Hil G. The National Kidney Registry: transplant chains—beyond paired kidney donation. *Clin Transplant*. 2009:253–264, at pp. 253–254. Reciprocal A/B and B/A means that the first pair had a donor of blood type A and a recipient of blood type B and the second pair had a donor of blood type B and a recipient of blood type A.
2. Rivero E. "Gift certificate" enables kidney donation when convenient and transplant when needed. UCLA Newsroom. July 11, 2016. Last accessed August 19, 2021.https:// newsroom.ucla.edu/releases/gift-certificate-enables-kidney-donation-when-convenient-and-transplant-when-needed
3. Ross LF, Rubin DT, Siegler M, et al. Ethics of a paired-kidney-exchange program. *N Engl J Med*. 1997;336:1752–1755.
4. Rapaport FT. The case for a living emotionally related international kidney donor exchange registry. *Transplant Proceed*. 1986;19(suppl 2):5–9.
5. Park K, Moon JI, Kim SI, Kim YS. Exchange donor program in kidney transplantation. *Transplantation*. 1999;67:336–338.
6. McLellan F. US surgeons do first "triple-swap" kidney transplantation. *Lancet*. 2003;362(9382):456.
7. Montgomery RA, Katznelson S, Bry WI, et al. Successful three-way kidney paired donation with cross-country live donor allograft transport. *Am J Transplant*. 2008;8:2163–2168.
8. These estimates are from Zenios S, Woodle ES, Ross LF. Primum non nocere: avoiding harm to vulnerable candidates in an indirect kidney exchange. *Transplantation*. 2001;72:648–654. Similar estimates were calculated by Segev DL, Gentry SE, Warren DS, Reeb B, Montgomery RA. Kidney paired donation and optimizing the use of live donor organs. *JAMA*.2005;293:1883–1890.

9. Melcher ML, Blosser CD, Baxter-Lowe LA, et al. Dynamic challenges inhibiting optimal adoption of kidney paired donation: findings of a consensus conference. *Am J Transplant.* 2013;13:851–860, at p. 851.
10. Veale and Hill, "The National Kidney Registry."
11. Kidney paired donation pilot program to begin matching in October. United Network for Organ Sharing. Oct 5, 2010. Last accessed 8/19/2021.https://unos.org/news/kidney-paired-donation-pilot-program-to-begin-matching-in-october/
12. One could say ABO-compatible, but due to inequities in waiting time of different ABO-candidates (with those of blood type O having one of the longest waiting times), one can justify limiting this variation to ABO-identical deceased donors so that not every list-paired recipient is eligible for an O-donor, only those candidates who are blood type O themselves.
13. Montgomery RA, Gentry SE, Marks WH, et al. Domino paired kidney donation: a strategy to make best use of live non-directed donation. *Lancet.* 2006;368:419–421.
14. Montgomery is quoted as stating: "And fairness is served because the last paired donor's kidney in the chain is allocated to the next compatible patient on the deceased donor waiting list." See, Hopkins performs historic "six-way domino" kidney transplant. Johns Hopkins Medicine. April 8, 2008. https://www.hopkinsmedicine.org/news/media/releases/hopkins_performs_historic_six_way_domino_kidney_transplant
15. Rees MA, Kopke JE, Pelletier RP, et al. A nonsimultaneous, extended, altruistic-donor chain. *N Engl J Med.* 2009;360:1096–1101. These NEADs are also referred to as "open chains" whereas chains that are terminated by allocating the last paired donor kidney to a candidate on the waitlist is known as a "closed chain." See Gentry SE, Montgomery RA, Segev DL. Controversies in kidney paired donation. *Adv Chronic Kidney Dis.* 2012;19:257–261.
16. National Kidney Registry. NKR Quarterly Reports. Paired Exchange Quarterly Reports. Q1 Results 2020. Published May 6, 2020. Last accessed 8/19/2021.https://www.kidneyregistry.org/pages/p608/Q12020.php
17. Veale and Hill, "The National Kidney Registry."
18. National Organ Transplant Act (NOTA), Pub L No. 98-507. Approved October 19, 1984, at 42 USC § 274e.
19. Charlie W Norwood Living Organ Donation Act, Pub L No. 110-144, 121 Stat 1814 (2007).
20. Krawiec KD, Rees MA. Reverse transplant tourism. *Law Contemp Problems.* 2014;77:145–173, at p. 151.
21. Simmons RG, Marine SK, Simmons RL. *Gift of Life: The Effect of Organ Transplantation on Individual, Family and Societal Dynamics.* New Brunswick, NJ: Transaction Books, 2002.
22. Ross LF. What the medical excuse teaches us about the donor as patient. *Am J Transplant.* 2010;10:731–736.
23. Melcher et al, "Dynamic challenges," at p. 852.
24. Of course, a prospective donor can change her mind. To minimize undue pressure, those donors who do not elect to be considered for paired exchanges and domino

chains upfront would not be recontacted but instead would have to recontact the transplant center personally and ask to be considered for paired exchange or domino chain donation. At that point, the living donor evaluation would proceed.

25. Department of Health and Human Services, Part II. Centers for Medicare and Medicaid Services. 42 CFR Parts 405, 482, 488, and 498. Medicare Program; Hospital Conditions of Participation: Requirements for Approval and Re-Approval of Transplant Centers to Perform Organ Transplants. *Fed Reg.* 2007;72(61):15198–15280. Of note, United Network for Organ Sharing (UNOS)/Organ Procurement and Transplantation Network (OPTN) modified its bylaws the same year. Appendix B, Section XIII, 2007. Updated in current UNOS/OPTN policy handbook in section 14.2 Independent Living Donor Advocate Requirements. Last updated 7/27/21. Last accessed 8/19/21.https://optn.transplant.hrsa.gov/media/1200/optn_policies.pdf

26. Ross et al, "Ethics of a paired."

27. Ross, "What the medical excuse."

28. Ross et al, "Ethics of a paired."

29. Cowan N, Gritsch HA, Nassiri N, Sinacore J, Veale J. Broken chains and reneging: a review of 1748 kidney paired donation transplants. *Am J Transplant.* 2017;17:2451–2457.

30. Serur D, Charlton M, Lawton M, et al. Donors in chains: psychosocial outcomes of kidney donors in paired exchange. *Prog Transplant.* 2014;24:371–374.

31. See, for example, the risk of vascular complications in directed donation: Osman Y, Shokeir A, Ali-el-Dein B, et al. Vascular complications after live donor renal transplantation: study of risk factors and effects on graft and patient survival. *J Urol.* 2003;269:859–862; and Lerman M, Mulloy M, Gooden C, et al. Post transplant renal vein thrombosis, with successful thrombectomy and review of the literature. *Int J Surg Case Rep.* 2019;61:291–293. There are also reports in the literature of the risk of early graft loss in paired kidney exchanges. See, for example, Gurkan A, Kacar S, Varilsuha C, et al. Exchange donor transplantation: ethical options for living renal transplantation. *Transplant Proc.* 2011;43:795–7; and Verbesey J, Thomas AG, Ronin M, et al. Early graft losses in paired kidney exchange. Experience from 10 years of the National Kidney Registry. *Am J Transplant.* 2020;20:1393–1401.

32. See, for example, Sanner MA. Exchanging spare parts or becoming a new person? People's attitudes toward receiving and donating organs. *Soc Sci Med.* 2001;52:1491–1499; and Sharp LA. Organ transplantation as a transformative experience: anthropological insights into the restructuring of the self. *Med Anthropol Q.* 1995;9:357–389.

33. Serur et al, "Donors in chains," at p. 373.

34. Serur et al, "Donors in chains."

35. Serur et al, "Donors in chains."

36. Organ Procurement and Transplantation Network, National Data. Last updated August 18, 2021. Last accessed August 19, 2021. https://optn.transplant.hrsa.gov/data/view-data-reports/

37. See, for example, Voiculescu A, Ivens K, Hetzel GR, et al. Kidney transplantation from related and unrelated living donors in a single German centre. *Nephrol Dial Transplant.* 2003;18:418–425; Ahmad N, Ahmed K, Kahn MS, et al. Living-unrelated donor renal transplantation: an alternative to living-related donor transplantation?

Ann R Coll Surg. 2008;90:247–250; and Simforoosh N, Shemshaki H, Nadjafi-Semnani M, Sotoudeh M. Living related and living unrelated kidney transplantations: a systematic review and meta-analysis. *World J Transplant.* 2017;7:152–160.

38. Waterman AD, Schenk EA, Barrett AC, et al. Incompatible kidney donor candidates' willingness to participate in donor-exchange and non-directed donation. *Am J Transplant.* 2006:6:1631–1638.

39. Rodrigue JR, Leishman R, Vishnevsky T, Evenson A, Mandelbrot DA. Concerns of ABO incompatible and crossmatch-positive potential donors and recipients about participating in kidney exchanges. *Clin Transplant.* 2015;29:233–241.

40. See Waterman, "Incompatible kidney"; and Rodrigue, "Concerns of ABO incompatible."

41. Steinberg D. Compatible-incompatible live donor kidney exchanges. *Transplantation.* 2011;91:257–260, at p. 258 (reference omitted). Ironically, blood safety studies find that "Directed donors had a significantly higher prevalence of positive tests for anti-HTLV-I (relative risk 2.32) and HBsAg (relative risk 1.99)." See Kruskall MS, Umlas J. Acquired immunodeficiency syndrome and directed blood donations: a dilemma for American medicine. *Arch Surg.* 1988;123:23–25; and Pink J, Thomson A, Wylie B. Infectious disease markers in autologous and directed donations. *Transfus Med.* 1994;4:135–138. One of the explanations is that data were flawed because they compared the prevalence of positive tests in directed donors (which involved 60%–70% first-time donors), compared to a much lower percentage of first-time donors in community volunteer donors, and repeat donors are known to be safer than first-time donors.

42. See, for example, Peng A, Vo A, Jordan SC. Transplantation of the highly human leukocyte antigen-sensitized patient: long-term outcomes and future directions. *Transplant Rev.* 2006;20:146–156; Montgomery RA, Lonze BE, King KE, et al. Desensitization in HLA-incompatible kidney recipients and survival. *N Engl J Med.* 2011;365:318–326; Marfo K, Lu A, Ling M, Akalin E. Desensitization protocols and their outcome. *Clin J Am Soc Nephrol.* 2011;6:922–936; Lo P, Sharma A, Craig JC, et al. Preconditioning therapy in ABO-incompatible living kidney transplantation: a systematic review and meta-analysis. *Transplantation.* 2016;100:933–942; and Huang E, Jordan SC. Kidney transplantation in adults: HLA desensitization. *UpToDate.* Literature review current through July 2021. This topic last updated January 8, 2021. https://www.uptodate.com/contents/kidney-transplantation-in-adults-hla-desensitization

43. See, for example, Montgomery RA. Renal transplantation across HLA and ABO antibody barriers: integrating paired donation into desensitization protocols. *Am J Transplant.* 2010;10:449–57l; Yabu JM, Pando MJ, Busque S, Melcher ML, et al. Desensitization combined with paired exchange leads to successful transplantation in highly sensitized kidney transplant recipients: strategy and report of five cases. *Transplant Proc.* 2013;45:82–7; and Pham TA, Lee JI, Melcher ML, et al. Kidney paired exchange and desensitization: strategies to transplant the difficult to match kidney patients with living donors. *Transplant Rev.* 2017;31:29–34.

44. Melcher et al, "Dynamic challenges."

45. See, for example, Simmons RG, Hickey K, Kjellstrand CM, Simmons RL. Family tension in the search for a kidney donor. *JAMA*. 1971;215:909–912; and Simmons RG, Klein SD. Family noncommunication: the search for kidney donors. *Am J Psychiatry*. 1972;129(6):687–692.

46. Ross, "What the medical excuse."

47. Sack K. 60 lives, 30 kidneys, all linked. *The New York Times*. February 18, 2012:A1. Last accessed August 19, 2021. https://www.nytimes.com/2012/02/19/health/lives-forever-linked-through-kidney-transplant-chain-124.html

48. See, for example, Rapaport, "The case" and Woodle ES, Daller JA, Aeder M, et al. Ethical considerations for participation of nondirected living donors in kidney exchange programs. *Am J Transplant*. 2010;10:1460–1467.

49. De Klerk M. The Dutch Living Donor Kidney Exchange Program. Thesis. Printed by Ridderprint offsetdrukkerij b.v., Ridderkerk; 2010. De Klerk discusses policies around Europe.

50. Klerk de M, "The Dutch," at p. 26.

51. Kranenburg LW, Visak T, Weimar W, et al. Starting a crossover kidney transplantation program in the Netherlands: ethical and psychological considerations. *Transplantation*. 2004;78:194–197.

52. Kranenburg L, Zuidema W, Vanderkroft P, et al. The implementation of a kidney exchange program does not induce a need for additional psychosocial support. *Transpl Int*. 2007;20:432–439.

53. Slaats D, Lennerling A, Pronk MC, et al. Donor and recipient perspective on anonymity in kidney donation from live donors: a multicenter survey study. *Am J Kidney Dis*. 2018;71:52–64.

54. Rapaport, "The case."

55. Cowan et al, "Broken chains."

56. Veale and Hil, "The National Kidney Registry" and Melcher ML, Veale JL, Javaid B, et al. Kidney transplant chains amplify benefit of nondirected donors. *JAMA Surg*. 2013;148:165–169.

57. See, for example, Dickerson JP, Procaccia AD, Sandholm T. Optimizing Kidney Exchange with Transplant Chains: Theory and Reality. In: *Proceedings of the 11th International Conference on Autonomous Agents and Multiagent Systems (AAMAS 2012)*. Conitzer, Winikoff, Padgham, van der Hoek, eds. June 4–8, 2012, Valencia, Spain; and Bray M, Wang W, Song PX-K, et al. Planning for uncertainty and fallbacks can increase the number of transplants in a kidney-paired donation program. *Am J Transplant*. 2015;15:2636–2645.

58. Rawls J. *A Theory of Justice*. Cambridge, MA: Belknap Press of Harvard University Press; 1971.

59. Actually, there were some exclusions in the Minnesota protocol to maximize the life-years gained by the nondirected donor, the ethics of which one of us discussed elsewhere. See Ross LF. Solid organ donations between strangers. *J Law Med Ethics*. 2002;30:440–445, at pp. 442–443.

60. It would be even fairer if the kidney were allocated to the candidate at the top of the waitlist using a national run, but this would take away the incentive of the transplant

center to engage Good Samaritan donors who present to their institution from participating in national paired exchanges or domino chains in order to ensure that their patients and their institution benefited directly from the Good Samaritan donor.

61. Liu W, Treat E, Veale JL, Milner J, Melcher ML. Identifying opportunities to increase the throughput of kidney paired donation. *Transplantation.* 2015;99:1410–1415, at p. 1410.
62. Liu et al, "Identifying opportunities."
63. Holscher CM, Jackson K, Thomas AG. Temporal changes in the composition of a large multicenter kidney exchange clearinghouse: do the hard-to-match accumulate? *Am J Transplant.* 2018;18:2791–2797.
64. Ross LF, Rodrigue J, Veatch RM. Ethical and logistical issues raised by the advanced donation program "pay it forward" scheme. *J Med Philos.* 2017;42:518–536, at p. 522 (references omitted).
65. Hawryluk, M. To give his grandson a kidney, grandfather creates organ transplant voucher. The Bulletin. Updated Feburary 4, 2020, Last accessed August 19, 2021. https://www.bendbulletin.com/lifestyle/health/to-give-his-grandson-a-kidney-gran dfather-creates-organ-transplant-voucher/article_051abbcd-8535-5f04-9d7a-5b6fe 0972ec1.html; and Ross et al, "Ethical and logistical."
66. Veale JL, Nassiri N, Capron AM, et al. Voucher-Based Kidney Donation and Redemption for Future Transplant. *JAMA Surg.* 2021 Jun 23;e212375. doi:10.1001/jamasurg.2021.2375. Online ahead of print. Last accessed August 20, 2021.
67. Ross et al, "Ethical and logistical," at p. 533.
68. Ross et al, "Ethical and logistical."
69. Ross LF, Woodle ES. Kidney exchange programs: an expanded view of the ethical issues. In: Touraine JL, Traeger J, Betuel H, Dubernard JM, Revillard JP, Dupuy C, eds. *Organ Allocation: Proceedings of the 30th International Conference on Transplantation and Clinical Immunology.* Dordrecht: Kluwer Academic Publishers; 1998:285–295.
70. Ross LF. The ethical limits in expanding living donor transplantation. *Kennedy Inst Ethics J.* 2006;16:151–172, at p. 156. Doubly altruistic is a poor word choice to the extent that we believe that emotionally related donors are not fully altruistic. See, Glannon W, Ross LF. Do genetic relationships create moral obligations in organ transplantation? *Cambridge Q Health Care Eth.* 2002;11:153–159.
71. Gentry SE, Segev DL, Simmerling M, Montgomery RA. Expanding kidney paired donation through participation by compatible pairs. *Am J Transplant.* 2007;7:2361–2370.
72. Durand C, Duplantie A, Fortin MC. Transplant professionals' proposals for the implementation of an altruistic unbalanced paired kidney exchange program. *Transplantation.* 2014;98:754–759.
73. Kranenburg LW, Zuidema W, Weimar W, et al. One donor, two transplants: willingness to participate in altruistically unbalanced exchange donation. *Transpl Int.* 2006;19:995–999.
74. Ratner LE, Rana A, Ratner ER, et al. The altruistic unbalanced paired kidney exchange: proof of concept and survey of potential donor and recipient attitudes. *Transplantation.* 2010;89:15–22.

75. Ratner et al, "The altruistic unbalanced."
76. Steinberg, "Compatible-incompatible," at p. 258.
77. Ross, "The ethical limits."
78. Ratner LE, Ratner ER, Kelly J, et al. Altruistic unbalanced paired kidney exchange at Columbia University/New York-Presbyterian Hospital: rationale and practical considerations. *Clin Transplant*. 2008:107–112.
79. Ross, "The ethical limits," at p. 158. Of note, I have changed the donor and recipient labels (eg, Donor 1) in the quote to match the donor and recipient labels in Figure 8.3. In the original article, Joel Feinberg's discussion about the difference between being harmed and being wronged was cited. See Feinberg J. *Harm to Others: The Moral Limits of the Criminal Law*. New York, NY: Oxford University Press; 1984, at pp. 34–35.
80. Gill JS, Tinckam K, Fortin MC, et al. Reciprocity to increase participation of compatible living donor and recipient pairs in kidney paired donation. *Am J Transplant*. 2017;17:1723–1728.
81. See, for example, Osman et al, "Vascular complications"; Lerman et al, "Post transplant"; and Haljamäe U, Nyberg G, Sjöström B. Remaining experiences of living kidney donors more than 3 yr after early recipient graft loss. *Clin Transplant*. 2003:17:503–510.
82. Fortin M-C. Is it ethical to invite compatible pairs to participate in exchange programmes? *J Med Ethics*. 2013;39:743–747, at p. 746.
83. Frosch DL, May SG, Rendle KAS, Tietbohl C, Elwyn G. Authoritarian physicians and patients' fear of being labeled "difficult" among key obstacles to shared decision making. *Health Affairs*. 2012;31:1030–1038, at p. 1030.
84. Frosch et al, "Authoritarian," at p. 1032.
85. Frosch et al, "Authoritarian," at p. 1030.
86. Although beyond the scope of this book, the compatible recipient may also feel deferentially vulnerable—both to the donor and to the donor's health care team (LDAT). This points to the importance of explaining all options upfront both to the donor and the candidate such that options not acceptable to either the donor or the recipient are not re-addressed after HLA and compatibility testing are done if that is what they chose. Of course, the potential donor can change her mind. This is discussed in reference 24.
87. Baines LS, Dulku H, Jindal RM, Papalois V. Risk taking and decision making in kidney paired donation: a qualitative study by semistructured interviews. *Transplant Proc*. 2018;50:1227–1235.
88. Clark E, Hanto R, Rodrigue JR. Barriers to implementing protocols for kidney paired donation and desensitization: survey of U.S. transplant programs. *Prog Transplant*. 2010; 20:357–365.
89. Cuffy MC, Ratner LE, Siegler M, Woodle ES. Equipoise: ethical, scientific, and clinical trial design considerations for compatible pair participation in kidney exchange programs. *Am J Transplant*. 2015;15:1484–1489.
90. Gentry SE, Montgomery RA, Segev DL. Kidney paired donation: fundamentals, limitations, and expansions. *Am J Kidney Dis*. 2011;57:144–151.

91. Gentry et al, "Kidney paired donation: fundamentals."
92. Ross and Woodle, "Ethical issues," at p. 1540. See also Ross and Woodle, "Kidney exchange programs."
93. Ross and Woodle, "Ethical issues," at p. 1540.
94. Cuffy et al, "Equipoise."
95. Rodwin MA. Strains in the fiduciary metaphor: divided physician loyalties and obligations in a changing health care system. *Am J Law Med.* 1995;21(2–3):241–257, at p. 251.
96. The concept of the veil of ignorance is an integral part of Rawl's theory of justice. See Rawls, *A Theory,* at pp. 136–142.
97. Ross and Woodle, "Ethical issues."
98. Sells RA. Paired-kidney-exchange programs. *N Engl J Med.* 1997;337:1392–1393.
99. Delmonico FL, Morrissey PE, Lipkowitz GS, et al. Donor kidney exchanges. *Am J Transplant.* 2004;4:1628–1634.
100. The OPTN/UNOS Kidney transplantation Committee explains:

    A list exchange variance was in effect in OPTN/UNOS Regions 1, 2, 5, 9 and 11 from 2001–2014, ending when the new Kidney Allocation System (KAS) was implemented in December 2014. Region 1 had the highest volume of list exchanges during this time. In 2004, the New England Organ Bank established the New England Program for Kidney Exchange (NEPKE) and expanded the standard list exchange variance to include list exchange chains in KPD. Three candidates received a deceased donor transplant from NEPKE list exchange chains. (references omitted)

    OPTN/UNOS Kidney Transplantation Committee. Allowing Deceased Donor-Initiated Kidney Paired Donation (KPD) Chains. OPTN. Last accessed August 19, 2021.https://optn.transplant.hrsa.gov/media/2219/kidney_pcconcepts_201707. pdf, at p. 7.
101. Melcher ML, Roberts JP, Leichtman AB, Roth AE, Rees MA. Utilization of deceased donor kidneys to initiate living donor chains. *Am J Transplant.* 2016;16:1367–1370.
102. Of note, in the NKR registry, Flechner and colleagues deny that donor-recipient pairs with recipients of blood type O and high sensitization accumulate, although they do acknowledge that:

    . . . the predominant characteristics of those unmatched candidates were 74% ABO blood type O and 29% cPRA = 100%. While the difficulty to find donors for these hard-to-match recipients has thus far depended on the entry of blood type O nondirected donors for chain initiation, future expansion of KPD via increasing network pool sizes, compatible pair enrollments, the possibility of deceased donor chain initiation, and global sharing may further expand these opportunities. (references omitted)

    See, Flechner SM, Thomas AG, Ronin M, et al. The first 9 years of kidney paired donation through the National Kidney Registry: characteristics of donors and recipients compared with National Live Donor Transplant Registries. *Am J Transplant.* 2018;18:2730–2738, at p. 2737

103. Ross and Woodle, "Ethical issues"; and Ross and Woodle, "Kidney exchange programs."
104. Delmonico et al, "Donor kidney exchanges."
105. Delmonico et al, "Donor kidney exchanges," at p. 1632.
106. Ross LF, Zenios S. Practical and ethical challenges to paired exchange programs. *Am J Transplant.* 2004;4:1553–1554, at p. 1554.
107. Rawls, *A Theory.*
108. Veatch RM. *Transplantation Ethics.* Washington, DC: Georgetown University Press; 2000. In the second edition of this book, which was co-authored by one of us (LFR), we discuss the controversy and agree that the ABO-incompatible list-paired exchange is not fair to those of blood type O.
109. Ackerman PD, Thistlethwaite JR Jr, Ross LF. Attitudes of Minority patients with end stage renal disease regarding ABO-incompatible list-paired exchanges. *Am J Transplant.* 2006:6:83–88.
110. Ackerman, "Attitudes."
111. Ackerman, "Attitudes."
112. On reflection, even ABO-compatible list-paired exchanges may create ethical issues, particularly if the person who would have matched to the deceased donor was an individual with an elevated PRA who had a very low likelihood of finding another match. While this issue goes beyond the scope of our book, we note that this argument starts with an assumption that a matched run candidate has some "ownership" of the kidney.
113. Delmonico et al, "Donor kidney exchanges," at p. 1633.
114. Delmonico et al, "Donor kidney exchanges," at p. 1633.

9

Expanding Living Donor Liver Transplantation

Case 9-1: It was the best of times.

On November 27, 1989, *The New York Times* detailed the plan for the first United States (US) liver transplant using a graft from a live donor. Gina Kolata wrote:

Surgeons at the University of Chicago are to perform the nation's first liver transplant from a living donor today, ushering in what is widely expected to be a new era in transplantation.

The surgical team, led by Dr. Christopher Broelsch, planned to remove a section of liver from a 29-year old Texas woman, Teresa A. Smith, and transplant it into her 21-month-old daughter, Alyssa.[1]

Twenty-five years later, on November 27, 2014, the Associated Press published an update. Alyssa Riggan and her mother were both doing well.[2] One of us (JRT) is quoted reminiscing about the procedure:

"I can tell you we were all extremely concerned about the safety of the mother, Teri, who was just a trouper throughout," Thistlethwaite said. "We were really thankful she got through the operation safely. The feeling when Alyssa's operation was finished was one of elation that it appeared to be a success. . . . It was a feeling we had really done something worthwhile that would help, not just this patient, but others as well."[3]

Case 9-2: It was the worst of times.

The media has also played a major role in publicizing when living donor liver transplantation (LDLT) goes awry. On January 15, 2002, *The New York Times* published the story of Mike and Adam Hurwitz:

The Living Organ Donor as Patient. Lainie Friedman Ross and J. Richard Thistlethwaite, Jr, Oxford University Press.
© Oxford University Press 2022. DOI: 10.1093/oso/9780197618202.003.0009

A healthy 57-year-old man died on Sunday at Mount Sinai Hospital in Manhattan from surgical complications after an operation in which he donated part of his liver to provide a transplant for his brother. The [recipient] brother, 54, is recovering.[4]

The following day, January 16, 2002, *The New York Times* reported that Mount Sinai was temporarily halting their LDLT program:

The hospital, which uses more living donors for liver transplants than any other hospital in the United States, said the operations for adult recipients would be stopped while it investigated the case of the 57-year-old man who died on Sunday, 3 days after donating part of his liver to his brother, 54. The brother survived.[5]

9.1 The History of Living Liver Transplant

In 1963, Thomas Starzl attempted 5 deceased donor liver transplants (DDLT)—the first on a child and the next 4 on adults—all with poor results.[6] After a self-imposed moratorium, his next 8 attempts in 1967 involved deceased donor liver grafts into pediatric recipients with half surviving more than 1 year.[7] However, it was not until the mid-1980s, with improvements in organ preservation and the development of effective immunosuppression that liver transplant became a viable therapeutic option.[8]

Between March 1971 and April 1998, Starzl and his team transplanted 808 children (<18 years of age).[9] However, young children were more likely to die on the deceased donor liver waitlist than their adult counterparts because of the lack of appropriately sized deceased donor grafts. This led to the development of 2 deceased donor liver techniques: reduced-size[10] (or literally trimming the graft to decrease its size) and split-liver[11] (where the 2 lobes of the liver can be given to 2 candidates, often the larger graft given to an adult and the smaller graft given to a child). These methods decreased but did not eliminate waitlist mortality for infants and children.[12] However, the split-liver technique paved the way for LDLT where 1 lobe remains in the donor and the other lobe serves as a living liver graft. The technique was first attempted with living donors for pediatric recipients in 1988 and 1989 in Brazil, but the recipients failed to survive beyond the early postoperative period.[13]

Russell Strong et al in Australia are credited with performing the first successful LDLT using a left lateral segment (LLS) from a mother to her son.[14] At the same time, the University of Chicago was developing a research protocol that was approved by the institution's institutional review board (IRB) to perform pediatric living donor liver transplantation (pLDLT). The University had decided to do the procedure under a research protocol because the outcomes for both the donors and the recipients were unknown. We (JRT was a member of the team) published the plan in the *New England Journal of Medicine* in 1989 to promote discussion within the liver transplant community regarding the ethical issues that the procedure raised.[15] We performed our first case later that year (see case 9-1) and published our first series of 20 cases 2 years later.[16]

Adoption of pLDLT in the US occurred slowly. As Cronin and colleagues explained:

> Only after the favorable results of this clinical trial had been published did several leading liver-transplantation programs in the United States, Europe, and Asia begin transplanting liver grafts from living donors into carefully selected children. Substantial technical modifications have improved the procedure, which is now usually effective and safe for both the recipient and the donor. More than 1500 such surgeries have been performed throughout the world. Only two donors have died, although it is possible that there have been unreported deaths among donors.[17]

The first successful LDLT between 2 adults was performed in Japan in 1993 using the donor's left lobe.[18] Because "[t]he smaller left hepatic lobe provides insufficient hepatic mass for most adult Americans, who are often physically larger than most Asians,[19] most US centers did not initially develop adult-to-adult living donor liver transplantation (aLDLT) programs.

A right lobe LDLT had been performed by the Kyoto group in 1992 for transplantation from an adult into a 9-year-old recipient. The right lobe was procured because the donor's left lobe vascular anatomy was not conducive to left lobe procurement and transplantation.[20] The first right hepatic lobe aLDLT was reported from a team in Hong Kong in 1996,[21] and the first one in the US was reported in 1998 by a team from the University of Colorado.[22] The Colorado team's success led to rapid development of aLDLT programs in the US, without many of the precautions taken in the development of pLDLT programs. We discuss the lack of precautions and their consequences in the next section.

9.2 Too Fast Too Soon? Death of a Living Donor

In 2000, a survey was developed and submitted to all US transplant centers to determine the number of programs performing or planning to perform aLDLT, the size and characteristics of these programs, and their criteria for evaluation of potential donors and recipients. Data were submitted by "84 of the 122 programs (69 percent) describing the results of 449 adult-to-adult transplantations."[23] These centers performed 2,878 liver transplantations in 1999, representing 62% of all liver transplantations performed in the US that year. Half of these programs (42 of 83 programs) already had performed at least 1 aLDLT, and 32 of the remaining 41 centers (78%) were planning to initiate an aLDLT within the next year. At the time of the survey, only 13 US centers had performed greater than 10 cases of aLDLT, and collectively these 13 centers had performed 80% of all aLDLTs. However, only 11% of liver transplant programs that responded to this survey had no intention of performing LDLT.[24]

Was this too fast too soon? In December 2000, the National Institutes of Health (NIH) and the American Association for the Study of Liver Diseases cosponsored a 2-day workshop entitled "Living Donor Liver Transplantation" to review the scientific, medical and nonmedical issues associated with LDLT.[25] The conference report attempted to summarize what was known about LDLT. The data about short- and long-term risks were scant. Mitchell Shiffman and colleagues created a table of complications based on 10 of the largest series that had been published, which found bile duct strictures to be the most common complication occurring in 3%–8% of all living donors.[26] Other complications were found in 2% or less of living donors. Liver function declines were found to be temporary with bilirubin and prothrombin time returning to normal within 3–5 days.[27] Mortality information was not available. Shiffman and colleagues explained:

Before this NIH-sponsored conference, reports regarding donor deaths had circulated in the transplant community. However, at the time of this meeting, no reports describing the events that contributed to donor mortality had been published. Mortality for donors undergoing left-lateral segmentectomy for pediatric recipients has been reported to be in the range of 0.1% to 0.2%. At this conference, one donor death was formally acknowledged of 123 adult LDLTs performed in Europe, and one donor death, of an estimated 400 procedures performed in the United States.[28]

The NIH report pointed out 3 concerns associated with the adoption of LDLT by US transplant programs. First, they noted the difference between how the transplant community proceeded with pLDLT versus aLDLT:

> Unfortunately, a similar path has not been followed for LDLT in adults. The adult operation was never studied in a formal protocol, and recipient indications were not formally defined. Despite this, the procedure has gained widespread popularity and has been embraced by both the medical and lay communities.[29]

Second, the NIH report expressed concern that there was no consensus regarding who were the appropriate recipients (those acutely ill versus those more clinically stable), what the appropriate living donor work-up should entail (with wide variation on the use of invasive testing), and what surgical technique should be used.[30] Third, the report lamented the lack of a "regulatory body or registry [that] currently tracks living donation and donor mortality."[31]

Six months after the NIH meeting, in an article published in *The New England Journal of Medicine,* David Cronin and colleagues at the University of Chicago expressed concern that many key aspects of the use of living donor grafts for aLDLT remained unclear. Specifically, they pointed to both the lack of agreement on both the technique that is most effective and that provides the greatest safety for donor and recipient, as well as the lack of clearly defined or standardized indications for the surgery.[32] They also expressed serious reservations:

> [T]he rapid proliferation of programs that perform transplantation in adults with the use of grafts from living donors (most of those in the United States have performed fewer than 10 procedures each) is alarming for an innovative, nonstandardized operation that places two people, one of whom is healthy, at risk.[33]

Their concerns were prescient, but misdirected. In 2002, a living donor death occurred at Mount Sinai hospital, the most experienced center in the US (see case 9-2). The negative publicity from this case led to a significant decrease in both the number of LDLT and the number of liver transplant programs that performed aLDLT in the US.[34] While 524 LDLT were performed in 2001 (including 112 pLDLT and 412 aLDLT), only 363 LDLT were performed in 2002 (including 73 pLDLT and 290 aLDLT) and it fell further in 2003 (total 322 LDLT including 68 pLDLT and 254 aLDLT). The number of LDLTs performed in the US remained under 300 for the next decade.[35] There has been a large upswing in the number of deceased and living liver transplants with LDLT since 2014, reaching its 2001 peak level of 524 LDLT in 2019.[36] Nevertheless, aLDLT is currently being performed only in 35 centers across the US and only 10 centers are performing more than 10 aLDLT annually.[37]

Who are the living liver donors? The majority of living liver donors in the US are first-degree relatives. According to the UNOS database, between January 1, 1988 and August 20, 2021, there have been 8127 LDLT involving 2111 adult children donating to their parents (26.0%), 1528 parents donating to their (mostly minor) children (18.9%), and 1060 siblings (13.0%) accounting for 57.8% of all LDLT. Another 420 (5.2%) living donors are spouses or life partners.[38] Data from Japanese transplant centers shows that in aLDLT, graft survival was highest in adult children donating to their parents, followed by siblings/spouses and lowest in parents donating to their adult children.[39] Similar results are shown in an international review on the importance of donor age (for both deceased and living donors) on graft survival.[40] These results may create some undue pressure on potential donors and will be explored in the vulnerabilities section 9.3.4.

9.3 Is It Ethical to Perform aLDLT?

We evaluate aLDLT using our living donor ethics framework which consists of 5 principles: (1) respect for persons, (2) beneficence, (3) justice, (4) vulnerabilities, and (5) special relationships creating special obligations.

9.3.1 Respect for Persons

The principle of respect for persons focuses on whether the living liver donor is acting autonomously and can give a voluntary and informed consent, free of undue pressure. Some ethicists objected to the original University of Chicago pLDLT protocol on the grounds that the "parents should not be offered the procedure because they will find it extremely difficult to refuse."[41] Arthur Caplan asked, "Does anyone really think parents can say 'No' when the option is certain death for their own son or daughter?"[42] George Annas also argued that "The parents basically can't say no."[43] These are valid concerns: a study of parents who donated to their children in chronic liver failure found that the parents admitted that their child's illness left them "no choice" such that they did not employ a reasoned decision-making process:

> Virtually all of the donors, 14 out of the 15 donors interviewed, reported that they never really made a decision to be a donor. Rather, agreeing to donate was an "automatic leap" they made upon first hearing of the possibility.[44]

As Robert Crouch and Carl Elliott noted, this threat to autonomy (coercion) "comes not from another person but from the agent" him- or herself.[45] And yet this "internal coercion" may not be inconsistent with autonomy. Mark Siegler and John Lantos, ethicists involved in the University of Chicago pLDLT protocol design, wrote:

> [the "internal coercion"] may be unavoidable but may also be indistinguishable, in many cases, from laudable psychological motivations for donation. In any case, this sort of coercion is not unique to organ transplantation. The need to balance selfishness and altruism is a universal feature of an individual's relationship with his or her family. Because this is a universal element of human interaction, we do not think that it invalidates voluntary consent.[46]

Empirical studies confirm the analysis offered by Siegler and Lantos. Christina Papachristou and colleagues found in in-depth interviews that "a complete absence of coercion on the decision to donate seems unrealistic because of the dynamics initiated by the life-threatening condition of the recipient."[47] Veronique Fournier and her ethics colleagues in France describe being invited to interview potential donors for LDLT (mainly parents), and coming to realize that their goal of determining whether the donor's consent was autonomous and free of coercion was "insufficient," if not misguided.

> . . . we gradually shifted the main focus of the pre-transplant screening interview away from the single goal of evaluating as external observers freedom of donor consent . . . but rather help them [the prospective donors] to clarify their own mind and decision. They use the meeting as

an opportunity to express their doubts and questions freely. It is valuable to them, because they tend to suffer from a lack of such outlets for their concerns, being reluctant to burden family and friends with questions other than those related to the recipient's survival, and they are unwilling to open up to clinical teams due to their fear they will be disqualified as good donors. Today, we are fully convinced that, the most appropriate role for an ethics team in LDLT is to empower and fully support donors.[48]

That is, Fournier and colleagues shifted to a more relational conception of autonomy in which the ethics team helps potential donors think about their own values and interests and supports them in their decision-making process both pre- and post-transplantation rather than focusing on whether to endorse or disqualify a potential donor because of expressions of anxiety, ambivalence, and even familial pressure.[49] Citing Lisa Anderson-Shaw and colleagues, Fournier and colleagues note that they now describe their role as one of "donor advocacy."[50]

To have an effective consent conversation, potential donors must be informed about the potential donor benefits and risks as well as the potential recipient benefits and risks (discussed under §9.3.2 Beneficence). A broad consent discussion requires that the transplant community do a better job of quantifying the benefits and risks of graft procurement from living liver donors (including differential risks of different procurement procedures). However, the consent process should be more robust than a provision of a litany of risks and benefits. The living donor advocate team (LDAT) which includes a living donor advocate (LDA) and other transplant professionals focused on the donor's well-being should not merely accept a potential donor's unreflective claim that donor benefits outweigh donor risks as an expression of authentic unalterable donor autonomy. Rather, the LDAT should engage with the potential donor in a shared decision-making process that helps her exercise her autonomy and make an informed decision consistent with her interests, beliefs, and values.[51] The transplant team should engage donors in a discussion of what impact the donation will have both short-term and long-term on relationships, jobs, and lifestyle, and what would happen if a serious adverse event occurred. We support a multi-step process in which the donor has discussions with various members of the LDAT who help ensure that the donor identifies and understands the range of risks and benefits, the meaning of donation for the donor, her motivations and how the donation fits into her life plans, and that she is aware of the therapeutic options that exist given the expanding non-transplant alternatives for some liver disease.[52]

Of course, LDLT involves 2 patients: the donor and the recipient. The recipient must also give consent and there may be some recipients who are not willing to accept a living liver donor graft because they may be unwilling to let a family member (the most likely living liver donor) to take such risks on their behalf.

9.3.2 Beneficence

In the context of LDLT, there must be a positive net balance of benefits over risks to the donor as well as to the recipient. The main donor benefit is psychological: the donor benefits from helping the recipient and the post-donation companionship. Even in the case of a failed transplant, the donor benefits from at least trying (eg, "I did all I could"). A Good Samaritan living liver donor with no ties to the recipient can benefit psychologically as well, knowing that an unknown recipient has been given another chance at life.[53]

The recipient benefit is obvious: liver transplantation is life-saving. In 2000, graft and recipient outcome survival were better with fewer biliary complications with DDLT (in which candidates received an entire liver) compared with recipient outcomes from a living liver lobe transplant.[54] In contrast, the Adult-to-Adult Living Donor Liver Transplantation (A2ALL) Consortium collected retrospective and prospective data from January 1998 through January 2014 and found better unadjusted survival in LDLT recipients. This survival advantage was attenuated after risk adjustment (hazard ratio = 0.98, $P = 0.90$) as LDLT recipients had lower mean model for end-stage liver disease (MELD) scores (15.5 vs 20.4); fewer received their liver transplant while they required treatment in the intensive care unit, or were even on an inpatient unit; and fewer were undergoing dialysis, were being ventilated, or had ascites.[55] Similarly, a retrospective study from the University of Pittsburgh in 2019 found that recipients who received a living donor graft at their center had better outcomes compared with those who received a deceased donor graft, although they admitted that "the 2 recipient groups are different with notably higher MELD scores and longer waiting times in the DDLT group."[56] Abhinav Humar and colleagues also noted similar findings from other studies:

[T]here have been now several single-center analyses, national data analysis, and multicenter analysis that have all demonstrated superior outcomes with LDLT versus DDLT, especially beyond a certain learning curve for the center. Despite this, very few centers have embraced the procedure, and it continues to be utilized by only a few programs in often selected situations, mainly in patients with lower acuity of illness.[57]

Recipient risks are common (~40% of recipients of living donor liver grafts in both the US and Europe).[58] The most common risk is a biliary complication which can be quite serious. Other serious risks include hepatic artery thrombosis and acute graft failure requiring retransplantation.[59]

For the donor, the main benefits are psychological: the psychological benefit of saving the recipient's life, enhanced self-esteem, and a positive impact on the donor-recipient relationship.[60] However, a positive impact is not assured. Some studies find new strain on the donor-recipient relationship because of recipient guilt and indebtedness but also distress about donor judgment regarding recipient lifestyle and adherence.[61] Others show that the psychological benefits are often dependent on recipient outcomes.[62]

Strong also proposed that the wide variation in reported donor complications in the literature was due to the "inconsistency in the definition of what constitutes a complication." However, as Strong explains, "This should not be the case, because the donor is an otherwise healthy individual who is undergoing surgery, not for his or her own benefit, but to save the life of another, and any adverse event is a complication."[63]

Two developments have improved the reporting of complications in living liver donors. First was the development of the Clavien system for surgical complications[64] and its adoption to living liver donation.[65] Second were the results from the A2ALL Consortium that studied 245 living liver donors and found that 148 donors (38%) had a total of 220 complications, with 82 donors (21%) having 1 complication and an additional 66 (17%) having 2 or more.[66] In comparison, a recent worldwide survey reported a donor morbidity rate of 24%, but these results must be interpreted with some hesitation given the potential for under-reporting bias in a voluntary survey.[67] These reports do make clear, however, that the extent of donor morbidity is significantly greater than many earlier studies reported.[68]

Although morbidity and mortality occur in all 3 donor partial hepatectomy methods (LLS, left lobe, and right lobe), donors of right lobe grafts have the most severe complications and the highest mortality rate and LLS donors have the lowest morbidity and mortality.[69] However, adult recipients of right lobe grafts have lower mortality, making the decision about which lobe to procure for an adult candidate a tension between donor safety and recipient survival.[70]

The A2ALL Consortium was an important step in the right direction and has increased our understanding of short-term risks, but long-term data are still lacking.[71] The Vancouver forum only recommended 1-year follow-up for living liver donors,[72] although UNOS now requires 2 years for all living donors.[73] There has been no attempt to identify and assess the occurrence and frequency of long-term donor risks despite 3 decades of pLDLT and 2 decades of aLDLT. One qualitative study in France found that many living liver donors supported a registry:

... to track the long-term effects of the donation procedure, because they still have some questions about it. Forty-four percent of donors wondered if having given a part of their livers will have any negative impact on their health in the future.[74]

Living liver donor registries are needed to inform the transplant community of the incidence of possible later occurring morbidities (such as bowel obstruction, biliary stricture, or vascular thrombosis) which otherwise may not be fully appreciated.[75]

Given incomplete knowledge of the risks to living donors in the global transplant community, the information on risks currently shared with the donor is, at best, a rough estimate and is probably presented differently at different centers. The potential living liver donor's understanding of risk is also compromised by the fact that they may not fully internalize the risks to which they are exposing themselves. As Owen Surman explains:

While donors may acknowledge risk, they expect and believe there will be a favorable outcome, because the surgeon's willingness to carry out the operation is taken as a tacit reassurance of their safety.[76]

There is far less information about the psychosocial complications of living liver donors than that of kidney donors, although what is known suggests increased stress and increased anxiety at least in the short term. Larry Goldman reported outcomes in the donors in the original pLDLT trial at the University of Chicago in the early 1990s. Of the 20 living liver donors to pediatric recipients, there were 2 marital dissolutions and 1 adjustment disorder within the short follow-up period (3–10 months, mean = 4 months).[77] The A2ALL consortium evaluated donor stress at 9 US liver transplant programs:

> The A2ALL consortium showed that 90% of donors felt positively about their donation, that most donors experienced high psychosocial growth, and that nearly 95% of donors reported they would make the decision to donate again if they could. Following donation, most donors had stable or even improved relationships with their spouses or recipients. However, psychological distress is common in both liver and kidney donors, and ~70% of liver donors have psychosocial symptoms attributed to donation for several months post-donation.[78]

It is critical that future research explores what can be modified to reduce this distress.

International psychosocial data are comparable to US data. A study in Germany by Marc Walter and colleagues assessed psychosocial stress in 46 liver donors 6 months after donation. They reported that 11% of the donors had an "enhanced perception of stress."[79] A survey from the Japanese Liver Transplantation Society was reported at the Vancouver Forum. They identified a significant number of donors (40%) who

> . . . expressed anxiety regarding their future health. This anxiety was independent of the extent of liver resection since left lateral segment donors were equally concerned when compared with right lobe donors.[80]

These results may still represent an underestimation because donors whose recipient died were noted to be more likely to be nonresponders lost to follow-up.

The international transplant community has failed to accurately document how many living donors have died peri-operatively which, as noted by Strong, is not an ambiguous event.[81] Several researchers have attempted to determine the total number of deaths of living liver donors worldwide. One study reported 14 deaths by March 2005,[82] another reporting 19 deaths between 1989–2006[83] and another study reported 23 deaths as of October 2012.[84]

Understanding risks and benefits is further complicated by the fact that most LDLT is being done in the context of emotional relationships such that there is debate whether each party (the donor and the recipient) should consider only their own risks and benefits or whether donors may consider recipient benefits and recipients may consider donor risks.[85] We now agree with Spital that donor risk:benefit and recipient risk:benefit must be calculated separately because the donor and recipient are individual patients and the donation and living donor transplantation must be evaluated as unique donor and recipient procedures. In addition, we acknowledge the moral agency of the transplant teams, which must also determine that the risk:benefit calculations are positive in order to justify performing each of these procedures.

Although the donor risk:benefit must be calculated separately from the recipient risk:benefit, this does not mean that the donor must only consider her own self-regarding benefits and risks. Donors morally can include other-regarding benefits and risks (ie, the benefits and risks to the recipient). One must understand the donor's decision within the context of an emotional relationship in living liver transplantation since almost three-fifths of all LDLT involve first-degree relatives and another 5.3% are spouses.[86] The interests of the self and the interests of loved ones are often not neatly separated in intimate relationships. As John Hardwig explains,

> In healthy intimate relationships, the Kantian distinction between altruistic, moral regard for the ends of others and egoistic pursuit of my own ends fails because the distinction between egoism and altruism ultimately makes no sense in this context.[87]

That is, a donor's well-being is intertwined with the well-being of her recipient. Donors have both self-regarding and other-regarding interests and goals that should be included in their donor risk: benefit calculation. However, this does not mean that one can simply add up benefits to donor and recipient and determine if they outweigh the risks to donor and recipient because donor and recipient are unique individuals who individually must decide how much weight to give to self-regarding and other-regarding interests when they balance their benefits and risks. The donor must believe that the psychological benefits she will get from donating plus the benefit she gets from recipient's clinical benefit outweigh the direct physical and psychological donor risks. Likewise, the recipient must believe that the clinical benefits he will get from accepting a living donor organ outweigh the psychological distress he may feel by willingly accepting the donor's decision to expose herself to clinical health risks—and this is true whether the donor is emotionally related or a stranger.[88] The recipient can refuse the offer (eg, if the recipient is not willing to let the donor take that amount of risk). While this is true for all living solid organ transplants, it is heightened for aLDLT because of the increased donor risk.

Finally, the donor and recipient must understand the alternative, which is to wait for a deceased donor graft. Waiting, however, may have a high risk of mortality. Demand greatly outpaces supply and over 1,000 candidates active on the deceased donor liver waitlist in the US has died every year since 1997,[89] and this number does not include those who are removed from the waitlist because they deteriorated while waiting.[90]

9.3.3 Justice and the Fair Selection of Donors

When examining the principle of fairness in the selection of living kidney donors, we examined the demographics of the living kidney donors. We noted greater acceptance of complex living kidney donors today than 20 years ago and wide inter-center variability in living kidney donor eligibility criteria (see chapter 4). There is also great variability in living liver donor eligibility, as detailed by Singh Soin and colleagues:

> Varying selection criteria for donor age, steatosis, preoperative liver biopsy, acceptable comorbid conditions, right versus left graft, type of right lobe graft (RLG), acceptable GRWR [graft-to-recipient weight ratio], among others. . . . [91]

This variability in selection criteria raises justice concerns. While 96% of all liver transplants employ a graft from a deceased donor, almost two-thirds of living liver donors are a first-degree relative or life partner. In part this may be due to preference of transplant teams. In a qualitative study of transplant professionals, Elin Thomas et al found that:

> Donations between emotionally related donor and recipients (especially from parents to their children) increased the acceptability of an LLD [living liver donor] compared with those between strangers. Most healthcare professionals (HCPs) disapproved of altruistic stranger donations, considering them to entail an unacceptable degree of risk taking.[92]

That a family is encouraged to look internally for a living liver donor raises issues of deferential vulnerability. How about as explored in 9.3.4.

Whereas most kidney transplant programs began accepting nondirected donors in the early 2000s, only a few programs accepted nondirected living liver donors. In their initial article about the nondirected living donor, Matas et al restricted the participation to kidney donation. Matas et al explained:

> As we gain more experience with transplanting parts of other organs from living donors, it is likely that the risks of donation will decrease. We will then need to reconsider our policy of restricting nondirected donation to kidney transplantation.[93]

Now that Good Samaritan kidney donors are widely accepted and both donor and recipient outcomes have been found to be excellent, some centers have begun to accept Good Samaritan living liver donors.[94] This is not permitted in all countries, and even in countries where it is legally permitted, not all centers are willing to procure Good Samaritan living liver grafts.[95] One reason not to permit Good Samaritan living liver donation is that the benefit argument based on intertwined lives is not valid when the living liver donor is a Good Samaritan liver donor (and depending on the program and the wishes of the donor and recipient, a personal relationship may never be allowed to develop). For example, the Good Samaritan liver protocol at the University of Toronto, one of the institutions with extensive experience with Good Samaritan liver donors, initially allowed for donors and recipients to meet if both agreed, but now requires anonymity to be consistent with Canadian law about deceased donors.[96] Anonymity is not always achieved, as some donors have identified themselves to candidates whom they selected because of media appeals or community news.[97] Those who support Good Samaritan living liver transplantation argue that Good Samaritan donors may get strong psychological benefit without this intimate relationship. And yet, even in those programs there is concern about the extent of the donor risks. This has led some programs to restrict (or at least preferentially recommend) Good Samaritan living liver donors to donate to young children who only need a LLS.[98] Of the 50 Good Samaritan donors described by the University of Toronto, 28 (56%) donated to young children and 22 (44%) donated to adults.[99]

9.3.4 Vulnerabilities

Let us consider the relevant vulnerabilities (see Table 3.3). Potential living liver donors who have capacitational vulnerability (due to age or cognitive impairment) should be uniformly rejected.[100]

Deferential vulnerability may exist in the context of living liver donation, given power relationships and role expectations, particularly in some countries and some cultures where only intrafamilial living donation is culturally acceptable. Family relationships are complex and the LDAT must explore the motivation to donate within the donor-recipient relationship and within the wider family context.[101] Pressure may be greatest on adult children because younger living liver donor grafts have a higher rate of graft survival.[102] At least 1 study has shown that adult children who donate to their parents show the highest mental stress and conflict.[103] To ensure that the donor does not feel undue pressure to donate, the potential donor must be given many opportunities to back out. The LDAT must also ensure that the donor's reasons will be kept confidential in terms of what all members of the LDAT and the recipient transplant team discuss with the recipient as well as others who support either the donor or recipient.

Living liver donors may be at significant risk of medical vulnerability "because of the presence of a serious health-related condition in the intended recipient for which there are no satisfactory or timely remedies." Although DDLT is a satisfactory remedy, and may even be preferable to LDLT for some patients and some conditions, there is an acute shortage of deceased donor livers. Depending on the etiology of the recipient's liver failure and its likely time course, it could be the case that the recipient will not be offered a deceased donor liver graft in a timely fashion. Waiting until the candidate is sick enough to get a high MELD score may decrease the likelihood that the deceased donor graft will function. The candidate may become too sick and get delisted. These possibilities put additional pressure on the potential living liver donor.

Situational vulnerability will be most acute in the setting of acute liver failure (ALF) where the "medical exigency of the intended recipient prevents the education and deliberation needed by the potential living donor to decide whether to participate." This situation will be discussed in the chapter 10. Even in the scenario of chronic liver failure, the gravity of the illness and the unpredictability of a deceased donor graft becoming available may override reluctance.[104]

Allocation vulnerability asks whether the potential donor is lacking in subjectively important social goods that will be provided as a consequence of participation as a donor. Here, when the potential living liver donor is well known to the candidate recipient, it is important to explore the donor's relationship to the recipient and the wider circle of family or friends to ensure that the donor is not agreeing to donate, despite serious reservations, on the premise that doing so will re-ingratiate her into that circle. Even a Good Samaritan donor may, whether consciously or not, be seeking approval and elevated stature among her own peer group through making what she believes is an extravagant philanthropic gift, a piece of herself to a stranger. At a minimum, the donor must understand that donation can have mixed effects on relationships and that there is no guarantee that donation will make up for past problems or resolve old conflicts.[105] Data show that unrealistic donor expectations are associated with worse psychological donor outcomes.[106] While these concerns apply to any living donation, it is important that it is explored in depth in the case of living liver donation because of the degree of donor morbidity associated with the procurement of living donor grafts.

Another important vulnerability in the case of aLDLT is infrastructural vulnerability. This was the case in the US in the early 2000s when many transplant programs elected to perform aLDLT despite the lack of "field strength"—a coin termed by Francis Moore, a pioneering surgeon, to refer to an institution's preparedness to undertake innovative procedures.[107] Most programs at the time lacked the field strength required for a successful LDLT program, which includes the personnel, expertise and resources to perform the operation and the ability and resources to provide the postoperative care necessary for both the living liver donors and their recipients. Moore rejected the argument that justified doing "remarkable and untried things. . . under the rubric of desperate remedies" and argued for a closer ethical examination.[108]

In 2016, the British Transplant Society (BTS) produced guidelines to develop aLDLT programs in the United Kingdom. BTS recommended limiting the number of transplant centers offering aLDLT in the UK to allow the limited number of programs to gain the experience required to ensure donor safety and good recipient outcomes.[109] Similarly, in an article entitled "Should living donor liver transplantation be part of every liver transplant program?" Zakiyah Kadry and colleagues examined the growth in the number of centers performing living donor liver transplantation in Europe and concluded that the answer should be "no":

The issue of donor safety is probably an excellent dissuasive factor for the initiation of aLDLT program. However, both institutional and peer reviewed oversights and self-regulation within the liver transplant community are necessary to maintain high standards, patient/donor safety as well as public trust.[110]

In the US, approximately 25% of liver transplant programs perform aLDLT, although most still perform less than 10 annually.[111] This low number of cases challenges the attainment and maintenance of necessary field strength.

This is not to ignore the fact that donor deaths have occurred in some of the most experienced LDLT centers.[112] While transplant programs are required to inform potential donors and recipient about their institution's recipient outcomes as well as comparative outcomes nationally, living donor outcomes including types and severity of complications are not collated and therefore not disclosed in any systematic manner. How well potential living donors understand the significance of this infrastructural vulnerability when electing to be a living donor is unclear.

9.3.5 Special Relationships Create Special Obligations

In this principle, we are focused on the relationship between the donor and the LDAT, and the role of the LDAT in helping potential donors consider and negotiate their vulnerabilities. As Fournier and colleagues learned from interviewing former living donor candidates:

> donors said that the ethical concerns about LDLT should not be limited to assessing the freedom of their consent, but should provide many other forms of support . . . donors expected an ethics team to support and strengthen their autonomy rather than challenge its quality and existence. They perceive their offer to be living donors as their best move as "ethical agents."[113]

The role of the LDAT is to promote the autonomy of donors, understood relationally, and to empower donors to engage in "risky" life-saving activities if such action is consonant with the donor's values, beliefs, and interests. Fournier and colleagues found that living donors need this support not just preoperatively but also postoperatively.[114] The need for long-term follow up is also important for donors whose recipients have a bad outcome. These donors are more likely to have a worse psychological outcome.[115] Long-term follow-up or including the ongoing availability of the LDAT is important because it affirm the transplant program's obligations to donors with whom the special relationship creates special obligations.

At least 1 study shows that living donors are willing to accept more risk and less likely benefit than a transplant program would permit.[116] However, the transplant team, as moral agents, are allowed to set limits on the amount of risk that donors may take. While competent adults should have the right to take risks, surgeons are also moral agents who should refuse to perform an LDLT if: (1) the likelihood of recipient benefit is too low to justify donor risk, (2) the risk to the donor is too high, (3) the team believes that the donor is not acting voluntarily or that the donor is experiencing undue pressure from outside sources, or (4) the transplant team or institution lacks the appropriate field strength to perform LDLT. That is, transplant professionals are moral agents and there may be situations where they can and should say "no," even when a potential donor states her willingness to proceed despite the risks.[117]

9.4 Conclusion

The adoption and expansion of pLDLT is a model of how innovative technologies should proceed. The transplant community identified a need (high mortality of young children on the liver waitlist) and attempted to solve it by developing new deceased donor graft techniques. Split-liver and reduced-size deceased donor graft techniques were controversial because they used liver grafts that were also needed by adults in end-stage liver disease. The transplant community then adapted the split-liver technique to potential living donors. After a successful (although brief) research protocol that showed low donor morbidity and mortality and excellent graft and recipient survival, pLDLT was widely adopted and led to the near eradication of mortality of young children on the deceased donor liver waitlist.

In contrast, the adoption of aLDLT in the US proceeded too quickly—expanding to too many centers without adequate field strength. While the expansion was halted and contraction occurred, in part due to a highly publicized living donor death, lost ground has been regained in the past 5 years.

Better living donor outcome data for both the donors and their recipients are still needed.

In the next chapter, we consider the ethical boundaries of LDLT by exploring the case of LDLT for ALF.

Notes

1. Kolata G. First U.S. liver transplant from live donor is set. *The New York Times*. November 27, 1989. Last accessed August 20, 2021.http://www.nytimes.com/1989/11/27/us/first-us-liver-transplant-from-live-donor-is-set.html

2. AssociatedPress.FirstUSlivertransplantrecipientmarks25thanniversary.*TheDailyNews*. November 27, 2014. Last accessed August 20, 2021.http://www.nydailynews.com/life-style/health/u-s-liver-transplant-recipient-marks-25th-anniversary-article-1.2026177

3. Associated Press, "First US liver," citing J. Richard Thistlethwaite.

4. Grady D. New Yorker dies after surgery to give liver part to brother. *The New York Times*. January 15, 2002. Last accessed August 20, 2021. http://www.nytimes.com/2002/01/15/us/new-yorker-dies-after-surgery-to-give-liver-part-to-brother.html

5. Grady D. Donor's death at hospital halts some liver surgeries. *The New York Times*. January 16, 2002. Last accessed August 20, 2021. http://www.nytimes.com/2002/01/16/nyregion/donor-s-death-at-hospital-halts-some-liver-surgeries.html

6. Otte JB. History of pediatric liver transplantation. Where are we coming from? Where do we stand? *Pediatr Transplant*. 2002;6:378–387.

7. Otte, "History," and Starzl TE, Groth CG, Brettschneider L, et al. Orthotopic homo-transplantation of the human liver. *Ann Surg*. 1968;168:392–415.

8. Starzl et al, "Orthotopic."

9. Jain A, Mazariegos G, Kashyap R, et al. Pediatric liver transplantation in 808 con-secutive children: 20-years' experience from a single center. *Transplant Proc*. 2002;34:1955–1957.

10. See, for example, Bismuth H, Houssin D. Reduced-sized orthotopic liver graft in he-patic transplantation in children. *Surgery*. 1984;95:367–370; Broelsch CE, Emond JC, Thistlethwaite JR, Rouch DA, Whitington PF, Lichtor JL. Liver transplantation with reduced-size donor organs. *Transplantation*. 1988;45:519–524; Broelsch CE, Emond JC, Thistlethwaite JR, et al. Liver transplantation, including the concept of reduced-size liver transplants in children. *Ann Surg*. 1988;208:410–420; and Emond JC, Whitington PF, Broelsch CE. Overview of reduced-size liver transplantation. *Clin Transplant*. 1991;5(2 part 2):168–173.

11. Otte JB, de Ville de Goyet J, Alberti D, Balladur P, de Hemptinne B. The concept and technique of the split liver in clinical transplantation. *Surgery*. 1990;107:605–612; and Emond JC, Whitington PF, Thistlethwaite JR, et al. Transplantation of two patients with one liver. Analysis of a preliminary experience with "split-liver" grafting. *Ann Surg*. 1990;212:14–22.

12. Murcia J, Vazquez J, Lopez SM, et al. Innovative techniques in pediatric liver. *Eur J Pediatr Surg.* 1996;6:152–154.

13. Raia S, Nery JR, Mies S. Liver transplantation from live donors. *Lancet.* 1989;2(8661):497.

14. Strong RW, Lynch SV, Ong TH, Matsunami H, Koido Y, Balderson GA. Successful liver transplantation from a living donor to her son. *N Engl J Med.* 1990;322:1505–1507.

15. Singer PA, Siegler M, Whitington PF, et al. Ethics of liver transplantation with living donors. *N Engl J Med.* 1989;321:620–622.

16. Broelsch CE, Whitington PF, Emond JC, et al. Liver transplantation in children from living related donors. Surgical techniques and results. *Ann Surg.* 1991;214:428–437, discussion at pp. 437–439.

17. Cronin DC 2nd, Millis JM, Siegler M. Transplantation of liver grafts from living donors into adults—too much, too soon. *N Engl J Med.* 2001;344:1633–1637.

18. Hashikura Y, Makuuchi M, Kawasaki S, et al. Successful living-related partial liver transplantation to an adult patient. *Lancet.* 1994;343(8907):1233–1234.

19. Trotter JF, Wachs M, Everson GT, Igal K. Adult-to_Adult Transplantation of the Right Hepatic Lobe from a Living Donor. *N Eng J Med.* 2002;346(14);1074–1082 at p. 1074.

20. Yamaoka Y, Washida M, Honda K, et al. Liver transplantation using a right lobe graft from a living related donor. *Transplantation.* 1994;57:1127–1130.

21. Lo CM, Fan ST, Liu CL, et al. Extending the limit on the size of adult recipient in living donor liver transplantation using extended right lobe graft. *Transplantation.* 1997;63:1524–1528.

22. Wachs ME, Bak TE, Karrer FM, et al. Adult living donor liver transplantation using a right hepatic lobe. *Transplantation.*1998;66:1313–1316.

23. Brown RS Jr, Russo MW, Lai M, et al. A survey of liver transplantation from living adult donors in the United States. *N Engl J Med.* 2003;348:818–825.

24. Brown et al, "A survey."

25. Shiffman ML, Brown RS, Jr., Olthoff KM, et al. Living donor liver transplantation: summary of a conference at The National Institutes of Health. *Liver Transpl.* 2002;8:174–188.

26. Shiffman et al, "Summary of a conference."

27. Shiffman et al, "Summary of a conference."

28. Shiffman et al, "Summary of a conference," at p. 179 (references omitted).

29. Shiffman et al, "Summary of a conference," at p. 181.

30. Shiffman et al, "Summary of a conference."

31. Shiffman et al, "Summary of a conference," at p. 179.

32. Cronin et al, "Too much, too soon."

33. Cronin et al, "Too much, too soon," at p. 1633.

34. OPTN (Organ Procurement and Transplantation Network) National Data. Updated August 19, 2021. Last accessed August 20, 2021. https://optn.transplant.hrsa.gov/data/view-data-reports/national-data/. Hereinafter referred to as OPTN Data.

35. OPTN Data.

36. OPTN Data.

37. Abu-Gazala S, Olthoff KM. Current status of living donor liver transplantation in the United States. *Ann Rev Med.* 2019;70:225–238. This is based on 2018 data.

38. OPTN Data.

39. Kubota T, Hata K, Sozu T, et al. Impact of donor age on recipient survival in adult-to-adult living-donor liver transplantation. *Ann Surg.* 2018;267:1126–1133.

40. Luė A, Solanas E, Baptista P, et al. How important is donor age in liver transplantation? *World J Gastroenterol.* 2016;22:4966–4976.

41. Crouch RA, Elliott C. Moral agency and the family: the case of living related organ transplantation. *Camb Q Healthc Ethics.*1999;8:275–287.

42. Crouch and Elliott, "Moral agency," citing Arthur Caplan at p. 276.

43. Crouch and Elliott, "Moral agency," citing George Annas at p. 276.

44. Crowley-Matoka M, Siegler M, Cronin DC 2nd. Long-term quality of life issues among adult-to-pediatric living liver donors: a qualitative exploration *Am J Transplant.* 2004;4:744–750, at p. 745.

45. Crouch and Elliott, "Moral agency," at p. 276.

46. Siegler M, Lantos JD. Commentary: ethical justification for living liver donation. *Cambr Q Healthc Ethics.* 1992;1:320–325, at pp. 323–324.

47. Papachristou C, Walter M, Dietrich K, et al. Motivation for living-donor liver transplantation from the donor's perspective: an in-depth qualitative research study. *Transplantation.* 2004;78:1506–1514.

48. Fournier V, Foureur N, Rari E. The ethics of living donation for liver transplant: beyond donor autonomy. *Med Health Care Philos.* 2013;16:45–54, at p. 45.

49. Fournier et al, "The ethics of living donation."

50. Fournier et al, "The ethics of living donation," at p. 45. Fournier et al are citing Anderson-Shaw L, Schmidt ML, Elkin J, Chamberlin W, Benedetti E, Testa G. Evolution of a living donor liver transplantation advocacy program. *J Clin Ethics.* 2005;16:46–57.

51. See, for example, Dy SM, Purnell TS. Key concepts relevant to quality of complex and shared decision-making in health care: a literature review. *Soc Sci Med.* 2012;74:582–587; and Tan JC, Gordon EJ, Dew MA, et al. Living donor kidney transplantation: facilitating education about live kidney donation—recommendations from a consensus conference. *Clin J Am Soc Nephrol.* 2015;10:160–167.

52. See, for example, Kren BT, Chowdhury NR, Chowdhury JR, Steer CJ. Gene therapy as an alternative to liver transplantation. *Liver Transpl.* 2002;12:1089–1108; Shijna S, Sato K, Tateishi R, et al. Percutaneous ablation for hepatocellular carcinoma: comparison of various ablation techniques and surgery. *Can J Gastroenterol Hepatol.* 2018:Article ID 4756147. Last accessed 8/20/2021. https://www.hindawi.com/journals/cjgh/2018/4756147/; and Liu M, Shah V. New prospects for medical management of acute alcoholic hepatitis. *Clin Liver Dis.* 2019;13:131–135.

53. Kisch AM, Forsberg A, Fridh I, et al. The meaning of being a living kidney, liver, or stem cell donor—a meta-ethnography. *Transplantation.* 2018;102(5):744–756.

54. Trotter JF, Wachs M, Everson GT, Kam I. Adult-to-adult transplantation of the right hepatic lobe from a living donor. *N Engl J Med.* 2002;346:1074–82; Abt PL, Mange KC, Olthoff KM, et al. Allograft survival following adult-to-adult living donor liver

transplantation. *Am J Transplant.* 2004;4:1302–1307; and Thuluvath PJ, Yoo HY. Graft and patient survival after adult live donor liver transplantation compared to a matched cohort who received a deceased donor transplantation. *Liver Transpl.* 2004;10:1263–1268.

55. See, for example, publications from the A2ALL Consortium: Olthoff KM, Merion RM, Ghobrial RM, et al. Outcomes of 385 Adult-to-Adult Living Donor liver transplant recipients: a report from the A2ALL Consortium. *Ann Surg.* 2005;242:314–323; Olthoff KM, Smith AR, Abecassis M, et al. Defining long-term outcomes with living donor liver transplantation in North America. *Ann Surg.* 2015;262:465–475; Freise CE, Gillespie BW, Koffron AJ, et al. Recipient morbidity after living and deceased donor liver transplantation: findings from the A2ALL Retrospective Cohort Study. *Am J Transplant.* 2008;8:2569–2579; and Olthoff KM, Abecassis MM, Emond JC, et al. Outcomes of adult living donor liver transplantation: comparison of the Adult-to-Adult Living Donor Liver Transplantation Cohort Study and the national experience. *Liver Transpl.* 2011;17:789–797.

56. Humar A, Ganesh S, Jorgensen D, et al. Adult living donor versus deceased donor liver transplant (LDLT versus DDLT) at a single center time to change our paradigm for liver transplant. *Ann Surg.* 2019;270:444–451, at p. 447.

57. Humar et al, "Adult living donor," at p. 444. Humar and colleagues acknowledge that some may object to the comparisons given the lack of risk adjustment. They respond:

> Although some may argue that this makes for an unfair comparison, this is the reality of what patients being evaluated for a transplant face. The option for them is not a LD [living donor] or a DD [deceased donor]. In actuality, the options are: moving forward with a LD if someone suitable is available or being placed on a waiting list and possibly moving forward with a transplant once they reach the top of the waiting list. If the potential waiting list mortality is factored into the analysis as one would do in an intent-to-treat analysis, then the results favor an LDLT even more. (Humar et al, "Adult living donor," at p. 447)

58. Samstein B, Smith AR, Freise CE, et al. Complications and their resolution in recipients of deceased and living donor liver transplants: findings from the A2ALL Cohort Study. *Am J Transplant.* 2016;16(2):594–602; and Sanchez-Cabus S, Cherqui D, Rashidian N, et al. Left-liver adult-to-adult living donor liver transplantation: can it be improved? a retrospective multicenter European study. *Ann Surg.* 2018;268(5):876–884.

59. Samstein et al, "Complications," and Sanchez-Cabus et al, "Left-liver."

60. Kisch et al, "The meaning."

61. See, for example, Thys K, Schwering K-L, Siebelink M, et al. Psychosocial impact of pediatric living-donor kidney and liver transplantation on recipients, donors, and the family: a systematic review. *Transpl Int.* 2015;28(3):270–280; and Simmons RG, Marine SK, Simmons RL. *Effect of Organ Transplantation on Individual, Family and Societal Dynamics.* New Brunswick, NJ: Transaction Books; 2002.

62. See, for example, Butt Z, Dew MA, Liu Q, et al. Psychological outcomes of living liver donors from a multicenter prospective study: Results from the Adult-to-Adult

Living Donor Liver Transplantation Cohort Study2 (A2ALL-2). *Am J Transplant.* 2017;17(5):1267–1277.

63. Strong RW. Living donor liver transplantation: an overview. *J Hepatobiliary Pancreat Surg.* 2006;13:370–377, at p. 373.

64. Clavien PA, Sanabria JR, Strasberg SM. Proposed classification of complications of surgery with examples of utility in cholecystectomy. *Surgery.* 1992;111:518–526.

65. Ghobrial RM, Saab A, Lassman C, et al. Donor and recipient outcomes in right lobe adult living donor liver transplantation. *Liver Transpl.* 2002;8:901–909; and Tamura S, Sugawara Y, Kaneko J, et al. Systematic grading of surgical complications in live liver donors according to Clavien's system. *Transpl Int.* 2006;19:982–987.

66. See, Beavers KL, Sandler RS, Fair JH, Johnson MW, Shrestha R. The living donor experience: donor health assessment and outcomes after living donor liver transplantation. *Liver Transpl.* 2001;7:943–947; Ghobrial RM, Freise CE, Trotter JF, et al. Donor morbidity after living donation for liver transplantation. *Gastroenterology.* 2008;135:468–476; and Abecassis MM, Fisher RA, Olthoff KM, et al. Complications of living donor hepatic lobectomy—a comprehensive report. *Am J Transplant.* 2012;12:1208–1217.

67. See Cheah YL, Simpson MA, Pomposelli JJ, et al. Incidence of death and potentially life-threatening near-miss events in living donor hepatic lobectomy: a world-wide survey. *Liver Transpl.* 2013;19:499–506.

68. Barr ML, Belghiti J, Villamil FG, et al. A report of the Vancouver Forum on the care of the live organ donor: lung, liver, pancreas, and intestine data and medical guidelines. *Transplantation.* 2006;81:1373–1385.

69. For morbidity, see Ross GR, Parekh JR, Parker WF, et al. Left hepatectomy versus right hepatectomy for living donor liver transplantation: shifting the risk from the donor to the recipient. *Liver Transpl.* 2013;19:472–481. For mortality, see Ringe B, Strong RW. The dilemma of living liver donor death: to report or not to report? *Transplantation.* 2008;85:790–793. Ringe and Strong estimate the donor death rate at 0.1 to 0.3% based on 14,000 living donor liver transplants performed worldwide, and calculate that mortality of right lobe donation may reach 0.5%.

70. Bathla L, Vargas LM, Langnas A. Left lobe liver transplants. *Surg Clin North Am.* 2013;93:1325–1342; and Roll GR, Parekh JR, Parker WF, et al. Left hepatectomy versus right hepatectomy for living donor liver transplantation: shifting the risk from the donor to the recipient. *Liver Transpl.* 2013;19:472–481.

71. Abu-Gazala and Olthoff, "Current status."

72. Barr, "Vancouver Forum," at p. 1377.

73. (OPTN) Organ Procurement Transplantation Network. See specifically Policy 14, Living Donation. Last updated 6/17/2021. Last accessed 8/20/2021. https://optn.transplant.hrsa.gov/media/1200/optn_policies.pdf

74. Fournier et al, "The ethics of living donation," at p. 51.

75. In the UK, there is a longitudinal living donor registry. As explained in a document co-authored by the British Transplant Society:

> Life-long follow-up is recommended after donor hepatectomy. For donors who are resident in the UK, this can be offered locally or at the transplant centre

according to the wishes of the donor, but such arrangements must facilitate the collection of data for submission to the UK Living Donor Registry.

British Transplant Society, British Association for the Study of the Liver. Living donor liver transplantation. July 2015. Last accessed 8/20/21. https://bts.org.uk/wp-content/uploads/2016/09/03_BTS_LivingDonorLiver-1.pdf, at p. 151.

In 2014, a new version of the Korean Organ Transplantation Registry (KOTRY) was launched that will follow living kidney and living liver donors prospectively for life. See Yang J, Jeong JC, Lee J, et al. Design and methods of the Korean Organ Transplantation Registry. *Transplantation Direct*. 2017;3(8):e191.

In the United States, Bertram Kasiske and colleagues proposed a longitudinal long-term living liver and living kidney registry. See Kasiske, BL, Asrani SK, Dew MA, et al. The Living Donor Collective: a scientific registry for living donors. *Am J Transplant*. 2017;17:3040–3048.

76. Surman OS. The ethics of partial liver donation. *N Engl J Med*. 2002;346:1038.
77. Goldman LS. Liver transplantation using living donors. Preliminary donor psychiatric outcomes. *Psychosomatics*. 1993;34:235–240.
78. Abu-Gazala and Olthoff, "Current status," at p. 232, references omitted but all refer to the A2ALL studies. Many of them are cited in reference 54.
79. Walter M, Papachristou C, Fliege H, et al. Psychosocial stress of living donors after living donor liver transplantation. *Transplant Proc*. 2002;34:3291–3292.
80. Barr et al, "Vancouver Forum," at p. 1377 citing data from the Japanese Liver Transplantation Society.
81. Strong, "Living donor," at p. 373.
82. Trotter JF, Adam R, Lo CM, Kenison J. Documented deaths of hepatic lobe donors for living donor liver transplantation. *Liver Transpl*. 2006;12:1485–1488.
83. Bramstedt KA. Living liver donor mortality: where do we stand? *Am J Gastroenterol*. 2006;101:755–759.
84. Cheah et al, "Incidence of death."
85. See for example, Spital A. Intrafamilial organ donation is often an altruistic act. *Camb Q Healthc Ethics*. 2003;12:116–118; Glannon W, Ross LF. Motivation, risk, and benefit in living organ donation: a reply to Aaron Spital. *Camb Q Healthc Ethics*. 2005;14:191–194, discussion pp. 195–198; and Cronin et al, "Too much too soon."
86. See text corresponding to reference 37.
87. Hardwig J. Should women think in terms of rights? *Ethics*.1984;94:441–455, at pp. 445–446.
88. Fournier et al, "The ethics of living donation." Fournier argues we need to pay more attention to recipient risk. See also Bailey PK, Ben-Shlomo Y, de Salis I, Tomson C, Owen-Smith A. Better the donor you know? A qualitative study of renal patients' views on "altruistic" live-donor kidney transplantation. *Soc Sci Med*. 2016;150:104–111.
89. OPTN Data.
90. OPTN Data.
91. Soin AS, Chaudhary RJ, Pahari H, Pomfret EA. A worldwide survey of live liver donor selection policies at 24 centers with a combined experience of 19 009 adult living

donor liver transplants. *Transplantation.* 2019;103(2):e39–e47, at p. 39. Variability is also described in Abu-Gazala and Olthoff, "Current status."

92. Thomas EH, Bramhall SR, Herington J, Draper H. Live liver donation, ethics and practitioners: "I am between the two and if I do not feel comfortable about this situation, I cannot proceed." *J Med Ethics.* 2014;40:157–162, at p. 157.

93. Matas AJ, Garvey CA, Jacobs CL, Kahn JP. Nondirected donation of kidneys from living donors. *N Engl J Med.* 2000;343:433–436, at p. 436.

94. See for example, Otte JB. Good Samaritan liver donor in pediatric transplantation. *Pediatr Transplant.* 2009;13:155–159; Reichman TW, Fox A, Adcock L, et al. Anonymous living liver donation: donor profiles and outcomes. *Am J Transplant.* 2010;10:2099–2104; and Raza MH, Aziz H, Kaur N, et al. Global experience and perspectives on anonymous nondirected live donation in living donor liver. *Clin Transplant.* 2000;34:e13836; Levy GA, Selzner N, Grant DR. Fostering liver living donor liver transplantation. *Curr Opin Organ Transplant.* 2016;21:224–230; Goldaracena N, Jung J, Aravinthan AD, et al. Donor outcomes in anonymous live liver donation. *J Hepatol.* 2019;71:951–959; and Wright L, Ross K, Abbey S, Levy G, Grant D. Living anonymous liver donation: case report and ethical justification. *Am J Transplant.* 2007;7:1032–1035.

95. Duvoux C. Anonymous living donation in liver transplantation: squaring the circle or condemned to vanish? *J Hepatol.* 2019;71:864–866.

96. Wright et al, "Living anonymous."

97. Goldaracena et al, "Donor outcomes," at p. 952.

98. Goldaracena et al, "Donor outcomes," at p. 952.

99. Goldaracena et al, "Donor outcomes."

100. One exception is the living liver domino donor who may be a child with a metabolic disease like maple syrup urine disease (MSUD) and donates his or her liver when undergoing liver transplantation as discussed in chapter 2.

101. Papachristou et al, "Motivation," and Abdeldayem H, Kashkoush S, Hegab BS, Aziz A, Shoreem H, Saleh S. Analysis of donor motivations in living donor liver transplantation. *Front Surg.* 2014;1:25. doi:10.3389/fsurg.2014.00025

102. See, for example, Kubota et al, "Impact of donor age" and Lué et al, "How important."

103. Erim Y, Beckmann M, Kroencke S, et al. Influence of kinship on donors' mental burden in living donor liver transplantation. *Liver Transpl.* 2012;18:901–906.

104. Papachristou, "Motivation."

105. Papachristou C, Walter M, Schmid G, Frommer J, Klapp BF. Living donor liver transplantation and its effect on the donor-recipient relationship—a qualitative interview study with donors. *Clin Transplant.* 2009;23:382–391.

106. Erim Y, Beckmann M, Valentin-Gamazo C, et al. Quality of life and psychiatric complications after adult living donor liver transplantation. *Liver Transpl.* 2006;12:1782–1790.

107. Moore FD. Three ethical revolutions: ancient assumptions remodeled under pressure of transplantation. *Transplant Proc.* 1988;20(1 suppl 1):1061–1067, at p. 1064.

108. Moore, "Three ethical revolutions," at p. 1064.

109. Manas D, Burnapp L, Andrews PA. Summary of the British Transplantation Society UK Guidelines for Living Donor Liver Transplantation. *Transplantation*. 2016;100:1184–1190, at p. 1186.

110. Kadry Z, McCormack L, Clavien P-A. Should living donor liver transplantation be part of every liver transplant program? *J Hepatol*. 2005;43:32–37, at p. 35.

111. Abu-Gazala and Olthoff, "Current status."

112. Abu-Gazala and Olthoff, "Current status" at p. 231.

113. Fournier et al, "The ethics of living donation," at p. 53.

114. Fournier et al, "The ethics of living donation," at p. 51.

115. Kisch et al, "The meaning," at p. 753 citing studies from living donor kidney, liver and stem cell donors.

116. Cotler SJ, McNutt R, Patil R, et al. Adult living donor liver transplantation: preferences about donation outside the medical community. *Liver Transpl*. 2001;7:335–340.

117. Elliott C. Doing harm: living organ donors, clinical research and *The Tenth Man. J Med Ethics*. 1995;21:91–96, at p. 95.

10

Living Donor Liver Transplantation
for Acute Liver Failure

Case 10-1: (This is a hypothetical case.)

Jane, an 18-year-old college freshman, presented 1 month ago to the student health clinic for fatigue and nausea during midterms. A pregnancy test was negative, and she was well hydrated and held down a meal in the emergency department. She was discharged without any medications, but she was told to return if her symptoms did not improve. Today she presents again with continued complaints of fatigue and nausea. She has experienced no change in weight, has had no recent ill contacts, and is not taking any medications. She denies drinking alcohol or using street drugs. She is visibly jaundiced with scleral icterus. At this visit, on further questioning, she has not taken any recent Tylenol or aspirin, but states she has been taking an herbal supplement for her fatigue that her paternal grandmother had sent from China. It is unlabeled and is sent to toxicology. While waiting for labs to come back, she becomes increasingly somnolent consistent with progressive encephalopathy and her lab values are consistent with acute liver failure (ALF). She is admitted to the intensive care unit (ICU) and her parents are called. They are divorced and live out of town.

Her parents arrive the next morning. The ICU physicians explain that her condition has rapidly progressed. She is being listed as Status 1A for a deceased donor liver transplant (DDLT) but it is uncertain whether a deceased donor liver will become available in time. Her mother asks what caused her liver to fail. Preliminary toxicology data suggest that the supplement she was taking from her grandmother contains large doses of carthamus tinctorius oil which has been linked to ALF.[1] Her mother asks if she can be a living liver donor, but she is very petite and the team does not believe she has adequate liver mass for donation. When her father offers to undergo a living donor evaluation, his new wife, visibly pregnant, objects loudly. He responds that it is his mother who sent the herbal supplements and he feels he owes it to his daughter.

The Living Organ Donor as Patient. Lainie Friedman Ross and J. Richard Thistlethwaite, Jr, Oxford University Press.
© Oxford University Press 2022. DOI: 10.1093/oso/9780197618202.003.0010

10.1 Acute Liver Failure

Acute liver failure (ALF), also known as fulminant hepatic failure (FHF), affects approximately 2000–3000 patients (adults and children) annually in the United States (US).[2] In the 1980s, mortality was greater than 90%,[3] but survival is now ~75% due to improvement in intensive supportive care, therapeutic interventions (eg, N-Acetylcysteine for acetaminophen toxicity), and the availability of liver transplantation.[4] The etiology of ALF differs between adults and children. Acetaminophen-toxicity accounts for over half of cases of ALF in adults;[5] approximately three-fourths of these cases are women with an average age of 37 years.[6] In children, almost half of the cases of ALF are indeterminate, and acetaminophen toxicity accounts for ~12% of cases (over 20% in adolescents).[7] Today, liver transplant for ALF accounts for approximately 8% of all liver transplants. The results of liver transplant for ALF have improved over the past few decades, but are not as good as the results seen in standard liver transplant (at least in the short term) and vary depending on the age of donor and recipient and the etiology of ALF.[8]

The diagnosis of ALF was an exclusion from the original University of Chicago pediatric living donor liver transplant (pLDLT) protocol performed between 1989 and 1991 to ensure that the donors (mainly parents) would have adequate time to reflect on the risks, benefits, and alternatives in order to give an informed consent for what was an experimental procedure.[9]

The first 3 reported cases of pLDLT for ALF were described by Koichi Tanaka and colleagues in 1994.[10] Adult-to-adult living donor liver transplant (aLDLT) for ALF followed quickly with the first report coming from Asia in 1996,[11] and in the US in 1997.[12] There were concerns early on regarding the high postoperative mortality rate of recipients in this setting.[13] In 2002, the New York State Health Department guidelines classified ALF as a contraindication for living donor liver transplant (LDLT).[14] However, with increasing experience and the use of larger right-sided grafts in adults, results improved and ALF became an accepted indication for LDLT for both adult and pediatric candidates.

In the US, LDLT for ALF is less common than it is in Asia because the US has a more robust DDLT program and US patients with ALF are placed as status I (highest priority) on the DDLT waitlist. The Adult-to-Adult Living

Donor Liver Transplant (A2ALL) Consortium involved 9 high-volume US liver transplant programs. Over a 9-year period, all patients "on the liver transplantation waitlist with a potential donor who underwent an initial history and physical examination, regardless of whether LDLT occurred" were enrolled in the A2ALL Consortium database.[15] Only 14 (1%) of the 1,201 potential LDLT recipients in this study had ALF.[16] Of the 14 patients with ALF, 10 received a LDLT, 3 received a DDLT, and 1 improved without a transplant. Recipient survival was 70% (7 of 10 patients) after LDLT and 67% (2 of 3 patients) after DDLT.[17] The A2ALL cohort study consortium reported on the outcomes:

> The complication rate of the recipients who underwent LDLT was similar to that of other recipients who underwent LDLT in the A2ALL study. Specifically, none of the patients had "small-for-size syndrome," and none required retransplantation.[18]

Donor complication rate was 50% in the setting of ALF, which was comparable to complication rate experienced by all donors in the A2ALL study (37.7%).[19]

The Acute Liver Failure Study Group (ALFSG) was established by the Food and Drug Administration (FDA) and the National Institutes of Health (NIH) in 1998 in order to develop and utilize a database and to develop an infrastructure to implement controlled trials of innovative therapies. Between January 1998 and July 2007, the ALFSG enrolled 1,147 patients at 23 clinical sites,[20] and by the end of 2013 ALFSG had enrolled more than 2,500 patients at 32 participating clinical centers.[21] Early outcomes data found patients in ALF did worse with LDLT than DDLT, but later outcomes with LDLT are comparable, if not better.[22] However, not all patients in ALF need a liver transplant. In the ALFSG registry, 617 of 1,696 (36%) of patients enrolled were listed for liver transplantation.[23] Over half of the listed patients who did not receive an organ recovered.[24] In pediatrics, the incidence of spontaneous recovery is even higher.[25]

The severe time constraints that ALF poses means that patients with ALF are usually listed for DDLT, and potential living donors are identified to begin the work-up for LDLT even before it is known whether a transplant will be necessary. Next we consider the ethical issues raised by living donation for ALF.

10.2 Ethical Analysis

In this chapter, we focus on the unique ethical issues raised by LDLT for ALF in children and adults. Our purpose is not to delve into the challenges of how to determine when or whether to list a patient in ALF for transplant, nor to evaluate whether LDLT or DDLT would be predicted to have better recipient outcomes for a particular patient. Rather we will focus on the issues that ALF raises for individuals who may be asked to serve as a living donor for a patient who is critically and acutely ill. The urgency of the situation means that the donor evaluation must be performed in hours to days, rather than weeks to months, which is the more typical time frame for a living liver donor evaluation. We will explore these issues using our living donor ethics framework which is based on 5 principles: (1) respect for persons; (2) beneficence; (3) justice; (4) vulnerabilities; and (5) special relationships creating special obligations.

10.2.1 Respect for Persons

This first principle focuses on informed consent and donor autonomy. The concern here is whether the threat of imminent death of a loved one prevents potential living donors from fully comprehending the benefits and risks of their decision to donate, and, even if they have a robust understanding, whether the life-threatening emergency interferes with their ability to make an informed and voluntary decision. That is, do donors facing the imminent death of a loved one have the ability to refuse the offer or request to serve as a living donor?[26]

One argument in favor of respecting the living donor's decision in the setting of a loved one with ALF is based on the fact that most living donors do not decide to donate based on a rational, well-considered, evidence-based analysis of the risks, benefits, and alternatives such that the short time frame has no real impact. The data have consistently shown that most donors make up their minds to volunteer to donate once they hear about the need, before beginning the donor evaluation. Carl Fellner and John Marshall described this finding in the early years of living donor kidney transplantation, before chronic dialysis was a realistic option:

> The answers were surprising. It appeared that not one of the donors weighed alternatives and decided rationally. Eight of the donors stated that

they made their decision immediately when the subject of the kidney transplant was first mentioned over the telephone "in a split-second," "instan-
taneously" or "right away." The other four said they just went along with
the tests hoping it would be someone else. They could not recall ever really
having made a clear decision yet they never considered refusing to go along
either and as it became clear towards the end of the selection process that
they were going to be the person most suited to be the donor, they finally
committed themselves to the act. However, this decision, too, still occurred
before the session with the team doctors in which all the relevant information and statistics were put before them and they were finally asked to
decide.[27]

In a later study, Fellner and Marshall also found that family members who
did refuse also refused "right away":

> by the same token for all those who refused to participate from the be-
> ginning, decision making is an early event preceding all information-gath-
> ering and clarification offered by the team.[28]

Larry Goldman, the psychiatrist involved in the University of Chicago
IRB-approved pLDLT protocol examined parental decision-making and
found that parents who agreed to participate made the decision immediately.[29] This was replicated in a California study where Bliss and colleagues
obtained the same results, even when the donors were Spanish-speaking
only, suggesting that the immediacy of the decision-making in the face of an
ill family member crosses cultural backgrounds.[30]

To the extent that donation is a split-second decision, even when the need
for transplant is not emergent, seeking voluntary consent on an emergent
basis may be no more or less coercive than decision-making in the setting
of less-emergent chronic organ failure, particularly when no comparable
alternatives exist. Yet, even if spontaneous nonreflective decision-making
is the norm, it is not ideal, and consent, specifically informed consent, may
be compromised. This raises the question of whether we should exclude all
living donors in the setting of ALF, let alone in other instances as well, when
their decision involves minimal reflection and deliberation.

The urgency of the health condition caused by ALF in the potential recipient does not allow the potential donor to solidify, better understand, and
affirm their decision over time.[31] While we agree that it may not be realistic

for potential living donors to make a fully informed and voluntary decisions, we do believe that competent adults can decide whether to donate a liver lobe in the setting of ALF for both a pediatric and adult recipient even if the decision is less rationally informed and established than one would theoretically like. We base this judgment, in part, on our understanding of voluntariness within a relational context. As Robert Crouch and Carl Elliott explain:

> If we are ever to get straight about the nature of voluntariness, we must recognize that moral and emotional commitments are not exceptional, are not constraints on freedom, but are rather a part of ordinary human life. More specifically, they are a part of ordinary *family* life that we must take seriously if we want to understand how family members can make free choices about organ donation.[32]

Safeguards, however, must be in place. The potential donor must have a thorough evaluation and engagement with the living donor advocacy team (LDAT), particularly social work and psychology team members, to ensure that the donor is truly willing to donate. Given the compressed time in which decisions must be made, institutions that perform LDLT for ALF will need to have members of the LDAT available to meet with potential donors once it is determined that a transplantation may be necessary. The LDAT needs to explore with potential donor(s) the emotional and psychological issues that donation raises and to ensure that all of the potential donors' questions are answered. The LDAT must empower the donor to halt the work-up and/or to self-exclude from further donor consideration at any time until the transplant is deemed unnecessary or until the emergent surgery is performed. The LDAT supports the donor's reflection on his or her decision by applying a relational conception of autonomy that does not just accept a competent patient's nonreflective decision as the final word, but rather engages the patient in thoughtful deliberation over several meetings in the time available.[33] Then, as long as the potential living donor fulfills all of the other medical and psychological criteria to which standard living liver donors are held, we believe that individuals can give an adequately informed consent for LDLT in the context of ALF.

Although not systematically collected, there are data to show that some adults do decline to serve as a living liver donor.[34] This is true even in countries where there is no deceased donor option,[35] and when the intended recipient is their young child.[36] In the original study at the University of

Chicago which excluded children with ALF, Goldman noted that 1 individual who completed the medical and psychiatric work up was rejected on medical grounds and 1 refused to donate despite an initial agreement.[37] In a more recent study of children with both chronic liver disease and ALF in Chile, Mario Uribe and colleagues also found that some parents chose not to donate:

LRLT [living related liver transplant] was proposed in 28 cases and performed in 17 (60.7%). The reasons for LRD [living related donor] rejection were: parent's fear of surgical complications in four cases; drug abuse in two; a mother without family support; medical reasons in two; and only one, due to anatomical reasons and in one case, cadaveric graft transplantation was performed while completing the father's evaluation.[38]

In this study, 7 of the 11 pediatric candidates whose living donor was excluded had ALF. While9 of these candidates "were transplanted with cadaveric organs . . . two patients with ALF died awaiting a liver."[39]

10.2.2 Beneficence

Again, in evaluating the risks and benefits of LDLT, one must consider the risks and benefits for the donor and the recipient individually, as well as the alternatives. The benefits of LDLT and DDLT for the candidate in acute (rather than chronic) liver failure are the same: the transplant is life-saving. The physical risks to living liver donors in the setting of ALF are similar to the risks for nonurgent living liver donation, although there may be additional psychological risks due to the sudden nature of the recipient's disease and the risk of imminent death.[40] Donor safety is always the top priority, even though the work-up is done more expeditiously:

Donor safety must still be the first priority in high-acuity situations. Careful screening for any conditions that represent increased risk to the donor is still essential. The same exclusion criteria that apply in elective situations must also apply in emergency cases, and no exceptions can be made to accommodate the needs of the recipient. No part of the donor evaluation should be skipped in the interest of time unless its omission can be clearly justified.[41]

That is, prospective donors must have a thorough medical and psychosocial evaluation, equal to the work-up done in the setting of chronic liver failure. They must also have liberal access to members of the living donor advocacy team (LDAT). While there is less opportunity for potential donors to fully explore issues of ambivalence (which are common) and other psychosocial issues because a final decision must be made in hours or days not weeks, multiple meetings should be held.

An important difference between chronic liver failure and ALF is the risk of rushing too soon to transplant or continuing medical therapy until it is too late. It is not always known whether the patient might recover and transplant would be unnecessary. There is no way of knowing the number of patients who received a transplant who would have recovered without it. However, the number of candidates in ALF who recover without undergoing transplantation must make one pause before taking a living donor to the operating theater. An LDLT performed rapidly may be life-saving, but it may override the chance of spontaneous recovery. Clearly a patient does better with his or her own liver because he or she can then avoid the risks of surgery and immunosuppression. However, waiting for a deceased donor liver raises the risk that an organ will not be available in time, or that by the time the organ is available, the patient has significantly deteriorated. Even if the patient is still eligible for a transplant, the likelihood of its success may be decreased. This is the crux of the tension of liver transplant for ALF.

Given that patients in ALF get priority status for a DDLT, the patient in ALF should undergo the work-up to be listed for a liver on the DDLT waitlist. Living donor alternatives should be considered simultaneously. If more than 1 potential living donor exists, several should be counseled and evaluated by the LDAT in parallel (rather than in the usual sequential method) in case 1 or more is ruled out. For the most part, initial testing can also be done in parallel, but most programs and families are likely to decide on a most likely candidate before imaging and other tests to examine liver anatomy are undertaken, which are usually performed sequentially and only if the initial donor's liver anatomy is inappropriate for a partial transplant hepatectomy or the initial donor requests not to continue the work-up. The potential living donors, in conversation with the LDAT, should be given the option of withdrawing at every stage of the work-up. The timing of living donor surgery must balance the risk of delay with both the chance that a deceased donor organ becomes available and the chance of spontaneous recovery.

The principle of beneficence in which benefits must outweigh risks can be met for living liver donors in the setting of ALF just as in the setting of chronic liver failure. There is, however, a need to develop even better prognostic tools to attempt to avoid unneeded transplants, whether the transplant is from a living or deceased donor.[42]

10.2.3 Justice

The main justice issues raised in the setting of ALF is the question of whether and when to offer transplantation as a therapeutic option. Once it is determined that a liver transplant may be necessary, time constraints result in simultaneously listing a candidate for a DDLT and performing a living donor work-up for eligible and willing potential living liver donors. The fair selection of living liver donors for patients in ALF would apply the same medical and psychosocial evaluations as living donors for patients in chronic liver failure. The variability in the criteria for living donors in the setting of chronic liver disease bodes poorly for the setting of ALF. While the medical work-up can be easily done in an abbreviated time course, the short time frame does not allow for potential donors to adopt better lifestyle health habits that will improve donor outcomes. The psychological assessment is also complicated by the lack of time for considered reflection.[43] It raises concerns regarding safety, quality, and justice.[44]

10.2.4 Vulnerabilities
The complete vulnerability taxonomy can be found in Table 3.3

Here we focus on those vulnerabilities that may be exaggerated by the constraints imposed by ALF. The biggest threat is the lack of time to work through psychosocial issues, which may exacerbate deferential, medical, and situational vulnerabilities.

Consider, first, deferential vulnerability. Adult children may act deferentially toward their parents and, therefore, acquiesce to serve as their living donor. While it may not be characteristic of liver transplantation in other countries, a study in India has shown that adult children are even more likely to be donors to their parents in the setting of ALF compared with the more chronic end-stage liver disease setting.[45] And yet, although not unique to ALF, the data show that adult children donating a liver lobe to their parents have more negative psychosocial issues than other donor-recipient relationship pairs, suggesting that their decision may be more of an expression of duty than of their actual preferences.[46] While this is not necessarily disqualifying, it does emphasize the importance of the role of the LDAT, and the need to provide the donor with psychological support both before and after the transplant.

Potential donors for ALF recipients may also be medically vulnerable because of "the presence of a serious health-related condition in the intended recipient for which there are only less satisfactory alternative remedies." Patients in ALF have a high death rate if not transplanted quickly, and even with the new US deceased donor liver allocation system that gives priority to those in ALF, a significant number of deaths still occur on the waitlist. The medical vulnerability of the candidate in ALF interferes with the potential donor's ability to provide a voluntary and informed consent because "the timing in organ donation is imposed by the needs of another and urgency creates additional pressure . . . which may compromise the autonomy of a potential donor."[47]

Another significant vulnerability is situational, in which the medical exigency of the intended recipient prevents the education and deliberation needed by the potential living donor to decide whether to participate as a living donor. In the setting of chronic liver failure, a significant number of potential living liver donors express ambivalence,[48] and some even feel a degree of pressure, or at least a lack of choice,[49] but there is time to work through these issues and to enable potential donors to address this vulnerability. In the setting of ALF and the tight timeline, this may not be possible. Living donors for patients with ALF express more stress than living donors evaluated for patients with chronic liver failure, although this has been shown to resolve post-transplant.[50]

Because the work-up must be done in a short period of time, transplant programs must ensure that all the steps involved in living donation in the chronic setting must be completed in a compressed time frame. This entails a complete clinical work up; counselling about risks, benefits, and alternatives; discussions with the LDAT to explore motivation, understanding of risks, and one's reaction to an adverse outcome; and engagement with other mental health professionals as indicated. Although best practice guidelines include a "cooling off period" to give the donor time to make a considered decision,[51] this is not possible in the setting of ALF. A compressed time frame may be inadequate to fully digest the information and reflect upon it. To minimize this vulnerability threat, expanded hours for access to mental health professionals is necessary. At minimum, members of the LDAT skilled in this area must be available throughout the emergency living donor evaluation process.

Finally, one must consider the infrastructural vulnerability—that is, whether the transplant programs have resources not only to address living liver donor clinical health issues but also psychological, social, and emotional issues preoperatively. Transplant programs need mental health professionals readily available during the compressed time period in which the donor work-up is being done and in which a decision needs to be made. Mental health resources should also be in place to help the donors postoperatively, particularly if there is an adverse recipient outcome. Also important is physical support for the donor during convalescence which needs to be evaluated and arranged by the LDAT pre-operatively given the high rate of living liver donor complications.[52]

Despite these vulnerabilities, we do believe that competent adults should be permitted to decide to be a living donor in the setting of ALF for both a pediatric and adult recipient, provided that the transplant program has the infrastructural resources and field strength to effectively evaluate, treat, and support the donor.[53]

10.2.5 Special Relationships Create Special Obligations

Throughout the book we have argued for the importance of an LDAT to support the potential living donor. Given the compressed time in which decisions must be made, institutions that perform LDLT for ALF will need to have mental health members of the LDAT available until the emergent surgery is performed in order to ensure that the donor's questions are answered, that the donor has the opportunity to reflect on his decision and the emotional and psychological issues that it raises, and that the donor has the opportunity to opt out. The LDAT must empower the patient to reflect on his decision and help him exercise his autonomy effectively, not just accept a competent patient's nonreflective decision as the final word. Within the time constraints, the potential donor and LDAT should engage in thoughtful deliberation. Then, as long as the living donor fulfills all of the criteria to which standard living liver donors are held, we believe that individuals can give an adequate consent for living donor transplantation.

However, the setting of ALF does make one think about the role for support even post-donation. While UNOS requirements for follow-up are mainly about physical health, it may behoove programs that do LDLT for ALF to incorporate some mental health services or referrals in their post-transplant follow-up care given the greater psychological stress that donors for candidates in ALF may experience.[54]

10.3 Denouement

In case 10-1, the most likely cause of ALF was from the herbal supplements sent by a grandparent from China. Michael Leise and colleagues explain the incidence of drug-induced liver injury (DILI):

> The incidence of DILI from herbal and dietary supplements varies by geography and patterns of herbal and dietary supplement use. It accounts for approximately 9% of the cases of DILI in the United States and up to 19% to 63% of the cases of DILI in Asian countries.[55]

The course of ALF in case 10-1 is consistent with DILI, which is often more likely to require liver transplantation for survival.[56]

In case 10-1, the patient is given status 1 priority on the DDLT waitlist but still may not get an appropriate offer in time. Her father's willingness to be a living donor is complicated by the fact that he has remarried and his new wife does not support the donation. Whether he is willing to create tension in his new family is something that the LDAT needs to address with him. Given the time constraints to adequately address these concerns, the potential donor needs as much information as possible regarding the likelihood of good donor and recipient outcomes, and he needs help in deciding what these outcomes mean for him, his daughter, his ex-wife, his new wife, and his infant-to-be. Family counseling should be available if he thinks this will help. The LDAT should help the donor consider the decision in a holistic context. He needs to understand the risks to which he is exposing himself. He needs to articulate how he will deal with the distress that this is causing his new wife. He needs to understand that a possible outcome for his daughter is acute graft failure with both small-for-size syndrome and vascular thrombosis being more common with LDLT than full-size DDLT. He needs to be counseled that if her living donor liver graft were to fail, she would then be re-listed for a deceased donor graft, which may not become available in time.

The father in case 10-1 must also understand that he is at risk for developing liver failure if too much of his liver is procured, although testing will be done to determine if he has adequate liver mass, and he will be excluded from donating if this risk is significant. As with all living liver donation, he needs to comprehend that although the risk of mortality is low, there is a relatively high risk (37.7%) of living liver donor complications.[57] The donor transplant team should also explain that if his daughter were to become too ill to survive while the work-up is still in progress, the team may decide to delist her from the deceased donor list and may not be willing to perform a LDLT. Surgeons will only expose a potential donor to risks for a third party if the third party is well enough to benefit from the procedure. Surgeons are moral agents who respect the principle of nonmaleficence—to not cause harm unless outweighed by expected benefit. The father needs to be assured that if he elects to back out of the donation, the transplant team will not tell others in the family why he is not being allowed to donate.

Ultimately the decision to donate belongs to the father who, as the potential donor, should make decisions in partnership with, and with the support of, the LDAT. Once it is decided that his daughter will need a transplant, arrangements should be made for his living donor evaluation and surgery, which should be carried out expeditiously. At this point there are 4 alternatives that could stop the living donor hepatectomy: (1) The candidate's condition acutely worsens and eliminates the transplantation option; (2) the candidate's condition improves such that her physicians would recommend a wait-and-see stance in terms of her need for a transplant; (3) the prospective donor might withdraw up until he is given anesthesia; and (4) a deceased donor organ becomes available that allows her to be transplanted in a time frame that doesn't further endanger her. In this last situation, the prospective donor can still decide that he wants to be the donor, but he would need to discuss this with his LDAT to clarify his reasons and reflect on his decision, and his LDAT would need to inform him about both the quality of the deceased donor organ and the fact that he could either be the "back-up" donor if the deceased donor transplant failed acutely or be re-evaluated as a donor if the deceased donor graft failed at a later date. The decision is his to make with the assistance and support of the LDAT.

Notes

1. de Ataide EC, Reges Perales S, de Oliveira Peres MA, et al. Acute liver failure induced by carthamus tinctorius oil: case reports and literature review. *Transplant Proc.* 2018;50:476–477.
2. Stravitz RT, Lee WM. Acute liver failure. *Lancet.* 2019;394:869–881.
3. Rakela J, Lange SM, Ludwig J, Baldus WP. Fulminant hepatitis: Mayo Clinic experience with 34 cases. *Mayo Clin Proc.* 1985;60:289–292.
4. See, for example, Reddy KR, Ellerbe C, Schilsky M, et al. Determinants of outcome among patients with acute liver failure listed for liver transplantation in the United States. *Liver Transpl.* 2016;22:505–515; and Lee WM. Recent developments in acute liver failure. *Best Pract Res Clin Gastroenterol.* 2012;26:3–16.
5. Yoon E, Babar A, Choudhary M, Kutner M, Pyrsopoulos N. Acetaminophen-induced hepatotoxicity: a comprehensive update. *J Clin Transl Hepatol.* 2016;4(2):131–142.
6. Rubin JB, Hameed B, Gottfried M, Lee WM, Sarkar M. Acetaminophen-induced acute liver failure is more common and more severe in women. *Clin Gastroenterol Hepatol.* 2018;16(6):936–946.
7. Squires RH Jr. Acute liver failure in children: etiology and evaluation. *UpToDate.* Literature review current through: July 2021. | This topic last updated: November 09, 2020.https://www.uptodate.com/contents/acute-liver-failure-in-children-etiology-and-evaluation. Updated Jan 13, 2020. Last accessed August 21, 2021.
8. Squires JE, McKiernan P, Squires RH. Acute liver failure: an update. *Clin Liver Dis.* 2018;22:773–805; and O'Grady JO. Timing and benefit of liver transplantation in acute liver failure. *J Hepatol.* 2014;60:663–670. Squires et al and O'Grady find that outcomes following liver transplant for ALF is improving, but the outcomes are on average worse than they are for patients receiving liver transplantation for chronic cholestatic diseases.
9. Broelsch CE, Whitington PF, Emond JC, et al. Liver transplantation in children from living related donors: surgical techniques and results. *Ann Surg.* 1991;214:428–437; discussion 437–439.
10. Tanaka K, Uemoto S, Inomata Y, et al. Living-related liver transplantation for fulminant hepatic failure in children. *Transplant Int.* 1994;7(suppl 1):S108–110.
11. Lo CM, Fan ST, Chan JK, Wei W, Lo RJ, Lai CL. Minimum graft volume for successful adult-to-adult living donor liver transplantation for fulminant hepatic failure. *Transplantation.* 1996;62:696–698.
12. Kato T, Nery JR, Morcos JJ, et al. Successful living related liver transplantation in an adult with fulminant hepatic failure. *Transplantation.* 1997;64:415–417.
13. Kam I. Adult-adult right hepatic lobe living donor liver transplantation for status 2a patients: too little, too late. *Liver Transpl.* 2002;8:347–349; and Testa G, Malago M, Nadalin S, et al. Right-liver living donor transplantation for compensated end-stage liver disease. *Liver Transpl.* 2002;8:340–346.
14. Novello AC. *New York State Committee on Quality Improvement in Living Liver Donation.* Troy, NY: New York State Health Department; 2002.

15. Campsen J, Blei AT, Emond JC, et al. Outcomes of living donor liver transplantation for acute liver failure: the Adult-to-Adult Living Donor Liver Transplantation Cohort Study. *Liver Transpl.* 2008;14:1273–1280, at p. 1274.
16. Campsen et al, "Outcomes of living donor."
17. Campsen et al, "Outcomes of living donor."
18. Campsen et al, "Outcomes of living donor," at p. 1277.
19. Campsen et al, "Outcomes of living donor," at p. 1277. Similar results were obtained by Urrunaga NH, Rachakonda VP, Magder LS, Mindikoglu AL. Outcomes of living versus deceased donor liver transplantation for acute liver failure in the United States. *Transplant Proc.* 2014;46:219–224.
20. Lee WM, Squires RH Jr, Nyberg SL, Doo E, Hoofnagle JH. Acute liver failure: summary of a workshop. *Hepatology.* 2008;47:1401–1415.
21. Reddy et al, "Determinants."
22. O'Grady, "Timing and benefit."
23. Reddy et al, "Determinants."
24. Reddy et al, "Determinants."
25. Squires JE, Rudnick DA, Hardison RM, et al. Liver transplant listing in pediatric acute liver failure: practices and participant characteristics. *Hepatology.* 2018;68:2338–2347.
26. Lo CM. Living donor liver transplantation for acute liver failure: no other choice. *Liver Transpl.* 2012;18:1005–1006.
27. Fellner CH, Marshall JR. Twelve kidney donors. *JAMA.* 1968;206:2703–2707, at p. 2704.
28. Fellner CH, Marshall JR. Kidney donors: the myth of informed consent. *Am J Psych.* 1970;126:1245–1251.
29. Goldman LS. Liver transplantation using living donors. Preliminary donor psychiatric outcomes. *Psychosomatics.* 1993;34:235–240.
30. Bliss A, Stuber ML. Giving life for the second time: a preliminary study of parental partial liver donation for pediatric transplantation. *Fam Syst Health.* 1999;17:217–228.
31. Abdeldayem H, Kashkoush S, Hegab BS, Aziz A, Shoreem H, Saleh S. Analysis of donor motivations in living donor liver transplantation. *Front Surg.* 2014;1:25. doi:10.3389/fsurg.2014.00025
32. Crouch RA, Elliott C. Moral agency and the family: the case of living related organ transplantation. *Camb Q Healthc Ethics.* 1999;8:275–287, at p. 278.
33. The function of the LDAT is discussed in detail in chapter 3, "Developing a Living Donor Ethics Framework."
34. See, for example, Valentín-Gamazo C, Malagó M, Karliova M, et al. Experience after the evaluation of 700 potential donors for living donor liver transplantation in a single center. *Liver Transpl.* 2004;10(9):1087–1096; Sharma A, Ashworth A, Behnke M, Cotterell A, Posner M, Fisher RA. Donor selection for adult-to-adult living donor liver transplantation: well begun is half done. *Transplantation.* 2013;95(3):501–506; and Weng L-C, Huang H-L, Lee W-C, et al. Psychological profiles of excluded living liver donor candidates: an observational study. *Medicine.* 2018;97(52):e13898.

35. Wahab MA, Hamed H, Salar T, et al. Problem of living liver donation in the absence of deceased liver transplantation program: Mansoura experience. *World J Gastroenterol.* 2014;20(37):13607–13614

36. Goldman, "Liver."

37. Goldman, "Liver."

38. Uribe M, Buckel E, Ferrario M, et al. Living related liver transplantation. Why this option has been discarded in a pediatric liver transplant program in Chile. *Transplant Proc.* 2005;37:3378–3379.

39. Uribe et al, "Why this option."

40. See, for example, Erim Y, Beckmann M, Kroencke S, et al. Psychological strain in urgent indications for living donor liver transplantation. *Liver Transpl.* 2007;13:886–895.

41. Marcos A, Ham JM, Fisher RA, et al. Emergency adult to adult living donor liver transplantation for fulminant hepatic failure. *Transplantation.* 2000;69:2202–2205, at p. 2205.

42. See, for example, Jin YJ, Lim YS, Han S, Lee HC, Hwang S, Lee SG. Predicting survival after living and deceased donor liver transplantation in adult patients with acute liver failure. *J Gastroenterol.* 2012;47(10):1115–1124; Kim TS, Kim JM, Kwon CHD, Kim SJ, Joh JW, Lee SK. Prognostic factors predicting poor outcome in living-donor liver transplantation for fulminant hepatic failure. *Transplant Proc.* 2017;49(5):1118–1122; and Chung HS, Lee YJ, Jo YS. Proposal for a new predictive model of short-term mortality after living donor liver transplantation due to acute liver failure. *Ann Transplant.* 2017;22:101–107.

43. Pamecha V, Vagadiya A, Sinha PK, et al. Living donor liver transplantation for acute liver failure: donor safety and recipient outcome. *Liver Transpl.* 2019;25:1408-1421.

44. Duerinckx N, Timmerman L, Van Gogh J, et al. Predonation psychosocial evaluation of living kidney and liver donor candidates: a systematic literature review. *Transpl Int.* 2014;27:2–18; and Nadalin S, Malago M, Radtke A, et al. Current trends in live liver donation. *Transpl Int.* 2007;20:312–330.

45. Pamecha et al, "Living donor."

46. Erim Y, Beckmann M, Kroencke S, et al. Influence of kinship on donors' mental burden in living donor liver transplantation. *Liver Transpl.* 2012;18:901–906.

47. Ross LF, Glannon E, Gottlieb LJ, Thistlethwaite JR. Different standards are not double standards: all elective surgical patients are not alike. *J Clin Ethics.* 2012;23:118–128, at p. 123.

48. See, for example, Weng L-C, Huang H-L, Tsai H-H, Lee W-C. Predictors of decision ambivalence and the differences between actual living liver donors and potential living liver donors. *PLoS One.* 2017;12(5):e0175672; and Pamecha V, Mahansaria SS, Bharathy KG, et al. Selection and outcome of the potential live liver donor. *Hepatol Int.* 2016;10:657–664.

49. Forsberg A, Nilsson M, Krantz M, Olausson M. The essence of living parental liver donation. *Pediatr Transplant.* 2004;8:372–380; and Otte J, Janssen M, Rosati M, Gonze D. Parental experience with living-related donor liver transplantation. *Pediatr Transplant.* 2004;8:317–321.

50. See, for example, Erim et al, "Psychological strain."
51. The Ethics Committee of the Transplantation Society. The consensus statement of the Amsterdam Forum on the care of the live kidney donor. *Transplantation.* 2004;78:491–492, at p. 492; and LaPointe Rudow D, Swartz K, Phillips C, Hollenberger J, Smith T, Steel JL. The psychosocial and independent living donor advocate evaluation and post-surgery care of living donors. *J Clin Psychol Med Settings.* 2015;22(2–3):136–149.
52. Samstein B, Smith AR, Freise CE, et al. Complications and their resolution in recipients of deceased and living donor liver transplants: findings from the A2ALL Cohort Study. *Am J Transplant.* 2016;16(2):594–602; and Sanchez-Cabus S, Cherqui D, Rashidian N, et al. Left-liver adult-to-adult living donor liver transplantation: can it be improved? a retrospective multicenter European study. *Ann Surg.* 2018;268(5):876–884.
53. Field strength is a concept proposed by Francis Moore and refers to the knowledge, training, and experience of those undertaking the innovation. See Moore FD. Three ethical revolutions: ancient assumptions remodeled under pressure of transplantation. *Transplant Proc.* 1988;20(1 suppl 1):1061–1067.
54. Erim et al, "Psychological strain."
55. Leise MD, Poterucha JJ, Talwalkar JA. Drug-induced liver injury. *Mayo Clinic Proc.* 2014;89(1):95–106 (references omitted).
56. See, for example, Lee, "Recent developments," and Reuben A, Koch DG, Lee WM, Acute Liver Failure Study Group. Drug-induced acute liver failure: results of a U.S. multicenter, prospective study. *Hepatology.* 2010;52:2065–2076.
57. See, Beavers KL, Sandler RS, Fair JH, Johnson MW, Shrestha R. The living donor experience: donor health assessment and outcomes after living donor liver transplantation. *Liver Transpl.* 2001;7:943–947; Ghobrial RM, Freise CE, Trotter JF, et al. Donor morbidity after living donation for liver transplantation. *Gastroenterology.* 2008;135:468–476; and Abecassis MM, Fisher RA, Olthoff KM, et al. Complications of living donor hepatic lobectomy—a comprehensive report. *Am J Transplant.* 2012;12:1208–1217.

PART 4

MORAL LIMITS TO EXPANDING LIVING DONORS

11

The Imminently Dying Donor

11.1 Introduction

Traditionally, living donors were very healthy, passed extensive physical and psychosocial evaluations, and gave a voluntary consent to donation. As the supply-demand gap grew, transplant programs became more accepting of less healthy donors. The medical restrictions concerning age, weight, and blood pressure, have all been loosened.[1]

This chapter focuses on the extreme case: whether and when individuals who have life-limiting conditions (LLC) should be considered for living organ donation. Specifically, we consider: (1) donation by individuals with advanced progressive severe debilitating disease for whom there is no ameliorative therapy; and (2) donation by individuals who are imminently dying or would die of the donation process itself. To understand the ethical issues that these cases raise, however, it is critical to distinguish the living donor with a shortened life expectancy from the deceased donor. We begin with a short description of deceased donor organ transplantation—from the determination of death to the procurement of organs according to the dead donor rule (DDR),[2] an ethical norm that values all human life and demands that persons are treated and cared for as living patients until death is declared. We then apply our living donor ethics framework (see Chapter 3) to cases described in the medical and medical ethics literature. While some of these scenarios could be ethical with appropriate safeguards, we explore and reject those scenarios that attempt to circumvent the DDR, which we believe is (or should be) inviolable out of respect for the dignity of all living beings.[3] Although circumventing the DDR may increase the number of living donor organs, it is unethical because it fails to give enough weight to the living donor as a patient in his or her own right—a patient who is medically vulnerable due to his or her own irreversible, irreparable, or degenerative health conditions.

The Living Organ Donor as Patient. Lainie Friedman Ross and J. Richard Thistlethwaite, Jr, Oxford University Press.
© Oxford University Press 2022. DOI: 10.1093/oso/9780197618202.003.0011

11.2 The DDR and Deceased Donor
Organ Transplantation

In the United States (US), the Uniform Declaration of Death Act states that death can be determined either by (1) irreversible cessation of circulatory and respiratory functions, or (2) irreversible cessation of all functions of the entire brain, including the brain stem.[4] In all cases of deceased donor transplantation, the donor must be dead and not merely dying. Only after death is declared do providers switch from treating the patient to focusing on the procedures necessary to prepare the decedent for organ donation. As Robert Arnold and Stuart Youngner explain regarding the implications of the DDR,

> persons must be dead before their organs are taken has two distinct connotations: 1. Patients must not be killed by organ retrieval; . . . and 2. Organs must not be taken from patients until they die.[5]

To be clear, the DDR is neither a law nor a regulation.[6] As David Rodríguez-Arias explains:

> John Robertson coined the expression "dead donor rule" to refer to a norm that organ donation policies have implicitly held since the beginning of multiorgan procurement, in the late 1960s. He characterized it as "a centerpiece of the social order's commitment to respect for persons and human life. It is also the ethical linchpin of a voluntary system of organ donation, and helps maintain public trust in the organ procurement system.[7]

Most deceased organ donors are declared dead by irreversible cessation of neurological function. A physician evaluates the patient to ensure that he or she lacks brain stem reflexes and fails an apnea test. The decedent is kept on the ventilator for organ oxygenation until organs are removed in the operating room. Both thoracic and abdominal organs can be procured.

In the case of death after irreversible cessation of cardio-circulatory function, there is a waiting time ("hands off" period) between the declaration of death and the procurement of organs to ensure auto-resuscitation does not occur.[8] Donation after circulatory death (DCD) is usually attempted in individuals who suffer a catastrophic injury (eg, from trauma or stroke), require life-sustaining treatment, and have a neurological prognosis inconsistent with recovery. Only after the decision is made to withdraw life-sustaining treatment is the option of DCD raised. This is referred to as "decoupling."[9] As Sam Shemie and colleagues from Canada who participated in the End-of-Life Conversations with Families of Potential Donors participants explain:

> this approach appears to help in avoiding perceptions that physicians have given up on patients prematurely or that physicians have a conflict of interest. It also gives families time to adjust to the shock of the death before considering donation.[10]

In the US, the decoupling is further achieved by the separation of personnel. Health care professionals care for the patient and work with the patient and families about goals of care and treatment plans, including treatment withdrawal. The organ procurement organization (OPO) team, on the other hand, discusses the options of postmortem organ donation, and if donation is authorized, the OPO team manages the body after death is declared.

The difference, then, between a living donor, even one with a life-limiting condition, and a deceased donor is two-fold. First, living donor organ transplantation involves 2 patients, a living donor and an intended recipient, whereas deceased donor organ transplantation involves only 1 living patient (the intended recipient). Second, the health care team caring for the living donor is responsible for the living donor as a patient in his or her own right. As we will discuss below, this team will be separate from the intended recipient's team and will include a living donor advocate (LDA) who will ensure that the donation is voluntary, informed, and consistent with the interests of the potential donor.

11.3 Living Kidney Donation From Donors With LLCs

The first two cases involve living organ donation by individuals with advanced progressive severe debilitating disease for whom there is no ameliorative therapy. Consider case 11-1, 1 of 5 case reports from the University Medical Center, Rotterdam, The Netherlands:

> Case 11-1: This patient [a 48-year-old man] was diagnosed with a stage III GOLD chronic obstructive pulmonary disease and severe emphysema. He was being treated by a pulmonologist, used a wheel chair because of respiratory insufficiency. In 2010, he requested and underwent psychosocial

screening for [non-directed] living donation. The reason for donation was based on his opinion that, at the moment, he was physically and mentally still healthy enough to donate a kidney. Moreover, he was aware of the fact that kidneys from living-donors function better than those from deceased donors. He reported: "By doing this I can give something back to society, just like my Mother would have done, because she was a really helpful person. I am sure she would have been proud of what I am going to do." Based on the interview and psychologic complaint questionnaire, no psychosocial problems were detected, and sense of reality was normal.[11]

The other 4 case reports in this article also involved persons with LLC who requested to serve as non-directed living donors: 2 had Huntington Disease but were judged to have the capacity to consent for donation, and 2 had recurrent brain cancers that were not thought to be transmissible by organ transplantation.[12]

The authors described 4 safeguards. First, "all donors are well informed and made the decision about unspecified donation by themselves."[13] The individuals voluntarily sought out the opportunity and gave an informed consent. Second, the donation was consistent with the donors' lives: all had previously registered in the Dutch organ donation register for deceased donation before stating interest in living donation. Third, the physicians consulted with the patients' independent medical specialists and found that "[n]one of them had an objection to the donor nephrectomy."[14] Fourth, all passed the psychological evaluation component of screening, just as their healthy donor counterparts had.[15]

The authors claimed that the 3-month post-donor nephrectomy evaluation by the transplant coordinator validated their decision to allow the individuals to serve as living donors. All of the donors stated that the donation lived up to their expectation and they would do it again. Although none reported abnormal post-nephrectomy pain or fatigue, and kidney function was stable, "the self-reported health status after donation had slightly decreased in two donors."[16] During the post-donation follow-up, 2 died by euthanasia, which is legal in the Netherlands (at 0.6 years and 4.9 years post-donation) and 1 died from his LLC (at 2.4 years post-donation). The other 2 were doing well in their last yearly medical follow-up.[17]

The case of W.B. (case 11-2) from Madison Wisconsin described by surgeons in *The Atlantic Monthly* contrasts with the cases from the Netherlands. W.B. was a 56-year-old previously healthy man who was recently diagnosed with amyotrophic lateral sclerosis (ALS) and had some compromised respiratory function. He approached the University of Wisconsin's transplant program as a prospective organ donor. As the surgeon-authors explain:

> Case 11-2: Initially, W.B. had assumed that he would arrange for his organs to be procured when he died, but then he read that kidneys from a living donor work better and last longer than kidneys from a deceased donor. For one thing, the death process takes a toll on organs, between the decreased flow of blood and oxygen and the release of inflammatory proteins. For another, kidneys that are removed after death inevitably endure "cold time"— when they are outside the body, on ice, without any blood flow at all.
>
> "Why not fork out a kidney before it becomes compromised by all the meds I am taking?" W.B. asked us when we met him in June.[18]

The Wisconsin surgeons refused to remove W.B.'s kidney because they were not sure that in his weakened condition he would tolerate the surgery or that, even if he tolerated the surgery, he would be able to be extubated. While W.B. was willing to assume those risks, and he had the support of his neurologist, the surgeons objected: "If we were to remove one of W.B.'s kidneys, and he died one, two, or even six months after surgery, his death would be a very public black mark on our program."[19]

How does the living donor ethics framework help evaluate the case reports from Rotterdam (case 11-1) and Wisconsin (case 11-2)?

Consider, first, the principle of respect for persons which is operationalized in the concept of informed consent. The individuals from Rotterdam and Wisconsin had decision-making capacity at the time they sought to be a living donor. All actively sought to donate, and their decision was consistent with other life decisions (eg, signing a donor card). The principle of respect for persons would support the voluntary and informed decisions of these patients.

However, this principle must be balanced against the other principles. The principle of beneficence would support donations provided that the benefits outweigh the harms. Whether living organ donation from a person with an LLC fulfills this principle is controversial. Some argue that the benefits of successfully being an organ donor outweigh the harms of undergoing surgery and the risks of postoperative complications even if one has only a short life-expectancy. They may also argue that the physicians may be harming someone like W.B. psychologically in thwarting his goals even as they protect him physically. Others argue that most of the benefit can be achieved by postmortem donation and one cannot justify taking a patient with an LLC to the operating room if the individual has a serious risk of an adverse outcome from the elective surgery, as might be expected in an individual with stage III GOLD chronic obstructive pulmonary disease (case 11-1) or ALS (case 11-2).

The third principle to consider is justice as fairness in the selection of living donors. Traditionally, living donors were adult biologically related family members. Today programs encourage patients to find living donors from a wider pool: spouses, friends, acquaintances located on social media, even strangers. Donors were traditionally very healthy to minimize both short-term perioperative risks and long-term health risks, although today programs accept less healthy individuals.[20] While long-term risks are of less concern in individuals with an LLC, some individuals with an LLC are at increased short-term risks (eg, W.B. was at risk of becoming ventilator dependent). If transplant programs were to encourage donations by persons with an LLC,[21] this would raise suspicions of discrimination and devaluation. However, in cases 11-1 and 11-2, the idea originated from the potential donors. W.B. approached the transplant center on his own volition, as did all of the individuals described in Rotterdam. In addition, all were seeking to donate non-directedly. These distinctions are important. The proposed donations are not the brainchild of transplant programs and/or potential recipients or recipient advocates expressing a devaluation of the lives of those with an LLC that would justify preferentially exposing them to donation risks because they have "less to lose." Rather, these cases involve individuals with LLC who autonomously proposed living donation to give additional meaning to their numbered days. Non-directed donation by individuals with an LLC is consistent with the principle of justice (although a campaign to encourage Good Samaritan donations from individuals with LLC would not be). It is fair because it treats all adults with decisional capacity equally in respecting their right to decide whether to serve as a living donor.

While the principles of respect for persons, beneficence, and justice are all consistent with respecting the donation request, such a conclusion raises discomfort in part because of the potential vulnerabilities of those with an LLC. Below we consider each of the vulnerabilities enumerated in chapter 3 (see Table 3.3).

The descriptions from Rotterdam (case 11-1) and Wisconsin (case 11-2), did not suggest that the potential donors had capacitational vulnerability.

All had the cognitive capacity to understand the risks and benefits and were able to give a voluntary informed consent. Nor were there any juridic (overriding authority who had an independent interest in the donation), deferential (patterns of behavior that may mask unwillingness), medical (serious health-related condition in the intended recipient), or situational (time pressure that would interfere with donor education or deliberation) vulnerabilities, as the idea to donate was their own. They had chronic illnesses that were life-limiting, but none were imminently dying.

We believe that the donors from Rotterdam and the potential Wisconsin donor possibly had allocational vulnerability—lacking in subjectively important social goods that would be gained by donation. Most were described as unfit for work, and several were quoted as saying that the donation would make them "useful," suggesting that they lacked social respect which they hoped could be gained by donating.[22] Individuals with an LLC must understand that donating to increase their perceived self-worth may backfire. Family members' responses may be mixed—some may view the donor as a self-sacrificing hero; others may think the donor is "crazy" or "reckless."[23]

The potential donors from Rotterdam and Wisconsin were also potentially socially vulnerable because of their illness and/or disabilities. The medical profession has a long history of abandoning dying patients, as do some friends and families.[24] Donation may be one way that these individuals seek to engage with their intimate relations out of a position of strength and not of vulnerability.

The threats of social and allocational vulnerability must be examined against the backdrop that these donors had approached the transplant programs on their own initiative. In both cases 11-1 and 11-2, the donor decided by himself that he (and society) would get more benefit from donating a kidney as a living donor rather than waiting until death, when declining health or the dying process might make the organs unusable for transplantation. Permitting living donation by individuals with an LLC empowered the individuals in Rotterdam to achieve the goal of helping a third party through organ donation at a time when they themselves felt that they had few other opportunities to contribute to society.

The fifth principle is the concept of special relationships creating special responsibilities adopted from Robert Goodin's work on *Protecting the Vulnerable*.[25] In living donor transplantation, the donor's health care team, known as the living donor advocate team (LDAT), consists of a living donor advocate (LDA), a nephrologist, a transplant surgeon and other health care professionals such as a social worker and a psychologist, when needed.[26] The LDAT is responsible for empowering prospective donors to address their vulnerabilities, and for protecting those who cannot by disqualifying them from donation. While all potential donors have potential vulnerabilities, when the potential donor has an LLC, some vulnerabilities may be exacerbated and different vulnerabilities may be at issue. The LDAT should ensure that the potential donor is acting consistently with his or her own values, is informed, has addressed potential vulnerabilities that may interfere with a voluntary decision, and has the right to withdraw from donating at any time.

Even if the LDAT determines that the donor is acting freely and without undue pressure, surgeons are moral agents. In the Wisconsin case, they stated that they have a responsibility to minimize harm. Leaving a donor ventilator-dependent postoperatively was not consistent with their interpretation of their obligations in the elective living donor setting.[27] The Wisconsin surgeons were also worried about institutional reputation.[28] While their decision may conflict with their patient's interest, it is important for the community of patients for whom they provide care. The Wisconsin surgeons, as moral agents, can and did refuse to accommodate W.B.'s desire to be a living donor. As Carl Elliott so eloquently explained: a physician as a moral agent decides "not simply whether a subject's choice is reasonable or morally justifiable, but whether he [the physician] is morally justified in helping the subject accomplish it."[29]

In sum, cases 11-1 and 11-2 describe cases in which competent adults request to serve as living donors. The donors differ from the standard non-directed donor because they are not healthy and have a short life-expectancy. While the potential donor with an LLC may be more socially and allocationally vulnerable, the donation may be consistent with his or her own life goals. A thorough living donor work-up, including evaluations by mental health providers and an LDA, is essential. While morally permissible for the Rotterdam physicians to respect the donation decisions by individuals with decisional capacity who have an LLC, the physicians in Wisconsin, as moral agents, were also within their right to refuse to take W.B. to the operating room if they thought they could leave him seriously worse off.

All the donors from Rotterdam and Wisconsin were seeking to donate non-directedly. Although not described in detail in this published manuscript, Yannick Rakké and colleagues in Rotterdam noted that they had also procured kidneys from 2 individuals with Huntington Disease who donated to specified recipients.[30] Directed living donation from individuals with an

LLC may generate deferential vulnerability concerns (for example, if the idea is proposed by another family member to whom the individual with the LLC is deferential). The need for an organ by a family member also raises concerns about medical and situational vulnerabilities. On the one hand, the individual with an LLC may be selected by the family as expendable, and the individual may feel pressured to donate quickly before his or her symptoms worsen and make him or her ineligible to be a living donor. On the other hand, the donor may also experience significant benefit in knowing that he or she has helped a family member, and it may increase his or her social standing within the family.[31] As such, potential directed donors with an LLC raise additional vulnerabilities compared to potential donors with an LLC who seek to donate non-directedly. Both require careful evaluation by an LDAT to assess donor understanding, voluntariness, and that the vulnerabilities are appropriately addressed.

Did Rotterdam go too far? We don't think so. Agreeing to accept donations from donors with LLC is consistent with the living donor ethics framework that we developed. While safeguards are necessary for all living donors, the potential donor with an LLC has additional vulnerability risks that require careful assessment by an LDAT. It will be an uncommon request, but its fulfillment may help individuals give meaning to their lives as they struggle to live with progressive and ultimately fatal debilitation. However, such donations should be limited to persons with decisional capacity who voluntarily and independently raise this option. Public endorsements or campaigns by transplant professionals to attract such candidates for either directed or non-directed donation should be avoided.

11.4 Pre-Mortem Donation From Individuals With LLCs

The next 4 cases involve living organ donation from individuals who are in the process of dying (pre-mortem donation). A case described by Paul Morrisey in the *American Journal of Bioethics* in 2012 explains why there is interest in pre-mortem donation from individuals who are authorized to be DCD donors (either from first-person authorization, as in case 11-3, or authorization from their family, as in case 11-4).

Case 11-3: A 28-year-old man suffered severe irreversible brain injury in an industrial accident but was not expected to progress to brain death.

The family and team agreed to withdrawal of treatment. The patient had a signed donor card and the family agreed to attempt donation after circulatory death (DCD). The family requested that upon procurement, one kidney would be allocated to a family member and agreed that the liver and second kidney would be allocated according to the wait list. Thoracic organ donation was not considered.[32]

Most DCD protocols require that the individual undergoes cardiorespiratory arrest within a given period of time after withdrawal of life support. If the potential donor survives for a longer time period, the organ retrieval procedure is aborted. In fact, even when potential DCD donors die within the allotted time, the number of organs actually procured and transplanted will depend on many factors. In the case described by Morrisey, procurement was not attempted:

> Upon extubation in the operating room, he maintained normal blood pressure and heart rate despite low oxygen saturations. After 60 minutes the transplant team requested further observation in the operating room for asystole. After an additional 30 minutes of hypotension and hypoxia, organ recovery was abandoned and the patient was returned to the intensive care unit. He died four hours later.[33]

The requirement that the patient be declared dead before donation may thwart potential donors from realizing their desire to donate. To circumvent this, Morrisey proposed that our current organ donation policies should be revisited in the situation of an elective withdrawal of life support for a neurologically devastated patient, and that the donor's surrogate be given the option of pre-mortem kidney donation:

> Case 11-4: The process begins as before with the identification of a suitable candidate for DCD: explicitly an individual with severe, irreversible brain injury. The family decides to withdraw life-sustaining treatments with the expectation of the patient's imminent death. A DNR [Do Not Resuscitate] order is entered. The family provides informed consent for kidney donation to be followed by end-of-life care. The patient is transported to the operating room for kidney recovery. Both kidneys are recovered via midline laparotomy with vascular control, equivalent to bilateral nephrectomy in a neurologically intact patient. General anesthesia and standard

analgesic care are administered, as would be given to a trauma victim with severe head injury undergoing surgery. The patient returns to the intensive care unit. A suitable interval from the operating room to the palliative care setting would enable the medical team to administer analgesia and sedation appropriate to end-of-life care without concern that an anesthetized patient is being extubated. End-of-life care is instituted according to the family's request, in a more relaxed time period without the requisite "rush" to organ retrieval following asystole required by DCD. This protocol enables the family to grieve and spend time with the decedent after death.[34]

Morrisey proposes that individuals with severe irreversible brain injury who are not expected to progress to brain death (and may die too slowly after extubation to meet DCD criteria) undergo pre-mortem bilateral kidney donation under anesthesia. After the procurement, the patient returns to the intensive care unit, gets appropriate palliative care, and then has treatment withdrawn.[35] Morrisey's article was followed by a number of commentaries. Smith and colleagues objected because Morrisey's proposal failed to protect the donor's interests, but, if Morrisey's proposal were modified to require first-person donor consent, then they would support it.[36] Wynn Morrison also supported the idea of pre-mortem donation in principle, but objected to the removal of both kidneys:

> The suggestion that bilateral nephrectomies be performed is the most ethically troublesome aspect of this protocol. The medical team's ability to predict, on an individual basis, the time frame within which a patient will die is imperfect. Removing both kidneys not only guarantees that the patient will die within a few weeks following the withdrawal when death otherwise might not have occurred, but iatrogenic renal failure also has the potential to complicate the symptom management of the dying patient.[37]

Removing only 1 kidney rather than both would allow the family to change its mind about treatment withdrawal without complicating the medical management of the patient.

In 2018, Christopher Zimmerman and colleagues at the University of Wisconsin at Madison did semi-structured interviews with families from their own center who had experienced a loved one's unsuccessful donation after cardio-circulatory death. They found that:

family members were accepting of donation before circulatory death for a single kidney, and many believed recovery of all organs was permissible because they believed the cause of death was the donor's injury, not organ procurement.[38]

In contrast, professional stakeholders from across the country were uniformly against the removal of all organs, but some were willing to "accommodate removal of a single kidney."[39]

Morrisey's proposal of removing both kidneys (or the Morrison revision of removing 1 kidney to avoid harm if the patient survived longer than expected) is one example of what has become known as imminent death donation (IDD). IDD entails procuring solid organs for organ donation while the patient is still living. It involves transforming the authorization to be a deceased donor under the Uniform Anatomical Gift Act[40] into an authorization for living donation (albeit from a dying patient). While the individual in case 11-3 has signed up to be a deceased donor, at the time of his injury, he had not made any attempts to be a living donor—whether as a Good Samaritan living donor or as a directed living donor to a family member. As the case is written, there was a family member with known end-stage renal disease and he had not initiated a living donor work-up. Thus, the proposal extrapolates that individuals who sign up to be a deceased donor are willing to be living donors, even though the patient had never made an effort to do so. It empowers surrogates to authorize living donation when, in fact, living solid living organ donors should require the first-person consent of the competent adult, and this requirement should be even more stringent when evaluating Good Samaritan living donation.[41]

Morrisey is not the only one to raise the issue of IDD. In 2014, 2 years after Morrisey's publication, the Ethics Committee of the United Network for Organ Sharing (UNOS) coordinated an intercommittee work group to consider the ethical implications of IDD—that is, "the recovery of a living donor organ immediately prior to an impending and planned withdrawal of ventilator support expected to result in the patient's death."[42] According to the Ethics Report, IDD applies to at least 2 types of potential donors:

(1) IDD might be applicable to an individual with devastating neurologic injury that is considered irreversible and who is not brain dead. The individual would be unable to participate in medical decision-making; therefore, decisions about organ donation would be made by

a surrogate or might be addressed by the potential donor's advanced directive.

(2) IDD might also be applied to a patient who has capacity for medical decision making, is dependent on life-support, has decided not to accept further life support and indicates the desire to donate organs prior to foregoing life support and death.[43]

Case 11-4 is an example of a potential type 1 IDD. An example of a type 2 IDD was described by Arnold and Youngner in 1993. The hypothetical case (case 11-5) involves a ventilator-dependent patient with ALS who has requested termination of life support, which is planned for the following day. In their hypothetical case, the patient then requests that prior to termination of life support he be taken to the operating room and be allowed to donate multiple abdominal organs under anesthesia. He would then be transported back to the intensive care unit where his ventilator would be disconnected at the arranged time, long before the patient would die from the organ removals.[44]

The UNOS Ethics Committee did not discuss the ethics of type 2 IDD, but focused exclusively on type 1 IDD and "ultimately determined that there could be circumstances where LD-PPW [living donation prior to planned withdrawal] may be ethically appropriate and justified by the potential benefits to donors, donor families and recipients."[45] However, 9 other UNOS committees objected to their proposal and the proposal was subsequently withdrawn.[46] Although the basis for their objections is not described, we agree with the nine other UNOS committees. We do not support type 1 cases of IDD on the grounds that this case empowers surrogates to convert a person's first-person authorization to serve as a deceased donor into a patient's willingness to be a living donor despite the fact that there is no potential medical or psychological gain for the patient himself.[47]

IDD is not the farthest point on the spectrum. Case 11-6 would involve an individual who is imminently dying (or his family) to ask the physicians not to wait for death to be declared before procuring organs. Instead the individual imminently dying (or his family) can ask the physicians to take the dying individual to the operating room on the ventilator and have all of his thoracic and abdominal organs removed under anesthesia (organ donation by euthanasia [ODE]).

ODE is different from organ donation after euthanasia. In countries where euthanasia is legal (eg, Canada, Belgium, and the Netherlands), donation after euthanasia is permitted. Like any other death after irreversible cessation of cardio-circulatory function, there is a "hands-off" waiting period after death is declared which means that the procurement is usually limited to the kidneys, and sometimes the liver, but the thoracic organs are often not usable. In ODE, the organs are procured in the operating room while the individual is still on the ventilator which means that all of the organs could be procured in a manner that allows for transplantation into eligible candidates.[48] Jan Bollen and colleagues in the Netherlands discuss growing support for combining these 2 procedures and some of the obstacles.[49] They acknowledge that ODE would require revisions to current legislation.[50]

Type 1 IDD limits which organs can be procured because the patient returns to the ICU alive before having life-sustaining treatment withdrawn.[51] In contrast, ODE would permit the procurement of all organs and would avoid what might be considered a charade of returning the imminent death donor to the ICU to remove cardiorespiratory support to allow death to proceed. As noted previously, many of the Wisconsin families who had authorized donation after cardio-circulatory death which was unsuccessful claimed that they would have supported the removal of all organs, although none of the transplant professionals did.[52] Some bioethicists also have argued in its favor.[53] Like the transplant professionals in Zimmerman's study, we believe it is morally wrong and violates the DDR, which we will explore in more detail below.

11.5 Ethics Framework for Imminent Death Donation

Case 11-3 is ethically straightforward because the family gives permission for the patient to become a DCD donor (which, in this case, we know is consistent with the patient's signed donor card). Case 11-4 is more ethically controversial because the patient's tragic condition was acute and the patient had no time to consider how he would want to be treated if he became severely brain injured and was not expected to recover. A proxy decision-maker, usually a family member, must decide what the patient would have wanted with respect to continuing or withdrawing life-sustaining medical therapies. The proxy can also authorize DCD donation if the proxy believes this is what the patient would have wanted. At minimum, the proxy would need to get court permission to authorize the incompetent patient to serve as a living solid organ donor.[54]

The living donor ethics framework can be used to evaluate IDD by an individual who lacks decisional capacity (case 11-4).

Consider the first 3 principles in the living donor ethics framework adopted from the *Belmont Report*: respect for persons, beneficence and justice.[55] Respect for persons requires that we respect the wishes of a patient with decisional capacity and protect those who lack capacity. Whether the patient in case 11-4 would have wanted to be a living donor and undergo surgery prior to treatment withdrawal is not known. Given his incapacity and lack of stated wishes, the principle of respect for persons requires protection even from well-meaning family members and transplant professionals, and thus the principle would not support donation. Pre-mortem donation is also not consistent with the principle of beneficence. The procurement would not be for his medical benefit and might even cause physical harm (eg, pain), without any potential psychological benefit. This contrasts with cases 11-1 and 11-2, in which the psychological benefit of being a donor was an important motivation for the individuals to serve as living donors. Given the lack of prior stated wishes in case 11-4 about living donation, it is hard to justify exposing him to any risks of pain or discomfort to benefit an unknown third party. Justice arguments also support limiting living organ donation to individuals who can provide their own voluntary and informed consent.

The fourth principle of the framework focuses on donor vulnerabilities. The potential donor's capacitational vulnerability in case 11-4 differentiates him from the donors in cases 11-1 and 11-2. The patient is also socially vulnerable because his neurological prognosis is poor, even if he were maximally treated. The data show that the severely disabled are frequently devalued.[56] The patient in case 11-4 also clearly has situational vulnerability: the severe brain injury prevents the education and opportunity to deliberate about whether to participate as a living donor. If there were a known potential transplant candidate in the family, the patient may also have medically vulnerability: the family may seek to procure the organ for their loved one pre-mortem to avoid the possibility of an aborted DCD donation due to the patient's prolonged survival after withdrawal of life support.

While cases of type 1 IDD do not necessarily violate the letter of the DDR (provided only 1 and not both kidneys are removed), we believe they do violate its spirit. The main reason for the individual to donate pre-mortem is because DCD may not come to fruition. In contrast, we believe that the harms of surgical intervention in the last hours of life—not for the benefit of the patient, but for the benefit of a third party, cannot be justified. As moral agents, transplant providers should invoke the DDR to protect dying patients. IDD is being done to circumvent the DDR, which protects dying patients because it requires pre-mortem care to be focused on the patient as a person (an end-in-oneself) and not solely as a potential source of organs (as merely a means to another's ends).[57] Thus, it is inconsistent with the special obligations that the LDAT has to potential donors with whom the LDAT has a special relationship. IDD also threatens public trust in the transplant and palliative care enterprises. We do not support type 1 IDD.

Type 2 IDD (case 11-5) differs from type 1 IDD (case 11-4) because the hypothetical individual in case 11-5 has decisional capacity and makes the request for and by himself. While this makes him less vulnerable, he is still quite socially vulnerable given his severe disability.[58] Again, IDD is only being considered because DCD may not be actualized due to many factors beyond the control of the patient and transplant team. Thus, type 2 IDD cases, like type 1 IDD, are ethically problematic because they also attempt to circumvent the DDR and the protections it affords to those who are dying. We do not support it.

Case 11-6 is slightly different than IDD, as described by the UNOS Ethics Committee, because in this case, the individual whose death is imminent does not die shortly after donation but, rather, the donation itself is the proximate cause of death. Case 11-6 challenges the premise of the DDR. It promotes organ procurement from individuals who are not dead but only "nearly dead" or "as good as dead."[59] That is, case 11-6 forces one to ask what protections the DDR provides in a case where life-sustaining treatment will be removed in the near future with imminent death expected.

The utilitarian asks whether the benefits of obtaining organs from dying patients before they die and violating the DDR outweighs the harms. While the donors (or their families) in these cases might say that the benefits outweigh the harms, we must ask what society at large would think and whether such actions would reduce public trust, not just in transplantation, but also in medical care of the dying. Some may be concerned that permitting donation by those with an LLC suggests that their lives are expendable, or at least that they are perceived as expendable by health care providers. Although procuring organs from the dying may increase organ procurement in the short run, the loss of public trust may cause fewer organs to be procured in the long run. Utilitarians may or may not support living donation by the imminently dying—depending on an assessment of the anticipated consequences, both intended and unintended. Other utilitarians may argue for at least a trial to determine what impact donation by the dying would have on the overall number of organs procured.

From a deontological or principle-based perspective, it is not enough to ask whether the benefits outweigh the harms, but to consider certain fundamental principles of bioethics that must be satisfactorily addressed. One such principle is whether ODE is consistent with respect for persons. Does it merely treat the living donor with very limited life expectancy as a means (a source of organs), or does it also consider the patient as a person or an end-in-him- or herself?[60]

There is also a logistical problem: transplant surgeons may not be willing to be the proximate cause of the patient's death. The DDR requires that patients are declared dead by health care providers not involved in the organ procurement. The DDR protects the dying patient's dignity and value by prohibiting the transplant procurement team's involvement until after the patient is declared dead.

What if transplant surgeons were willing to take patients to the operating room and procure their organs as a form of physician-assisted suicide? Currently it is not legal, and we believe that ODE should remain illegal. It circumvents important safeguards: the separation of patient care and patient care decisions from organ procurement as well as the separation of the determination of death from organ procurement.[61] These separations are important. They ensure respect for the dying patient and maintain patient and community trust in the transplant endeavor and the medical system more broadly.

In sum, the DDR helps to ensure respectful and appropriate care for the dying. There is value in maintaining a clear division of responsibilities between end-of-life care and organ procurement with 2 separate medical teams involved.

11.6 Conclusion

We began by considering cases of individuals with decisional capacity who are currently "healthy enough" to donate organs despite having an LLC. We then proceeded to the living donor who was imminently dying and the potential for IDD, and lastly the case of the person who seeks to die by organ procurement (see Table 11.1). The appearance of these cases in the literature implies some degree of legitimacy that makes them worthy of examination.

Table 11.1 Summary of Cases

Case	Case description	Is the outcome ethical?
11-1	First-person consent for living donation by individuals with decisional capacity and a life-limiting condition (LLC) (Rotterdam)	Yes. Living donation is permissible provided that patient vulnerabilities are adequately explored and patient gives an informed and voluntary consent. (It is also permissible to exclude individuals with an LLC if the LDAT does not believe that their vulnerabilities can be adequately addressed.)
11-2	First-person consent for living donation by individuals with decisional capacity and an LLC (Wisconsin)	Yes. Transplant team as moral agents can decide that the risk of harm is too great despite consent. (Other transplant teams may decide that the risks are surmountable and that donation is permissible with appropriate first-person consent.)
11-3	DCD with surrogate consent	Yes. Surrogates can consent when decision is consistent with prior wishes of decedent. Consistent with DDR.
11-4	Pre-mortem donation authorized by surrogates for a patient who is imminently dying (possibly followed by DCD)	No. Fails to respect the dignity and value of the dying patient by attempting to circumvent the DDR.
11-5	First-person pre-mortem donation (possibly followed by first-person consent to DCD)	No. Fails to treat the donor as a patient first. Exposes vulnerable individuals to unnecessary harms by attempting to circumvent the DDR.
11-6	Organ donation euthanasia authorized by first-person or surrogate consent	No. Removes protections from a vulnerable class of people. Inconsistent with DDR.

This table was first printed in Ross LF and Thistlethwaite JR. Living Donation by Individuals with Life-Limiting Conditions. *J Law Med Ethics*. 2019 (Spring);47: 112–122, Table 2: Summary of Cases on p. 121. Revised and modified with permission.

Abbreviations: DCD = donation after cardio-circulatory death; DDR = dead donor rule; LDAT = living donor advocate team; LLC = life-limiting condition.

They force us to ask whether such cases represent a permissible step along what admittedly could become a slippery slope or whether they are themselves a step too far in our quest to expand the organ donor pool.

Our answers are case dependent. Case 11-3 is a classic example of DCD and raises no red flags (provided adequate time has elapsed after cessation of circulation to ensure both that auto-resuscitation cannot occur and that cerebral brain function has ceased).[62] Cases 11-1 and 11-2 are cases of living donation in individuals with LLC who have decisional capacity and are not imminently dying. Living donation is being considered as a viable option because of the primacy placed on the principle of respect for persons in modern Western bioethics. In cases of living donation, the LDAT must evaluate all of the potential donor's vulnerabilities. When the potential living donor has an LLC, some of these vulnerabilities are augmented. As Elliott stated, the transplant physicians must decide not only whether the decision to donate is reasonable but whether they should participate.[63] As we saw in cases 11-1 and 11-2, different transplant physicians will come to different decisions about the morality of organ procurement from particular individuals with LLCs.

IDD (cases 11-4 and 11-5) and ODE (case 11-6) violate the DDR, which protects the dying by requiring that "Organs must not be taken from patients until they die."[64] To date, there are no reports in the literature describing the actual performance of IDD or death by organ procurement, and we believe they would represent a step too far.

Notes

1. Bia MJ, Ramos EL, Danovitch GM, et al. Evaluation of living renal donors: the current practice of US transplant centers. *Transplantation* 1995;60:322–327; and Mandelbrot DA, Pavlakis M, Danovitch GM, et al. The medical evaluation of living kidney donors: a survey of US transplant centers. *Am J Transplant.* 2007;7:2333–2343.
2. The phrase the "dead donor rule" (DDR) was coined by John Robertson. See Robertson JA. The dead donor rule. *Hastings Cent Rep.* 1999;29(6):6–14.
3. We employ the DDR as a bright line to distinguish donation from dead persons under the responsibility of the Organ Procurement Organization (OPO) and donation from dying individuals or individuals with LLC (the focus of this chapter) who are patients in their own right.

    We assert our position of the inviolability of the DDR—that the procurement of organs from deceased donors should only occur after the donor is pronounced dead (and in the case of donation after cardio-circulatory death, after a hands-off period). We acknowledge that the inviolability of the DDR is challenged by some in the transplant and ethics communities. Some argue that brain death does not equal death of the whole person so that donation after neurological death fails to conform to the DDR. Some therefore want to challenge brain death being synonymous with death of the person; others want to challenge whether it is critical that the whole brain is dead. There is also disagreement about whether those declared dead by cardio-circulatory death meet the criteria for death of the whole person (especially if there is a short hands-off period). Finally, there are those who argue that the DDR may thwart the autonomy and nonmaleficence interests of an individual who wants to be a donor. We will not explore these debates further as it goes beyond the focus of our book. For those interested, see Arnold R, Youngner S. The dead donor rule: should we stretch it, bend it, or abandon it? *Kennedy Instit Ethics J.* 1993;3:263–278; Truog R, Miller F. The dead donor rule and organ transplantation. *N Engl J Med.* 2008;359:674–675; Glannon W. The moral insignificance of death in organ donation. *Camb Q Healthc Ethics.* 2013;22(2):192–202; Truog RD, Miller FG, Halpern SD. The dead-donor rule and the future of organ donation. *N Engl J Med.* 2013;369(14):1287–1289; Shah SK. Rethinking brain death as a legal fiction: is the terminology the problem? *Hastings Cent Rep.* 2018;48(6 suppl 4):S49–S52.

4. National Conference of Commissioners on Uniform State Laws. Uniform Determination of Death Act. Drafted July–August 1980, approved by the American Medical Association October 19, 1980 .Approved by the American Bar Association February 10, 1981. Adopted by the states throughout 1981. Last accessed August 21, 2021.http://people.bu.edu/wwildman/courses/thth/projects/thth_projects_2003_lewis/udda.pdf

5. Arnold and Youngner, "The dead donor rule," at pp. 264–265.

6. Sade RM. Brain death, cardiac death, and the dead donor rule. *J S C Med Assoc.* 2011;107:146–149, at p. 147.

7. Rodríguez-Arias D. The dead donor rule as policy indoctrination. *Hastings Cent Rep.* 2018;48(6 suppl 4):S39–S42, citing Robertson, "The dead donor rule" at p. 6.

8. Ethically, the hands-off period between the cessation of pulse and respiration and procurement must ensure that cortical brain function has also ceased. One would not want to declare a person dead, nor to procure their organs, if still conscious. This is discussed in Veatch RM, Ross LF. *Defining Death: The Case for Choice.* Washington, DC: Georgetown University Press; 2016, at pp. 76–78.

9. The first mention of decoupling in the literature can be found in von Pohle WR. Obtaining organ donation: who should ask? *Heart & Lung.* 1996;25(4):304–309. Von Pohle found:

> When a dedicated representative from the local organ procurement organiza-
> tion, rather than the physician, presents the option of donation and decouples
> the discussion of death by neurological criteria from the presentation of the op-
> tion of donation, the rate of donation significantly increases. (p. 309)

10. Shemie SD, Robertson A, Beitel J, et al. End-of-life conversations with families of potential donors: leading practices in offering the opportunity for organ donation. *Transplantation.* 2017;101(5S-1):S17–S26, at p. S19.

There is some controversy about whether decoupling increases the rate of organ donation. Laura Siminoff and colleagues argue it does not and that it is unnecessary. See for example, Siminoff LA, Agyemang AA, Traino HM. Consent to organ donation: a review. *Prog Transplant.* 2013;23(1):99–104. Like Shemie and his Canadian colleagues, Shah and colleagues from the US southeast argue that it does. See Shah MB, Vilchez V, Goble A, et al. Socioeconomic factors as predictors of organ donation. *J Surg Res.* 2018;221:88–94.

We support the practice of decoupling because it creates a sharp line between dying patients and dead individuals. We argue for the decoupling process to ensure respectful and appropriate care for the dying patient (person), regardless of its impact on organ donation rates. We also support the practice because it reduces the appearance of any conflict of interest. It is critical for the medical community to maintain the community's trust that health care professionals taking care of a dying patient in their intensive care units are doing their best to restore health or alternatively giving compassionate palliative care when appropriate. It is also critical that patients and families trust the transplant teams who arrive to do deceased donor organ procurement and see that the surgeons respectfully stand by until the patient's care team determines death has occurred, even in the case of DCD. Lack of a sharp line between terminal care and organ retrieval has the potential to lead to mistrust of the organ procurement process and concern that the dying patient's interests are being pushed aside to maximize organ procurement to help other individuals. The absence or modification of decoupling could even decrease the desire of families to give permission for deceased donation.

11. Rakké YS, Zuidema WC, Hilhorst MT, et al. Seriously ill patients as living unspecified kidney donors: rationale and justification. *Transplantation*. 2015;99:232–235, at p. 234.
12. Rakké et al, "Seriously ill."
13. Rakké et al, "Seriously ill," at p. 234.
14. Rakké et al, "Seriously ill," at p. 233.
15. Rakké et al, "Seriously ill."
16. Rakké et al, "Seriously ill," at p. 234. The authors do not provide any additional information.
17. Rakké et al, "Seriously ill," at p. 234.
18. Mezrich J, Scalea J. As they lay dying. *The Atlantic*. April 2015. Last accessed August 21, 2021.http://www.theatlantic.com/magazine/archive/2015/04/as-they-lay-dying/386273/.
19. Mezrich and Scalea, "As they lay."
20. See Mandelbrot et al, "The medical evaluation."
21. Denu RA, Mendonca EA, Fost N. Potential yield of imminent death donation. *Am J Transplant*. 2018;18:486–491.
22. See Rakké et al, "Seriously ill."
23. Challenor J, and Watts J. "It seemed churlish not to": How living non-directed kidney donors construct their altruism. *Health*. 2014;18:388–405; and Jacobs CL, Roman D, Garvey C, et al. Twenty-two nondirected kidney donors: an update on a single center's experience. *Am J Transplant*. 2004;4:1110–1116.
24. See, for example, Back et al, "Abandonment"; Koon, "Meet"; and Pohl JM, Given CW, Collins CE et al. Social vulnerability and reactions to caregiving in daughters and daughters-in-law caring for disabled aging parents. *Health Care Women Int*. 1994;15:385–395.
25. Goodin RE. *Protecting the Vulnerable: A Reanalysis of Our Social Responsibilities*. Chicago, IL: University of Chicago Press; 1985
26. LaPointe Rudow D. The living donor advocate: a team approach to educate, evaluate, and manage donors across the continuum. *Prog Transplant*. 2009;19:64–70; and Steel JL, Dunlavy A, Friday M, et al. The development of practice guidelines for independent living donor advocates. *Clin Transplant*. 2013;27:178–184.

27. Mezrich and Scalea, "As they lay."
28. Mezrich and Scalea, "As they lay."
29. Elliott C. Doing harm: living organ donors, clinical research and *The Tenth Man*. *J Med Eth*. 1995;21:91–96, at p. 95.
30. Rakké et al, "Seriously ill," at p. 234.
31. See, for example, Jacobs C, Johnson E, Anderson K, et al. Kidney transplants from living donors: how donation affects family dynamics. *Adv Ren Replace Ther*. 1998;5: 89–97; Jacobs CL, Gross CR, Messersmith EE, et al. Emotional and financial experiences of kidney donors over the past 50 years: The RELIVE Study. *Clin J Am Soc Nephrol*. 2015;10:2221–2231; and Simmons RG, Marine SK, Simmons RL. *Gift of Life: The Effect of Organ Transplantation on Individual, Family and Societal Dynamics*. New Brunswick, NJ: Transaction Books; 2002.
32. Morrisey PE. The case for kidney donation before end-of-life care. *Am J of Bioeth*. 2012;12(6):1–8, at p. 1.
33. Morrisey, "The case."
34. Morrisey, "The case," at p. 2.
35. While not mentioned by Morrissey, it is clear that if the patient dies quickly enough after treatment is withdrawn, he would support the family's authorization to return the person to the operating room for DCD procurement of other organs.
36. Smith MJ, Rodríguez-Arias D, and Ortega I. Avoiding violation of the dead donor rule: the costs to patients. *Am J Bioeth*. 2012;12(6):15–17.
37. Morrison W. Organ donation prior to death—balancing benefits and harms. *Am J Bioeth*. 2012;12(6):14–15, at p. 15.
38. Zimmerman CJ, Baggett ND, Taylor LJ, et al. Family and transplant professionals' views of organ recovery before circulatory death for imminently dying patients: a qualitative study using semistructured interviews and focus groups. *Am J Transplant*. 2019;19(8):2232–2240, at p. 2232.
39. Zimmerman et al, "Family and transplant."
40. Uniform Anatomical Gift Act (1987, revised 2006).
41. There are rare exceptions to the requirement that living donors give a first-person informed consent to donation. For example, several dozen children have served as living solid organ donors as we discussed in the chapter on minor children (chapter 5). There have also been several court cases where plaintiffs have sought court permission to allow adults who lack decisional capacity to serve as living kidney donors. The results have been mixed with some courts permitting such donations, especially if the donation is to a first-degree biological relative with whom the incapacitated adult has a significant relationship. No court has ever given permission for an incapacitated adult to serve as a Good Samaritan donor and we do not believe that it should be permitted. See, for example, Cheyette C. Organ harvests from the legally incompetent: an argument against compelled altruism. *Bost Coll Law Rev*. 2000;41:465–515. National Conference of Commissioners on Uniform State Laws. Revised Uniform Anatomal Gift Act (2006). (Last revised or Amended in 2009). On the web at: uaga_final_aug09. pdf (donornetworkwest.org). Last accessed August 18, 2021.

42. Bolton L, OPTN/UNOS Ethics Committee. Ethical considerations of imminent death donation. OPTN. 2016. Last accessed Augusg 21, 2021.https://optn.transpl ant.hrsa.gov/media/1918/ethics_ethical_implications_of_idd_20160815.pdf, at p. 1. Hereinafter referred to as OPTN/UNOS Ethics Committee, "Ethical Considerations."

43. OPTN/UNOS Ethics Committee, "Ethical considerations," at p. 1.

44. See Arnold and Youngner, "The dead donor" at p. 271. Technically the individual could then have additional organs removed as a DCD donor if he were to die within the allotted time after the ventilator was withdrawn.

45. See OPTN/UNOS Ethics Committee, "Ethical considerations," at p. 1.

46. See OPTN/UNOS Ethics Committee, "Ethical considerations," at p. 2.

47. Interestingly, in their delineation of types of IDD cases, the UNOS Ethics Committee did consider the possibility that an individual might request IDD in their advance directive although they did not address it further. The problem with a request to be an IDD in an advance directive is that a critical component of the LDAT relationship with a living donor is to discuss the risks, benefits, and alternatives and to give the individual the right to renege up until the moment that the patient undergoes anesthesia. At the University of Chicago (where JRT worked and LFR still works), the living donor would be asked to confirm his or her willingness to undergo the surgery immediately pre-operatively. The person who states willingness to donate in an advance directive but who lacks consciousness at the time the surgery is scheduled would be unable to complete this final step and therefore would not be allowed to serve as a living donor.

48. See, for example, Ely EW. Death by organ donation: euthanizing patients for their organs gains frightening traction. *Intensive Care Med.* 2019;45:1309–1311; and Bollen J, Ten Hoopen R, Ysebaert D, van Mook W, van Heurn E. Legal and ethical aspects of organ donation after euthanasia in Belgium and the Netherlands. *J Med Ethics.* 2016;42(8):486–9.

49. See, for example, Bollen J, Ten Hoopen R, Ysebaert D, van Mook W, van Heurn E. Legal and ethical aspects of organ donation after euthanasia in Belgium and the Netherlands. *J Med Ethics.* 2016;42(8):486–9; and Bollen J, Shaw D, de Wert G, et al. Organ donation euthanasia (ODE): performing euthanasia through living organ donation. *Transplantation.* 2020;104(suppl 3):S298.

50. Bollen et al, "Legal and ethical"; and Bollen et al, "Organ donation euthanasia (ODE)."

51. Again, additional organs could be procured if the individual were willing to be a donor after cardio-circulatory death and he were to die within the allotted time after the ventilator was withdrawn. However, this would preclude thoracic organs (heart and lungs), which could be procured by ODE.

52. Zimmerman et al, "Family and transplant."

53. In addition to Bollen and colleagues (see reference 49), see also Miller FG, Truog RD. *Death, Dying and Organ Transplantation: Reconstructing Medical Ethics at the End of Life.* New York, NY: Oxford University Press; 2012; and Wilkinson D, Savulescu J. Should we allow organ donation euthanasia? Alternatives for maximizing the number and quality of organs for transplantation. *Bioethics.* 2012;26:32–48.

54. Nygren SL. Organ donation by incompetent patients. *Univ Chic Leg Forum.* 2006;Article 16. Last accessed August 21, 2021.http://chicagounbound.uchicago.edu/uclf/vol2006/iss1/16

55. The National Commission for the Protection of Human Subjects of Biomedical and Behavioral Research. *The Belmont Report: Ethical Principles and Guidelines for the Protection of Human Subjects of Research.* Washington, DC: Government Printing Office; 1978.

56. Gill CJ. Disability, constructed vulnerability, and socially conscious palliative care. *J Palliat Care.* 2006;22:183–189; and Stienstra D, and Chochinov HM. Vulnerability, disability, and palliative end-of-life care. *J Palliat Care.* 2006;22:166–174.

57. Kant I. *Grounding for the Metaphysics of Morals,* 1785, translated by Ellington JW. Indianapolis, IN: Hackett Publishing; 1981.

58. See Gill, "Disability"; and Stienstra and Chochinov, "Vulnerability."

59. See Miller and Truog, *Death, Dying,* at pp. 144–147.

60. Kant, *Grounding.*

61. Kotloff RM, Blosser S, Fulda GJ, et al. Management of the Potential organ donor in the ICU: Society of Critical Care Medicine/American College of Chest Physicians/Association of Organ Procurement Organizations consensus statement. *Crit Care Med.* 2015;43:1291–1325.

62. See, Veatch and Ross, *Defining Death,* at pp. 76–78.

63. Elliott, "Doing harm," at p. 59.

64. Arnold and Youngner, "The dead donor" at pp. 264–265.

12

Challenging (Organ and Global) Boundaries

Case 12-1: This case is quoted verbatim from Ana-Marie Torres et al.

We were approached by a patient (donor-L) whose mother was on dialysis and was waitlisted for kidney transplantation. The mother had nephrotic syndrome from biopsy-proven fibrillary glomerulonephritis and the daughter was deferred from kidney donation because of concern over her risk of being afflicted with the same condition later in life, especially given documented cases of an autosomal dominant inheritance. Donor-L proposed a bi-organ exchange based upon the Dickerson article. Donor-L had no proteinuria/hematuria and had adequate renal reserve. Magnetic resonance imaging and computed tomography scan demonstrated liver anatomy conducive to donation. Because of donor-L's small physique and her recipient's blood type, finding an exchange donor took 18 months. The eventual kidney donor (donor-K) desired to donate a portion of her liver to her sister, who had primary biliary cirrhosis. Evaluation revealed that donor-K's left lobe was < 30% of her liver volume. Right lobe donation was ruled out because of insufficient residual mass in her left lobe. Donor-K's left lobe did not have enough mass for the intended recipient (graft weight/standard liver volume = 32%). After discussion of the possibility of a bi-organ exchange, donor-K desired evaluation for possible kidney donation. Following standard evaluation for donor-K, involving a team separate from the medical personnel who evaluated donor-L, donor K was cleared. The novel nature of the organ exchange was explained to all 4 patients. . . .[1]

The Living Organ Donor as Patient. Lainie Friedman Ross and J. Richard Thistlethwaite, Jr, Oxford University Press.
© Oxford University Press 2022. DOI: 10.1093/oso/9780197618202.003.0012

Case 12-2: This case is quoted verbatim from Michael Rees and colleagues.

In October 2013, a 31yearold Filipino man, FM, developed ESRD and initiated hemodialysis via central venous catheter. FM and his wife, FW, were employed at the time of his diagnosis with an annual income of $4000 (average 2012 Philippine family income was $4950). In the Philippines, the cost of hemodialysis (without government-sponsored coverage, i.e., PhilHealth) is $100 per session, the cost of a dialysis catheter is $100, and the cost of erythropoietin is $30 per dose. Consequently, the yearly cost for ESRD treatment exceeded the couple's annual income. . . . Transplantation was considered, but the couple could not afford the procedure and subsequent immunosuppression.

Kidney transplantation in the Philippines is conditionally available through a government sponsored program (PhilHealth), but immunosuppression is not covered, so FM was deemed financially ineligible. FM was, however, eligible for a PhilHealth-sponsored program that paid for up to 45 dialysis sessions per year, which FM began using in July 2014. At that time, they were offered the opportunity to participate in a GKE [Global Kidney Exchange] transplantation sponsored by the Alliance for Paired Donation (APD). FW had blood type (BT-) O, and FM had BT-A without donor specific antibodies (DSAs); thus, their barrier to transplantation was financial, not immunological. . . .[2]
. . .

The first GKE transplantation was performed January 22, 2015 as part of a three-way NEAD [nonsimultaneous extended altruistic donation] chain. The chain has been extended over the first year to provide 11 total transplantations, and a bridge donor now waits to continue the chain.[3]

12.1 History of Two Novel Expansions of Organ Exchanges

In this chapter we examine 2 novel expansions of living donor organ exchanges: bi-organ (also known as trans-organ) exchange involving a living liver donor (donor-L)-kidney recipient (recipient-K) and a living kidney donor (donor-K)-liver recipient (recipient-L) exchange (case 12-1) and global kidney exchange (GKE) between a living kidney donor-recipient pair from a low- to middle-income country (LMIC) and living kidney donor-recipient pair(s) from a high-income country (HIC) (case 12-2).

The history of liver-kidney exchange is quite recent. In 2017, 2 computer scientists, John Dickerson and Tuomas Sandholm, published an article that they describe as "the first foray into the theory and computational methods necessary to set the groundwork for a fielded nationwide liver or multi-organ exchange."[4] They explained:

> In this paper, we begin by exploring the idea of large-scale liver exchange, and show on demographically accurate data that vetted kidney exchange algorithms can be adapted to clear such an exchange at the nationwide level. We then propose cross-organ donation where kidneys and livers can be bartered for each other. We show theoretically that this multi-organ exchange provides linearly more transplants than running separate kidney and liver exchanges. This linear gain is a product of altruistic kidney donors creating chains that thread through the liver pool; it exists even when only a small but constant portion of the donors on the kidney side of the pool are willing to donate a liver lobe.[5]

In the same year, Benjamin Samstein et al from New York published an article to the *American Journal of Transplantation* on the ethics of trans-organ paired exchange.[6] The authors seemed to be unaware of the Dickerson and Sandholm publication as they did not cite it. When Torres and colleagues wrote up their case report (case 12-1) a few months later, they cited both of these articles.

While the bi-organ donor transplant crosses the organ-specific boundary of kidney paired exchange (KPE) and its variants (which were discussed in great detail in chapter 8), the second case crosses a different boundary. The ethics, legal, and logistical issues of "reverse transplant tourism" (RTT) now referred to as a "global kidney exchange" (GKE) involves a kidney paired exchange between a donor-recipient pair from an HIC and a LMIC country. It was first introduced by Michael Rees, a urologist and transplant surgeon at the University of Toledo and Kimberly Krawiec, a professor of law at Duke University in a journal entitled *Law and Contemporary Problems* in 2014.[7] In 2017, Rees and colleagues published a case report in the *American Journal of Transplantation* (see case 12-2). GKE focused on incompatible living donor-recipient kidney pairs from HICs like the United States (US) who were unable to undergo directed donation but were willing to participate in an exchange or chain involving a living donor-recipient pair from a LMIC who were unable to undergo directed donation because of poverty (what Alexander Wiseman and John Gill referred to as "financial incompatibility" in their editorial accompanying the *American Journal of Transplantation* article[8]). The plan was for the LMIC donor-recipient pair to come to the US, participate in a chain, and then return to their country of origin with $50,000 in an escrow account for future care of the transplant recipient. Rees and colleagues specifically sought donor-recipient pairs from LMICs because the $50,000 could go much further there than it could in the US or other HIC (where it would last for 2–3 years at most).[9] They acknowledged that there was no long-term plan for the recipient after the money ran out (and it could run out quickly if complications were to develop), and no plan for donor resources or follow-up. They viewed the exchange (or chain) as a win for both the HIC because transplants improve quality of life, quantity of life, and are cost-saving compared to dialysis and for the LMIC because the candidate got a transplant and funding for follow-up care that would otherwise have been inaccessible.[10]

In this chapter, we examine the ethical controversies raised by these novel expansions using our living donor ethics framework (see chapter 3).

12.2 Evaluating Case 12-1: Are Bi-Organ Exchanges Ethical?

12.2.1 Beneficence

Although we usually begin with the principle of respect for persons, in this case study we begin with beneficence. Beneficence focuses on the risks and benefits for the donor(s), recipient(s), and donor-recipient pair(s). In case 12-1, both donors were voluntarily seeking to be living organ donors for their family members and they had both determined their willingness to accept the physical risks to improve their mother's/sister's health. Their candidates were on the deceased donor waiting list. Whether the candidates had sought alternative living donors is not mentioned. While the kidney candidate could remain on dialysis indefinitely, the liver candidate had no other clinical options. The kidney candidate's daughter (donor-L) is willing to take on the greater risk of living liver donation to help provide her mother with a kidney. She has decided that the physical benefit to her mother and the psychological benefit to herself outweigh the risks. The liver transplant candidate is being asked to accept a liver lobe from a stranger that is available now and avoids her getting sicker on the waitlist. Her sister (donor-K) now only has to donate a kidney which is safer and she states she is willing to do so. Both candidates express willingness to accept the exchange organ, and do not express concern about their family member's decision. Each donor and recipient calculate the benefits to outweigh the risks for themselves as individuals.

The bi-organ exchange raises a unique ethical issue about the unbalanced nature of the donor risks (and, some might argue, the unbalanced nature of recipient benefit).

The different physical risks from living kidney and living liver donation were described in chapter 1. Although Samstein et al claim that the "morbidity and mortality rates of live donor nephrectomy and live donor hepatectomy are becoming increasingly comparable,"[11] this is not the case for adult-to-adult living liver donor transplantation. While this may be true for left lateral segment living liver donation for a recipient child, living lobar donation as needed for adult-to-adult living liver transplantation involves significantly more risks than does living kidney donation even at the institutions that have large living liver donor programs as seen in the A2ALL data.[12] If the ethics depends on comparable risks, then the bi-organ exchange is not an ethical option at this time. Donating a kidney is much less risky than donating a whole liver lobe, especially in the short term.

The recipient benefits also seem unbalanced because the kidney candidate has dialysis as a viable alternative while waiting for a deceased donor organ. In contrast, the liver candidate had already "undergone a transjugular intrahepatic portocaval shunt for variceal hemorrhage, complicated by hepatic encephalopathy and severe pruritus with a model for end stage liver disease-sodium score of 19 at time of listing."[13] Her only option is to undergo a deceased or living donor liver transplant. Her need is more time-sensitive.

12.2.2 Respect for Persons

Both Torres and colleagues who described the actual case and Samstein et al who explored the ethics of such bi-organ exchanges argue that respect for persons supports the exchange if the donors and recipients are competent; have been informed of the risks, benefits and alternatives; and are capable of making informed decisions free of undue influence.[14]

The case report described by Torres et al clearly shows that donor-L was well informed and willing to participate. She proposed the option to the transplant team. Donor-K had already been worked up for living liver donation so clearly was willing to accept even more risk than the team would now ask her to do. The extent to which she would want to participate in an exchange had not necessarily been discussed prior to her disqualification as a living liver donor. Donor K seems to get the better end of the deal—a lower risk for herself (kidney rather than liver lobe donation) to ensure that her sister receive a living liver transplant. Although she was being asked to donate an organ that would expose her to less risk (kidney rather than liver lobe), the option did make it harder for her to be excluded from serving as a living organ donor at all. The possibility of a bi-organ paired exchange may take away the medical excuse from future potential kidney and liver donors, particularly from those who are medically excluded for organ-specific reasons (and not for more general medical reasons like a recent history of cancer). When we proposed the KPE (see chapter 8), we were concerned that exchanges took away the potential donor's excuse of ABO or crossmatch incompatibility, because there would be a recipient with whom the individual would be compatible, allowing for an exchange. The bi-organ paired exchange now further limits the medical excuse by saying that even if your kidney anatomy (eg, horseshoe kidney) or genetic risks (of kidney disease) would preclude you from kidney donation, those concerns may not place you at greater risk for liver disease and your liver anatomy may be acceptable for donation. This means that a potential living donor who is ruled out for one organ donation could be asked to donate a different organ as part of a bi-organ exchange. This increases the risk of undue pressure and requires an examination of the vulnerabilities that such an exchange would need to address as discussed 12.2.4.

The option of bi-organ exchanges also raises another autonomy concern: the ability to withdraw at a later time. Samstein and colleagues note that bi-organ exchanges may reduce the willingness of the donor's family to believe that the medical excuse is valid:

> The fact that trans-organ donation presents potential donors with more opportunities to be eligible and makes it harder to provide a medical excuse that satisfies family members and allows potential donors to refuse to donate without being blamed, calls for attention to the ways in which various pressures on donors might invalidate consent and for the development

of procedures that ensure that potential donors are acting voluntarily. This would require not only a complete medical and psychosocial evaluation of potential donors, but also social changes that can make the option of declining to donate to a loved one more acceptable.[15]

In KPE, best practices suggest that these options should be discussed early, even before human leukocyte antigen (HLA)-typing. This provides the living donor advocate team (LDAT), the team dedicated to the well-being of the donor, to gauge the potential donor's willingness to donate, and willingness to consider alternative donation options if unable to donate directly.[16]

An important reason why some candidates and their potential living donors do not participate in KPE is medical mistrust.[17] If bi-organ exchanges were to become common, the option to change the organ donated needs to be raised very early in the process, at the time of being worked up for living directed organ donation, particularly if there is the chance that the alternative organ carries greater risk (eg, from kidney to liver lobe). Stakeholder attitude about this type of discussion needs to be studied before a program is implemented to ensure that it does not reduce a willingness to donate any organ.

12.2.3 Justice

In this book we have focused on justice in terms of fairness in donor selection.[18] Fairness does not permit an over-reliance on vulnerable groups. Fairness also does not exclude members of vulnerable groups (eg, prisoners) if they can adequately address the threats that challenge their ability to give a voluntary and informed consent. Fairness in living donor selection requires the donation to be voluntary. Fairness also requires the transplant team to refuse to exploit those who may be so desperate that they are willing to sell their organs (see chapter 14). The National Organ Transplant Act (NOTA) of 1984 specifically prohibits the buying and selling of organs:

it shall be unlawful for any person to knowingly acquire, receive, or otherwise transfer any human organ for valuable consideration for use in human transplantation if the transfer affects interstate commerce.[19]

In 2007, the Charlie Norwood Act amended this statement by adding, "The preceding sentence does not apply with respect to human organ paired donation."[20] The amendment was written to permit kidney exchanges between 2 emotionally related donor-recipient kidney pairs who were either ABO or crossmatch incompatible. It was quickly interpreted to cover kidney chains. Some also claim that it covers compatible donor-recipient kidney pairs, which facilitates longer chains, but these variants are not addressed in the actual legislation.[21] Case 12-1 is the first case to ask whether the Charlie Norwood Act was meant only to cover same-organ donor-K-recipient-K exchanges and same-organ donor-L-recipient-L exchanges or whether can be more broadly interpreted to include bi-organ exchanges involving different human organs. One concern with this broader interpretation that it could lead to exchange/bartering of other goods (eg, your kidney for the cost of your mother's cancer treatment). It could become a nonmonetary form of exchange of items of "valuable consideration."

An alternative conception of justice, not used in this book, focuses on maximizing benefit for the greatest number (utilitarianism). For example, Dickerson and Sandholm, both nonclinicians, propose combining both living kidney and living liver lobe donor-recipient pairs in a single chain to potentially expand living donor transplants of both organs in order to save more lives (interpreting justice in a utilitarian way).[22] This proposal ignores the differential risks that bi-organ chains would ask their donors to accept and how such options would be offered so as to promote autonomy and not put potential donors in a position where it is hard to refuse.

Another justice concern is how transplant programs propose bi-donor organ transplant exchanges to potential exchange donors and still ensure that potential donors have the ability to refuse. That is, how can a transplant program offer the bi-donor organ exchange without leaving the potential donors with the sense that donation of one organ if not another has become inevitable if she wants to help her intended recipient. In this case, donor-L raised the option herself, suggesting she was not vulnerable to the suggestions of others, but was highly informed and resourceful. The fact that it took 18 months to find an appropriate exchange pair, even though that bi-organ exchange donor was being asked to accept less risk,[23] suggests that without aggressive promotion of bi-organ exchanges by transplant teams (which we do not support), it would likely be exceedingly rare. We do not support aggressive promotion because of the vulnerability concerns that they raise.

12.2.4 Vulnerabilities

Let us consider those vulnerabilities most relevant to bi-donor exchange donors. (The full taxonomy can be found in Table 3.3) The first is deferential. For some potential donors it will be difficult not to take up the alternative offer that is proposed by the transplant team (you are not eligible to donate a kidney to your mother but you could donate a liver lobe to a stranger in exchange for the stranger's donor giving your mother a kidney). To minimize this vulnerability, if bi-organ donation were to become an accepted option, discussions prior to a living donor work-up would have to explain all of the options, including bi-organ donation, that the potential donor could consider if no living donor were found suitable for directed donation. This solution parallels our recommendation about introducing upfront the participation of compatible kidney pairs into paired kidney exchanges and domino kidney chains even before it is determined whether the donor and recipient are compatible. In chapter 8 we proposed describing the inclusion of compatible pairs into paired exchanges and domino chains before compatibility testing (analogous to making choices behind the veil of ignorance [24]) to minimize any sense of undue pressure. Similarly, if bi-organ donor exchanges were an accepted option, the LDAT would need to explain to potential organ donors that such exchanges would only be re-considered if re-proposed by the potential donors. The practice of the LDAT taking a passive role after introducing the option of bi-organ exchanges is similarly to minimize the undue pressure that donors may experience to participate in these exchanges as a last resort. Avoiding undue pressure would be particularly important for potential kidney donors who might be asked to donate living liver lobes instead of a kidney, which potentially involves significantly greater risks of morbidity and mortality.[25]

We believe that mentioning the bi-organ donation option upfront may not be sufficient to protect potential donors from the vulnerabilities these exchanges raise. First, the potential living kidney donor may be deferentially vulnerable, and may not feel empowered to say no to health professionals when these options are introduced, and so may find themselves being re-contacted. This approach also entails some risk, as it may scare off some potential donors: "I wanted to find out if I could give my brother a kidney and the next thing you know they wanted my liver." This can exacerbate distrust.[26]

The potential donor may also feel medically vulnerable, having been selected, in part, "because of the presence of a serious health-related condition in the intended recipient for which there are only less satisfactory alternative remedies?" This is particularly true if the kidney donor's paired candidate is low on the waitlist, there are no other potential living kidney donors in the candidate's network, and the potential paired recipient is doing poorly on dialysis. It would also hold if the liver donor's paired candidate has a health condition that may cause ineligibility in a short period of time (example, hepatocellular carcinoma with tumors at the top end of the Milan size and number criteria).

Third, the social situation of potential donors may make them infrastructurally vulnerable. One factor is low health literacy such that the potential donor has not developed the ability to understand the risks and benefits that the donation of different organs entail.[27] This could be exacerbated by the unexpected nature of the request by the LDAT. The LDAT must have the training, the skills, and the resources necessary to help the donor understand what these exchanges entail, using simple and clear-cut language, aided by decision aids or other pictorial means if necessary. Unless these resources and support are available, the potential donor may not be able to fully evaluate the risks and benefits and make a decision consonant with their beliefs and values.

12.2.5 Special Relationships Create Special Responsibilities

The final principle in our framework is that "special relationships create special responsibilities," which we developed from Goodin's work entitled *Protecting the Vulnerable*. As we noted in chapter 3, the central argument of Goodin's book is that "we bear special responsibilities for protecting those who are particularly vulnerable to us."[28] We owe special responsibilities to potential living donors because we are considering exposing them to physical risks for the physical benefit of a third party. This does not mean that the LDAT should protect potential donors from all risks. However, in the case of bi-organ exchanges, we might be proposing that potential donors take on more risks than they had initially bargained for. At minimum, proposing bi-organ exchanges will require broad transparency about a number of aspects of the bi-organ exchange option. First, there are the different risks taken by the 2 donors. Second, both the donor and the recipient must be made aware of the anticipated donor outcomes (morbidity and mortality) for the different organs using both national data if available and data from the institution where the donations will take place. Third, there needs to be separate LDATs for each potential donor to ensure that all vulnerabilities and other threats to a voluntary and informed consent are addressed. Fourth, any member of the LDATs must have the authority to cancel (or at least defer) a bi-organ exchange if either donor is uncomfortable with the exchange.

The LDAT's special relationship to potential bi-organ exchange donors requires a reconception of autonomy and consent in order to empower potential donors to address their vulnerabilities in a shared decision-making process. Donor-L, who in case 12-1 proposed the bi-organ exchange, recognizes that she is taking greater risks than she would take if she were donating a kidney. The fact that she proposed the exchange, rather than it being offered to her, may make this case ethically permissible because it removed any real or perceived pressure or coercion from the transplant team.

We do not believe that bi-organ exchange is or ought to be adopted more widely. While voluntariness and willingness are not a concern in this case study, this option could put pressure on other families where family members have been ruled out for one organ but might then be asked to consider being worked up for a different organ for a different recipient in a bi-organ exchange. The suggestion of this option by an authority figure places too much pressure on prospective living donors by suggesting that they ought to pursue living donation by any means and at any cost to help their intended recipient.

12.3 Evaluating Case 12-2: Are Global Kidney Exchange Programs Ethical?

The Filipino couple who participated in the first GKE swap at the University of Toledo as described by Rees and colleagues in the *American Journal of Transplantation* was immunologically compatible and could, therefore, successfully be transplanted without the swap. The couple was financially unable to do so because of their poverty and their government's inability to provide the necessary resources.[29] The authors acknowledge that this exchange may not be permitted under NOTA because the Filipino couple was provided not only with their transplant but $50,000 in an escrow account. The escrow account would provide immunosuppression for almost 10 years if there are minimal or no recipient complications.[30] In fact, the authors concede that the reason to enroll a donor-recipient pair from an LMIC is that the same money would last for a much shorter time if the donor-recipient pair came from an HIC but lacked the financial resources.[31]

The publication by Rees and colleagues was accompanied by an editorial by Alexander Wiseman and John Gill, 2 transplant physicians, who challenged the legality of the concept of "financial incompatibility," stating that at minimum the "expansion of GKE would probably require amendment of NOTA."[32] The authors expressed moral concerns as well: "even if an individual derives benefits from a transaction, this in itself does not justify the transaction."[33] They expressed concern that the Filipino couple was chosen "based on their likelihood of facilitating other transplants" which they argued "commodifies the donor and recipient."[34] Wiseman and Gill further noted that "the Filipino donor kidney was potentially undervalued given the disproportionate benefit to American patients" and that "the limited post-transplant care provided to the Filipino recipient [was] probably inequitable."[35]

Since the publication of their article, Rees and colleagues have presented data at the American Transplant Congress in which they described 3 donor-recipient pairs, 2 from the Philippines and 1 from Mexico, all of whom had O-blood type donors and A-blood type recipients. The first donor-recipient pair from an LMIC led to 12 transplants (11 for US recipients).[36] The other 2 donor-recipient pairs from an LMIC led to "a total of 11 transplants and both have bridge donors scheduled to continue each chain."[37]

Francis Delmonico and Nancy Asher were direct in their condemnation: "To target economically underdeveloped countries to solicit donors when there is no assurance about the ultimate care of the living organ donor (or the absence of coercion) is unethical."[38] They pointed out that both Mexico and the Philippines (the countries from which the first 3 GKE LMIC donor-recipient pairs were selected), have problems with black market organ sales.[39]

Let us evaluate the GKE using the living donor ethics framework we developed in chapter 3.

12.3.1 Respect for Persons

Rees and colleagues argue that the LMIC donor-recipient pair are competent adults who act autonomously in deciding whether to participate. Francesca Minerva and colleagues agree, arguing that:

Lurking behind all the arguments against the GKE is the assumption that people who are poor are incapable of autonomous choices. So, if they appear to choose to act in ways that benefit not only themselves, but people in HICs, they must have been coerced, exploited, or commodified. Given the history of relations between HICs and LMICs, these sentiments are partly understandable and are a sufficient reason for providing safeguards to prevent harm to vulnerable people from LMICs.[40]

Statements by ethics committees from various international organizations are less convinced that the consent of the donors and recipients is ethically sufficient. They question whether the members of the donor-recipient pair from the LMIC are really who they say they are. The Declaration of Istanbul Custodian Group (DICG) statement noted that "Many of the countries from which poor donors and recipient would be drawn to participate in the GKEP are struggling to combat domestic organ trafficking," and they were not convinced that transplant programs in developed countries would be able to ascertain that there was no forged documentation regarding relationships given language, cultural, and community knowledge.[41] The International Society of Nephrology and the World Health Organization (WHO) Task Force on Donation and Transplantation of Human Organs and Tissues came to the same conclusions.[42]

12.3.2 Beneficence

According to Rees and colleagues, the argument in favor of GKE is that the benefits outweigh the risks for each donor and recipient. The objection by many transplant bodies is the concern of exploitation. The DICG stated that "Exploitation occurs when someone takes advantage of a vulnerability in another person for their own benefit, creating a disparity in the benefits gained by the two parties."[43] The DICG was very critical of (1) the severe imbalance of benefits, "helping the rich over the poor"; (2) the lack of infrastructure to ensure adequate follow-up care for the recipients, even with the $50,0000 in escrow; and (3) the lack of any plan for the follow-up of the donor. Rather they declared it "a new case of international organ trafficking."[44] The WHO task force also expressed concern that such a program will interfere with a country's obligation "to strive towards self-sufficiency in meeting the needs of its people in organ donation and transplantation."[45] The WHO task force asserts:

GKE proposal may have a negative impact on the development of local sustainable donation and transplantation programmes in LMICs as well as on initiatives to build ethically sound KPE programs with robust regulatory oversight.[46]

12.3.3 Justice

The justice concern focuses on fairness. The international transplant community was strongly negative in its ethical evaluation. They noted that the benefits of the program flow disproportionately to patients in developed countries.[47]

A second justice concern is how the participants are selected. There are many donor-recipient pairs in LMIC who cannot afford transplantation. The first 3 pairs involved donors of blood type O and candidates of blood type A. They are probably immunologically compatible and could donate directly. It is doubtful that the LMIC donor-recipient pair was selected fairly. Lottery (equal respect for all persons), or selection of the "worst off" (Rawlsian prioritization) would have been fair selection processes[48] but, instead, selection seems to have been designed to maximize benefit to HIC programs. The donor-recipient pairs were selected based on likely compatibility with donor-recipient pairs in exchange and chain registries where O-donors are always in short supply.

A third justice concern is whether it is fair to give a lump sum payment to donor-recipient pairs from LMIC and not compatible donor-recipient pairs in the US (an HIC) who participate in KPE or domino chains who also catalyze multiple transplants and reduce the costs for insurance companies (including the US government). While such a payment would seem to violate NOTA as it currently reads, if a loophole to permit payments for GKE is allowed, the claim by US compatible pairs to receive a similar benefit would need to be evaluated. This could lead to a back door means of legitimizing payment for all organs, an ethical issue we discuss in depth in the next chapter.

12.3.4 Vulnerabilities

Multiple vulnerabilities apply to living donors from LMIC (see Table 3.3). First, there may be juridic or deferential vulnerability (or both). Whether the donor (or donor-recipient pair) feels compelled to donate due to official (juridic) or more cultural (deferential) authority to the health care team who did the initial work-up in the LMIC and helped with the logistics that enabled them to travel to the HIC and participate in the GKE. Clearly an LDAT supplemented by a professional translator with cultural and linguistic competencies should be involved—before they fly to the HIC.

The donors are socially vulnerable because poor residents of LMICs are often a group whose rights and interests have been socially disvalued. The social vulnerability of the donor-recipient pair is of serious concern given that they are often from lower socioeconomic and educational backgrounds. More concerning is whether the donor is truly emotionally related to the recipient or is a stranger being "exploited" by organ traffickers (which would signify serious social and/or allocational vulnerability). Again, the cultural and language barriers cannot be overstated. As the WHO task force stated: "the detection of possible cases of human trafficking for the purpose of organ removal may be particularly difficult when evaluating and accepting nonresident living donors."[49]

Poor donor-recipient pairs from the LMIC may experience medical and/ or situational vulnerabilities because the recipient-candidates may have no real option for renal replacement therapy other than GKE.

Finally, there is infrastructural vulnerability, as was clearly noted in the international statements. The transplant infrastructure for the donor-recipient pair from the HIC ensures follow-up care for both the donor and recipient. LMIC transplant recipient follow-up care may not be as good as available in the HIC, and may be more difficult to attain even with the $50,000 payment that is meant to pay for follow-up care and immunosuppression because of problems related to distance to the transplant center, lack of transplant center resources, or lack of health care providers with necessary clinical experience. While the $50,000 may last as long as 10 years in some countries if there are no recipient medical issues, complications may lead to rapid use. There is no guarantee for dialysis or re-transplant if the paired kidney were to fail. Finally, the provision of the $50,000 lump-sum may be in violation of NOTA.[50]

Another serious infrastructural barrier is the language barrier, which may make it difficult to be certain that they have been given adequate information to deliberate about whether or not to participate as a living donor. By the time the LMIC donor-recipient pair arrives in the US, it may be too late for the donor to feel that he or she can withdraw and the LDAT may not be able to communicate in a way that would inform them of the donor's reluctance or unwillingness to proceed. The language barrier may be further compounded by low health literacy that exists in many LMIC.[51]

A second concern is that if GKE were to become commonplace, it unintentionally may function as a disincentive for the local development of transplant infrastructure in the LMIC.

The third and most serious concern is the failure of GKE to treat the LMIC donor fully as a patient. The money given to the donor-recipient pair from the LMIC is expected to be used for the follow-up care of the transplant recipient. Neither funds nor resources are provided to the donor, and it is not clear that the infrastructure necessary for donor follow-up exists in the LMIC despite potential long-term health consequences of unilateral nephrectomy.[52] There are also no resources provided for recouping donor salary. Proposed in July 2019 by presidential executive order here in the United States,[53] final rules to remove financial disincentives to living organ donation were published in the *Federal Register* in September 2020.[54] It is not clear if it would apply to a foreign donor or how it would be provided.

12.3.5 Special Relationships Create Special Obligations

As moral agents, transplant teams should refuse to participate in GKE because they cannot ensure that (1) the living donor is not a victim of organ trafficking; and (2) there is adequate infrastructure for follow-up care in the LMIC for both the donor and recipient. Instead, transplant programs should refuse to participate in GKE and defer to the DICG position:

> Health authority in both HICs and LMICs should make clear that the statutes and regulations which prohibit exchanging organs for something of value preclude the acceptance of the GKEP [Global Kidney Exchange Program] in their countries.[55]

In their original article, Krawiec and Rees argued that the GKE was ethical and legal because neither participant in a GKE swap could successfully transplant without the swap.[56] This argument is false. Financial incompatibility is not a clinical issue, but rather a global political and economic equity problem. The solution is not for HIC to benefit from the disparity while claiming charity, but to develop global solutions that help LMIC develop self-sufficient programs for ESRD.

The donor-recipient pairs in the GKE were ABO-compatible and the panel reactive antigen (PRA) of the first LMIC recipient was 0% (the others have not yet been reported).[57] Clinically the LMIC donor-recipient pair was able to participate in a direct transplant. While the LMIC recipient benefited from participating in the GKE, the LMIC donor-recipient pair was used as a means to provide clinical benefit to 1 or more HIC donor-recipient pairs and to provide financial benefit (cost-saving) to the HIC insurance companies (including the US government). If GKE were to become a viable program, some of that cost-saving may serve to compensate the companies that coordinate these exchanges. Both Michael Rees and Susan Rees have financial relationships with these companies.[58]

We believe that GKE violates NOTA and should be prohibited. It fails to consider the donor as a patient in his or her own right.

12.4 Conclusion

In summary, both bi-organ transplants and GKE were proposed and implemented by well-meaning transplant professionals, but whether the Norwood Act of 2007 was meant to include such exchanges is legally unclear. Neither program should continue until these legal issues are addressed. But even if legally addressed, the ethical challenges that they raise remain. Bi-organ transplants and GKE are often unjust because they challenge the fair selection of donors. These exchanges raise significant deferential and infrastructural vulnerability challenges that threaten the donor's ability (autonomy) to provide a voluntary and informed consent.

Notes

1. Torres A-M, Wong F, Pearson S. Bi-organ paired exchange—sentinel case of a liver-kidney swap. *Am J Transplant*. 2019;19:2646–2649.
2. Rees MA, Dunn TB, Kuhr CS, et al. Kidney exchange to overcome financial barriers to kidney transplantation. *Am J Transplant*. 2017;17:782–790, at p. 783
3. Rees et al, "Overcome financial," at p. 785, (references omitted).

4. Dickerson JP, Sandholm T. Multi-organ exchange. *J Artif Intell Res.* 2017;60:639–679, at p. 640.
5. Dickerson and Sandholm, "Multi-organ," at p. 639.
6. Samstein B, de Melo-Martin I, Kapur S, Ratner L, Emond J. A liver for a kidney: ethics of trans-organ paired exchange. *Am J Transplant.* 2018;18:1077–1082.
7. Krawiec KD, Rees MA. Reverse transplant tourism. *Law Contemp Probl.* 2014;77:145–173.
8. Wiseman AC, Gill JS. Financial incompatibility and paired kidney exchange: walking a tightrope or blazing a trail? *Am J Transplant.* 2017:17(3):597–598. To be clear, GKE refers to exchanges between a donor-recipient pair from an LMIC and a donor-recipient pair from an HIC. It does not refer to all kidney paired exchanges that occur across country borders as may be seen in Eurotransplant, for example, because these exchanges, like kidney paired exchanges performed in the US across state borders, do not involve a transfer of resources to a financially challenged donor-recipient pair. A description of the increased number of kidney transplants made possible by crossing country lines coordinated through Eurotransplant can be found in Biró P, Haase-Kromwijk B, Andersson T, et al. Building kidney exchange programmes in Europe—an overview of exchange practice and activities. *Transplantation.* 2019;103(7):1514–1522.
9. Rees et al, "Overcome financial," at p. 787.
10. Rees et al, "Overcome financial."
11. Samstein et al, "Trans-organ," at p. 1080.
12. For the risks of living liver donation, see, for example, Olthoff KM, Abecassis MM, Emond JC, et al. Outcomes of adult living donor liver transplantation: comparison of the Adult-to-Adult Living Donor Liver Transplantation Cohort Study and the national experience. *Liver Transpl.* 2011;17(7):789–797; and Abecassis MM, Fisher RA, Olthoff KM, et al. Complications of living donor hepatic lobectomy—a comprehensive report. *Am J Transplant.* 2012;12:1208–1217.
13. Torres et al, "Bi-organ," at p. 247.
14. Torres et al, "Bi-organ," and Samstein et al, "Trans-organ."
15. Samstein et al, "Trans-organ," at p. 1080.
16. See, for example, Melcher ML, Blosser CD, Baxter-Lowe LA, et al. Dynamic challenges inhibiting optimal adoption of kidney paired donation: findings of a consensus conference. *Am J Transplant.* 2013;13:851–860, at p. 851. The practice to raise the issue of domino chains and paired exchanges upfront is discussed in more detail in chapter 8.
17. Rodrigue JR, Leishman R, Vishnevsky T, Evenson A, Mandelbrot DA. Concerns of ABO incompatible and crossmatch-positive potential donors and recipients about participating in kidney exchanges. *Clin Transpl.* 2015;29:233–241.
18. Rawls J. *A Theory of Justice.* Cambridge, MA: Harvard University Press; 1971.
19. National Organ Transplantation Act (NOTA), Pub L No. 98-507. Approved October 19, 1984, at 42 USC § 274e.
20. National Organ Transplantation Act, as amended by the Charlie W Norwood Living Organ Donation Act, Pub L No. 110-144, 121 Stat 1814 (2007).
21. Healy K, Krawiec KD. Custom, contract, and kidney exchange. *Duke L J.* 2012;62(3):645–670.

22. Dickerson and Sandholm, "Multi-organ."
23. In the article, Torres and colleagues provide a minimal explanation: "Because of donor-L's small physique and her recipient's blood type, finding an exchange donor took 18 months." Torres et al, "Bi-organ," at p. 2646.
24. The concept of the veil of ignorance is an integral part of Rawl's theory of justice. See Rawls, *A Theory of Justice*, at pp. 136–142.
25. The risks of unilateral nephrectomy and living lobar hepactectomy are explored in detail in chapter 1. For kidney risks, see references 12–17 and for liver risks, see references 18–24.
26. See, for example, Rodrigue et al, "Concerns."
27. The literature on health literacy of living donors is scant. See, for example, Dageforde LA, Petersen AW, Feurer ID, et al. Health literacy of living kidney donors and kidney transplant recipients. *Transplantation*. 2014;98:88–93; and Gordon EJ, Mullee J, Skaro A, Baker T. Live liver donors' information needs: a qualitative study of practical implications for informed consent. *Surgery*. 2016;160:671–682.
28. Goodin RE. *Protecting the Vulnerable: A Reanalysis of Our Social Responsibilities.* Chicago, IL: University of Chicago Press; 1985, at p. 109.
29. Rees et al, "Overcome financial."
30. Rees et al, "Overcome financial," at p. 158.
31. Rees et al, "Overcome financial."
32. Wiseman and Gill, "Financial incompatibility," at p. 597.
33. Wiseman and Gill, "Financial incompatibility," at p. 597.
34. Wiseman and Gill, "Financial incompatibility," at p. 597. In this same vein, one might see the $50,000 payment to an exchange donor as precedent for all other potential compatible donors entering exchange programs: Why should being a foreigner from a LMIC qualify them to receive this payment more than other potential compatible exchange donors who might also facilitate many other transplants that would not otherwise happen?
35. Wiseman and Gill, "Financial incompatibility," at p. 597.
36. Rees M, Dunn T, Rees S, et al. Global kidney exchange. 2016;16(suppl 3). Last accessed August 22, 2201.https://atcmeetingabstracts.com/abstract/global-kidney-exchange/
37. Rees M, Dunn T, Rees S, et al. Global kidney exchange. *Am J Transplant*. 2017;17(suppl 3). Last accessed August 22, 2201. https://atcmeetingabstracts.com/abstract/global-kidney-exchange-2/
38. Delmonico FL, Ascher NL. Opposition to irresponsible global kidney exchange. *Am J Transplant*. 2017;17:2745–2746, at p. 2745.
39. Delmonico and Ascher, "Opposition," at p. 2745.
40. Minerva F, Savulescu J, Singer P. The ethics of the Global Kidney Exchange programme. *Lancet*. 2019;394:1775–1778, at p. 1777.
41. Statement of the Declaration of Istanbul Custodian Group [DICG] concerning ethical objections to the proposed global kidney exchange program. Last accessed August 22, 2021. https://www.theisn.org/wp-content/uploads/2020/07/ISN_DICG_Summary_Final.pdf
42. International Society of Nephrology (ISN). Summary of Ethical Objections to Global Kidney Exchange. https://www.theisn.org/images/ISN_DICG_Summary_Final.

pdf; and WHO Task Force on Donation and Transplantation of Human Organs and Tissues. Position statement on the proposal for a global kidney exchange. August 2018. Last accessed August 22, 2021. https://www.who.int/transplantation/donation/GKE-statement.pdf?ua=1

43. DICG, "Ethical objections," at p. 3.
44. DICG, "Ethical objections," at p. 5.
45. WHO Task Force, "Ethical objections," at p. 5.
46. WHO Task Force, "Ethical objections," at p. 5.
47. See, DICG, "Ethical objections," and WHO Task Force, "Ethical objections."
48. The equity argument in support of prioritizing those who are worst off is based on the arguments of John Rawls' in *A Theory of Justice*. We have applied this conception of justice in other chapters (see chapters 7 and 8) and in other manuscripts in which we discuss a fair allocation of deceased donor organs.
49. WHO Task Force, "Ethical objections," at p. 4.
50. Krawiec and Rees, in "Reverse transplant tourism," argue that GKE does not violate NOTA:

> When considering the extent to which RTT withstands common objections to inducements, it is important to remember one important difference between RTT and other inducement schemes that might qualify as valuable consideration under NOTA: RTT does not provide an inducement to donate an organ. Rather, RTT provides an inducement for someone who, in a perfect world free of financial and immunological barriers, would altruistically donate an organ to a friend or family member, to instead donate that same organ to someone else. Once this is recognized, it becomes clear how and why RTT does not run afoul of standard objections to inducements to donate. (p. 165)

We find this interpretation unconvincing.

51. Malaga G, Cuba-Fuentes MS, Rojas-Mezarina L, et al. Strategies for promoting health literacy at the primary care level: focusing on realities of a low and middle income country like Peru. *Ann Public Health Res*. 2018;5(2):1074. https://www.jscimedcentral.com/PublicHealth/publichealth-5-1074.pdf
52. See, for example, Muzaale AD, Massie AB, Wainwright J, McBride MA, Wang M, Segev DL. Long-term risk of ESRD attributable to live kidney donation: matching with healthy non-donors. *Am J Transplant*. 2013;13(suppl 5):204–205; Mjoen G, Hallan S, Hartmann A, et al. Long-term risks for kidney donors. *Kidney Int*. 2014;86:162–167; and Maggiore U, Budde K, Heemann U, et al. Long-term risks of kidney living donation: review and position paper by the ERA-EDTA DESCARTES working group. *Nephrol Dial Transplant*. 2017;32:216–223.
53. United States Department of Health and Human Services. HHS launches President Trump's "Advancing American Kidney Health" initiative. July 10, 2019. Accessed August 22, 2021.https://www.hhs.gov/about/news/2019/07/10/hhs-launches-president-trump-advancing-american-kidney-health-initiative.html
54. Health Resources and Services Administration (HRSA), Health and Human Services Department (HHS). Removing Financial Disincentives to Living Organ Donation. 42 CFR 121. *Fed Regist*. 2020;85:59438–59445. Published

September 22, 2020. Became effective October 22, 2020. Last accessed august 22,   2021.https://www.federalregister.gov/documents/2020/09/22/2020-20804/ removing-financial-disincentives-to-living-organ-donation

55. DICG, "Ethical objections," at p. 7.
56. Krawiec and Rees, "Reverse transplant tourism," at p. 147.
57. Rees et al, "Global kidney exchange (2016)."
58. Of note, in the manuscript by Rees et al, "Overcome financial," at p. 789, the authors acknowledge that they, too, may benefit from the widespread adoption of GKE:

> Michael Rees, Susan Rees, and Alvin Roth have an ownership interest in Rejuvenate Healthcare, LLC that may gain or lose financially as a result of this publication. Jonathan Kopke, Susan Rees, and Laurie Reece were compensated for their work for the Alliance for Paired Donation. Dr. Rees is the noncompensated CEO of the Alliance for Paired Donation.

13

Organ Markets

Case 13-1: The case of the conscientious senator (copied verbatim from Benjamin Hippen et al[1]).

Senator Alexis Murray is a member of the Senate's Committee on Health, Education, Labor, and Pensions, which is holding a hearing on a bill that will permit payment of up to $10,000 plus reimbursement of expenses to living kidney, liver, or lung donors. Senator Murray listens to testimony by a few individuals and by representatives of organizations that either support or oppose the bill. He is particularly struck by the story told by George Cranford, a computer repair technician.

Mr. Cranford's 25-year-old daughter, Karen, has diabetic nephropathy and has suffered from end-stage renal disease for five years. On renal dialysis, she has had frequent bloodstream infections, several of which have been nearly fatal. She is currently hospitalized, recovering from her latest methicillin-resistant staph aureus infection. The recurrence rate of such infections is high, and the mortality rate is between 50 and 75%. Karen is an only child; her parents and other relatives are unsuitable to donate a kidney. She is waiting for an organ from a deceased donor, but her place on the waiting list makes it likely that she will be among the 9,000 patients who die each year because of the shortage of organs for transplantation.

Mr. Cranford has several friends and acquaintances who have said that they have considered donating a kidney for Karen, but have decided not to do so because of concerns about lost income from time away from work, the possibility of losing their jobs, possible health consequences from having only one kidney, and the stress, pain, and physical risks of the donor operation. He expresses the belief that these concerns could be outweighed by the offer of an award of some kind, such as payment for health insurance, an income tax credit, or cash payment of a few thousand dollars. If some of his friends and perhaps many others around the country could be persuaded by such incentives to donate a vital organ, thousands of lives could be saved each year.

The Living Organ Donor as Patient. Lainie Friedman Ross and J. Richard Thistlethwaite, Jr, Oxford University Press.
© Oxford University Press 2022. DOI: 10.1093/oso/9780197618202.003.0013

13.1 Introduction

The case posed here was published as a debate between one of us (LFR) and Benjamin Hippen, a transplant nephrologist, and moderated by Robert Sade, a transplant surgeon. While it was posed as a hypothetical case, there have been numerous attempts to permit organ sales in the United States (US). In 1983, Virginia physician D. H. Barry Jacobs founded International Kidney Exchange, which offered to broker contracts between patients with end-stage renal disease (ESRD) and people willing to sell 1 kidney.[2] In response, the National Organ Transplant Act (NOTA) of 1984 included a provision that made it illegal to buy or sell organs in the US.[3]

In the hypothetical case 13-1, Mr. George Cranford is a computer repair technician whose 25-year-old daughter, Karen has ESRD and is currently doing poorly on dialysis waiting for a deceased donor organ. According to Mr. Cranford, several friends and acquaintances would donate a kidney for Karen but have declined to do so because of concerns about lost income from time away from work, the possibility of losing their jobs, possible health consequences from having only 1 kidney, and the stress, pain, and risks of donation. Mr. Cranford expresses the belief that these concerns could be outweighed by the offer of a financial reward of some kind.

Karen's story is sad, but so is the story of every individual in ESRD on dialysis. There are many such cases; the demand for solid organs for transplantation greatly exceeds their supply. Although NOTA made the buying and selling of organs illegal in the US in 1984, and the World Health Organization recommended a similar ban in 1991[4] (which was reaffirmed in 2010),[5] there is some support for a kidney market in academic circles.[6]

We argue that the market is not an ethical means to mitigate the shortage of organs for transplantation. In the original manuscript, one of us (LFR) argued for this position using the bioethical framework developed by Beauchamp and Childress.[7] Although Art Matas, a transplant surgeon from Minnesota, has used these principles to argue that a market is ethical,[8] one of us (LFR) showed why he and other pro-marketers have misrepresented these principles.[9] In this chapter, we now show, drawing heavily from this earlier publication, how our living donor ethics framework (see chapter 3) further strengthens the arguments against an organ market.[10]

13.2 Living Donor Ethics Framework

13.2.1 Respect for Persons

Supporters of a market for kidneys argue that the principle of autonomy means that individuals have the right to do as they please with their own bodies. As long as individuals sell their kidneys voluntarily, without coercion, they should be free to do so.[11] Market supporters also argue that by allowing individuals to either gift their kidneys or sell their kidneys, they are giving the potential sources (donors and vendors) of organs more choices. This enhances the autonomy of the organ suppliers.[12]

There are several arguments about why autonomy—or, more accurately, respect for autonomy—does not support an individual's right to sell a kidney. First, the organ market supporters ignore the fact that the principle of autonomy, like all guiding bioethics principles, is not absolute.[13] There are moral constraints on autonomy as is noted in the well-known aphorism: "The right to swing my fist ends where the other man's nose begins."[14] One moral constraint on autonomy is harm to others. Critics might argue that the harm to the organ vendor is to herself, not to others. They might object that protecting individuals from harming themselves is paternalistic and assumes that the physicians, the state, or some other third party knows what is better for the individual than the individual herself. The state does, in fact, place limits on autonomy to protect individuals from themselves. We have public health policies that require seatbelts. More significantly, the US government does not allow individuals to sell themselves into slavery. One reason that respect for autonomy does not support organ selling is based on the moral dignity of the individual;[15] another reason is based on the concern that the individual is not acting voluntarily or is being coerced due to unjust circumstances.[16]

Second, respect for autonomy, particularly respect for autonomy understood relationally[17] as we do throughout this book, permits one to challenge an individual's decision, not only when it will harm her, but also when it is contrary to the individual's best interest. There are many reasons why an individual may make a decision that is contrary to his or her interests: misinformation, miscalculation, coercion, or undue influence. Relational autonomy requires health care professionals to go beyond the mere disclosure of clinical facts and instead, through bi-directional discussion, translate information into concepts comprehensible and empowering to patients to help them make a well-deliberated decision consonant with their own reflective values, beliefs, and preferences.[18]

Third, the argument that permitting organ markets promotes autonomy is based on the false premise that more choices enhance autonomy. Those who are willing to sell their organs are those who are living in extreme poverty. The option to sell their organs makes them worse off. It is not that the poor person is wrong in their determination that selling their kidney is their best option when vending is legal, but rather that society is wrong to make organ sale a legal option. As Debra Satz has argued, if kidney sales are widespread, moneylenders may come to view kidneys as collateral, making it more difficult to obtain loans for those unwilling to risk having to part with a kidney.[19]

This argument—that the option to vend is what is harmful—does not depend on whether selling is bad or harmful to the sellers, nor whether the seller is correct in her assessment that selling her kidney is in her best interest. It depends on the claim that the social or legal pressure to sell an organ is harmful. In other words, the option to vend—not vending itself—is what threatens one's ability to make a decision free from undue pressure. If one believes that individuals who are willing to sell their kidneys are not acting voluntarily, it would be morally imperative to prohibit them from doing so.

The empirical data support this. In a review of the literature, Julian Koplin shows that outcomes for kidney vendors are poor in countries with black markets, as well as where the buying and selling of organs was (or is) legal.[20] Allison Tong and colleagues performed a systematic review of qualitative studies evaluating outcomes of kidney sellers and found that they not only remain in poverty but also lose "dignity, sense of purpose, respect, relationships and livelihood."[21]

Fourth, the argument that autonomy should allow a vendor to sell his or her kidney ignores another moral constraint on the vendor's autonomy: the need for third-party procurement of her kidney. Even if an individual were to argue that she has the right to sell her kidney, the transplant surgeon is also a moral agent who has the right to say that she is not willing to harm the potential organ source (it would be inaccurate to call them donors) for financial ends. While the surgeon may be willing to perform the same procedure if the potential organ source were donating a kidney to her brother freely without constraints, the surgeon's personal integrity may prohibit her from maiming another's body purely for economic gain.[22] (This will be further explored in the principle on special relationships 13.2.6.)

We also question whether those in the transplant community who support an organ market truly believe they are promoting the autonomy of those who are willing to vend. With colleagues, we surveyed transplant professionals about autonomy and risk in the organ market debate. We found that 20% of respondents supported a living kidney market but only 10% supported a living liver lobe market. Only half the number of physicians who support a kidney market support a market in liver lobes because of the amount of risk a living liver lobe resection entails.[23] If the debate were truly about autonomy, the solution would be not to prohibit the sale of the liver lobe, but rather to appropriately compensate for the significantly greater risk of morbidity and mortality. In short, the solution would be pay the living liver lobe vendor more.

Second, most market supporters do not discuss a free organ market. The US debate about a market in organs assumes that the organ sales will be covered under the Social Security Amendment of 1972 (Public Law 92-603 section 299I) which funds virtually all Americans for renal replacement therapies including dialysis and kidney transplantation.[24] Having insurance companies (including the federal government) pay for the organs, rather than the individuals with ESRD, avoids the situation in which only the rich can buy organs. Rather, under US government regulation, insurers (and the US government itself through Medicare) would be co-opted to pay vendors for kidneys from poor people in order to provide for kidney transplants for the rich and poor alike! The theoretical basis for this proposal is that it would be cost-saving for both the government and the insurance companies.[25] Gary Becker and Julio Elías have shown that a price tag of US $20,000 for a living donor kidney is fair given the risks of morbidity and mortality,[26] but a reward of up to $90,000 would still be cost-saving.[27]

Ignoring the financing, proponents of an organ market reject a free market (on grounds of its potential to be exploitative) and focus instead on a regulated market, often a restricted regulated market limited to US citizen-vendors.[28] Such a market offers a single price for a living kidney, even though, in a free market, a young tall healthy White male between the ages of 18 and 30 could demand a higher price than other potential donors because these kidneys have the longest graft survival. A restricted market also prevents oversupply, which might lead some potential sources to sell their kidneys for less than the US $20,000 proposed by Becker and Elías or the US $10,000 proposed in case 12-1.

Most people who support a regulated market restricted to US citizen-vendors believe they are protecting both recipients and vendors. They are protecting kidney candidates from the greater risks of infectious diseases seen in potential vendors from abroad.[29] They claim to be protecting the vendors because an unrestricted market price of US $20,000 or US $10,000 would bring a surfeit of potential organ vendors from developing countries for whom the dollar amount would be an undue inducement. A global kidney market, then, would be exploitative. It would allow people to buy and sell things under conditions of inequality which interferes with voluntary negotiations.[30] The reason to restrict the US market to US vendors sidesteps the global economic injustices that exist. If vendors were not restricted to US citizens, an organ's market value could fall to less than US $1,000.[31] This may not be a large enough incentive for Mr. Cranford's friends, but US $1,000 goes a long way in some poorer countries. There is something offensive about the US government buying kidneys from abroad. However, once it is legal to buy and sell organs in the US, it will be difficult to prevent sales across borders.

By rejecting a free market, proponents of a regulated market completely undermine their own argument. Like the market opponents, they actually place constraints on the autonomy of both vendors and recipients. They are limiting the right of a vendor to do as she pleases. Thus, market proponents and opponents only disagree on where to draw the line. Market opponents reject any payment incentive scheme, although they support reimbursement schemes that would make donating financially neutral for the donors.[32] Proponents like to draw the line on how much autonomy to give a seller based on a fixed payment level they believe is economically feasible without any concern, on one hand, for the free choice of the seller and, on the other hand, for the seller's vulnerability. They thus choose an arbitrary, self-serving place on the slippery slope that reduces the seller from a patient for whom they care to an organ source, a commodity that best serves their own, but not the seller's, purposes. The principle of respect for autonomy does not justify organ vending whether as a free market or an externally manipulated regulated market.

The argument against a market is made even stronger when one realizes that our framework uses the principle of respect for persons and not the principle of respect for autonomy. As we explained in chapter 3 (section 2), respect for persons goes beyond a negative conception of autonomy that focuses on a person's right not to be interfered with, and incorporates a relational autonomy that entails a more bidirectional decision-making process in which health care professionals actively engage the potential donor not only in discussions about risks and benefits but also in goals and values. In the context of procuring an organ from a living person, respect for autonomy focuses on the individual's right to self-determination whereas respect for persons focuses on the individual as a patient and the utilization of a shared decision-making process. The principle of respect for persons rejects an organ market because it fails to respect the organ source as a patient.

13.2.2 Beneficence

Market proponents also argue that beneficence supports a market because thousands of individuals die each year on the kidney transplant waitlist. Transplant professionals are, therefore, acting in the best interest of the patients in ESRD by allowing the sale of kidneys. With respect to minimizing harms, the supporters of a market note that we allow emotionally related living donors to donate a kidney. If the risks to kidney donors are considered acceptable when given voluntarily, the risks do not change when money is involved.[33] Finally, market proponents point out that a utilitarian conception of justice would support any means to increase organ procurement and save lives. Therefore, if a market would reduce the organ shortage (and there are good reasons to believe it would),[34] then a market is moral. They do not deny that inequalities exist but argue that the market will allow individuals with less resources to try to improve their situation by vending their kidneys through a voluntary market.[35]

So where is the fallacy in their arguments? The argument that beneficence requires physicians to help treat the thousands of patients in organ failure at any price fails because it ignores the fact that in transplantation with living sources, the vendor or donor becomes a patient as well.[36] We have a moral obligation to protect all living organ sources. Procuring an organ from a desperate vendor is not necessarily in the vendor's best interest. One has to prove first that selling body parts improves individual well-being. It may be more reasonable to reject social policies that do not ensure an adequate safety net that safeguard impoverished individuals from seeking organ vending as their only solution.

The concerns of harm cannot be pushed aside on the grounds that we take kidneys from volunteers and judge those harms as acceptable. There is a social consensus that living kidney donation offers psychosocial and emotional benefits to the donor that outweigh the physical risks. This explains an important distinction between exposing a living donor to the risks of surgery and the long-term clinical (and psychosocial) risks of unilateral nephrectomy while opposing the exposure of a paid donor to these same risks: we believe that a donor gains significant psychological benefits by aiding an emotionally related family member or friend (and, yes, sometimes a stranger).[37] Data (from Iran and India) show that paid vendors do not reap the benefits they expected (improved financial circumstances).[38] The data also show that they experience many emotional and social harms in the stigma that they face for having sold part of their body.[39]

These harms are not limited to the vendors. Michael Sandel argues that society is made worse off if it permits the commodification of body parts. The harm accrues not only to the vendor but to the rest of us who permit vulnerable individuals to sell their kidneys.[40] The argument from commodification holds that market valuation has a degrading effect on certain goods and practices if they are bought and sold, even if fair bargaining positions were to exist (a most unlikely position).

In sum, organ vending cannot be justified by the principle of beneficence.

13.2.3 Justice

Those who support an organ market argue that it is consistent with a utilitarian conception of justice that seeks to maximize the greatest good for the greatest number. This is true, however, only if we assume that the current crisis in end-stage renal failure is inevitable. A utilitarian conception of justice could be interpreted to require a focus on prevention in order to maximize benefit (prevention or delay of renal failure) and to minimize harm (by obviating the need to have living donors in the first place through both prevention and improvement in deceased donor organ procurement). Utilitarians might also reject an organ market because of the long-term harms that it can unintentionally cause. Although a market may provide societal gains by improving the life-years of those individuals already on dialysis, society may be harmed overall if more people end up with ESRD. Those at risk of needing a transplant themselves include the vendors, the recipients who no longer fear loss of a transplanted organ because there is an abundance of organs available for re-transplantation, and society at large that has failed to employ the preventive methods that are known to be effective (eg, control of diabetes and hypertension).[41] Finding more organs to treat end-stage organ disease must be balanced by a renewed focus on our public health/preventive health mission to reduce organ failure in the first place. Such a practice would do more to maximize overall health.

Most justice theorists would argue that in organ transplantation, as in many areas of medicine, we need to consider the distribution of goods (distributive justice) and not just the maximization of goods. One widely accepted theory of distributive justice is egalitarian justice, best associated with the work of John Rawls.[42] Egalitarian justice would permit policies that increase organ transplantation using living vendors if this policy would be accepted behind a veil of ignorance where one was not aware of one's personal traits but did have knowledge about the social and political state of affairs.[43] That is, behind the veil of ignorance, the person would not know their role in society, or their financial, educational, or social status. The individual would know that demand for organs greatly outstripped supply but would not know if she were healthy or an individual with ESRD, a family member of a person in ESRD, or a healthy but impoverished person without good job opportunities. Behind the veil, the rational Rawlsian individual would adopt policies to increase organ transplants provided that the new policies were not harmful to those who are already "worst off."[44] A market in organs would be most attractive to those who are "worst off" and who may see this as the only way to alleviate their poverty. A kidney market would then be understood to be exploitative and not permissible. Market proponents who seek to restrict the kidney market to US citizens concede this point by restricting vendors to "worst off" individuals in the US who are, on the whole, not as badly off as those from impoverished nations abroad. However, if kidney vending were to be legalized in the US, it is likely that other countries could quickly follow suit, as developing world organ markets currently have been constrained by international policy positions that proscribe it. In addition, once begun, it would be hard to restrict trade across borders. A US kidney market could do great harm to the "worst off" in countries that follow the American lead and permit organ sales in their own countries. Once markets develop, it will be hard for countries to prevent their poor citizens from seeking to sell their organs in better paying nearby nations.

Finally, we consider organ vending in the context of social justice. In a liberal society that values human rights and the dignity of man, an egalitarian conception of justice is the most appropriate conception of justice for public policy.[45] Where great disparities exist in wealth and opportunities, a claim that poor people should have the right to sell their kidney as 1 more option to escape poverty implicitly admits that the privileged don't need to do so. Worse, it denies any social responsibility that others may have to prevent such a tragic option.[46] Eduardo Rivera-Lopez eloquently explains,

> When we feel that the rest of us are (even minimally) responsible for that behavior [willingness to sell a kidney because of poverty], we have lost the moral authority to justify the permission of that behavior by appeal to an alleged concern for the autonomy of the individual or for the well-being of the community.[47]

A living organ market is inconsistent with a liberal society whose policies are based on an egalitarian justice framework. We are harmed as a society by a kidney market because it perpetuates an unjust socioeconomic system that disproportionately harms those who are financially and socially vulnerable.

13.2.4 Vulnerabilities of Mr. Cranford's Friends

Different vulnerabilities apply to different people due to their personal traits and their social situations. We first consider the vulnerabilities that may be associated with Mr. Cranford's friends, and in the next section we consider the vulnerabilities of the more typical vendor described in the literature to-date: a desperately poor person who lives in a low- to middle-income country. (The complete vulnerability taxonomy can be found in Table 3.3.)

The vulnerabilities of Mr. Cranford's friends are similar to the vulnerabilities experienced by individuals who altruistically choose to donate to a friend or acquaintance (see chapter 3). While Mr. Cranford's friends express sympathy for him and his daughter, none has agreed to begin the living donor work-up. Mr. Cranford hopes that a small financial incentive might get them to do so. We doubt it. It is likely that the inaction of Mr. Cranford's friends is an expression of their ambivalence, not a willingness that is being thwarted by financial need. A policy to pay Karen's father's friends may resolve any stress and financial burden incurred, but it does not address the risk of death which is a real but rare event, nor the other possible morbidities, including an increased risk of later developing ESRD themselves. If Mr. Cranford's friends really thought about the morbidity and mortality risks, the costs incurred for time off work, and travel expenses, along with the incentive they would find enticing, they would probably conclude that $10,000 is too small an amount, particularly in a country where future health care access is not guaranteed. For any friend with severe financial needs, the issue of undue influence of a monetary donor payment should be disqualifying.

Friends usually come from a similar socioeconomic status. We assume his friends have good jobs with health insurance and would self-identify as middle-class. In what ways are they vulnerable? Some of his friends may express deferential vulnerability to their bosses in the workplace, but Mr. Cranford is not their boss. Some of his friends may be allocationally vulnerable if they have heavy credit card debt or school tuitions; these friends could use the $10,000 and the admiration of their friends, but they also have other financial options (a second job, a second mortgage, or a loan from a family member or friend). There is no good reason to believe that this $10,000 incentive will be enough to convince them to donate, given the risks as well as the other costs of donation. An organ source should be informed that those who undergo living nephrectomy incur costs. In a 2014 Canadian study, the researchers reported that:

> Work and home productivity losses occurred in over 80% of subjects [. . .], and lost wages was reported by 47% of donors. In those who experienced loss of pay, the average number of days and income lost were 20 and $4567, respectively; for all donors average lost wage was $2144. Total workforce productivity loss that includes time off work with and without pay (i.e. vacation, sick leave, employment insurance) for all donors was $6729 [. . .].[48]

Similarly, a study of US living donors reported in 2015 found that

> Similar to Klarenbach et al., we found that most LKDs [living kidney donors] incurred direct and/or indirect costs, with one-third experiencing a net financial loss >$2500 and 20% with a loss >$5000. Considering that the median monthly household income for our LKD cohort was $5200, some potential LKDs may harbor some reservation about a potential loss that is the equivalent of 1 month of income.[49]

A more recent multi-site study in Canada and Australia, the Donor Nephrectomy Outcomes Research (DONOR) Network, also found that living donors incurred significant expenses.[50]. For some, the $10,000 will be a break-even or a small incentive at best, not an allocational boon. Donor financial neutrality has a lot of support,[51] but its aim is to prevent donor financial harm and not to offer financial gain. Mr. Cranford is hoping it could motivate his colleagues.

13.2.5 Vulnerabilities of the More Impoverished Organ Source

Impoverished individuals who consider organ vending face different vulnerabilities. We assume any policy to permit organ buying and selling in the US would restrict vendors to competent adults who can deliberate and decide whether or not to sell 1 of their own kidneys; that is, they are not capacitationally vulnerable. Still, one must acknowledge that even cognitively intact individuals who have decision-making capacity may have difficulty making decisions under conditions of extreme financial stress.

Potential vendors are juridically vulnerable (liable to the authority of others who may have an independent interest in that donation). In an ethnography of organ vendors in Bangladesh, Monir Moniruzzaman describes:

> When surgeries were conducted in India and other countries, brokers often seized sellers' passports, which meant they could not return to Bangladesh without relinquishing their organs. . . .[52]

Others are beholden to loan sharks who may pressure them to repay debts.[53] Even if they are not juridically vulnerable, some of these vendors will be deferentially vulnerable to their family's financial needs or to those to whom they owe money.

Data about international vendors show that they are all quite poor and mostly of low educational attainment. While some have proposed restricting selling to those above a certain income threshold to avoid the desperate seller,[54] there are no data to show that small incentives will be enough to actually encourage others to sell given the risks and potential stigma associated with it. Multiple surveys around the world suggest some support for financial incentives that might lead to a greater supply of organs from persons of greater means and education than current vendors.[55] However, whether this would come to fruition is questionable at best because many hypothetically state their willingness to donate to a stranger on a survey,[56] but between 1998 and 2020, UNOS has documented less than 3,300 Good Samaritan donors (over 90% donated a kidney, but the number also includes liver and lung donors) in the US.[57]

Vendors are also allocationally vulnerable since they are promised "important social goods that will be provided as a consequence of participation as a donor." And yet, in a thematic synthesis of the qualitative research available about vendors, Tong and colleagues found they are often debased by the deception of the brokers, stigmatized by their community, and rejected by family: "Not only do they remain in poverty, they lose dignity, sense of purpose, respect, relationships, and livelihood."[58]

A major vulnerability concern for those who sell their organs is infrastructural—knowing whether the political, organizational, economic, and social context of their care setting has the integrity and resources needed to manage living donation process and follow-up. In Iran, where kidney vending is legal, supporters acknowledge that there is no long-term follow-up of vendors and that that the program "neither has enough life-changing potential nor has enough long-term compensatory effect, resulting in long-term dissatisfaction of some donors."[59] In the US, transplant programs are only required to provide 2 years of follow-up care for living donors (and the care that is financially covered is limited to health issues arising from the surgery or the health risks that derive from having only 1 kidney), even though many of the health risks may not develop for decades.[60] There is no reason to believe we will take better care of vendors.

In sum, those who have served as living vendors appear to be vulnerable in many ways.

13.2.6 Special Relationships Create Special Obligations

In the context of organ vending, this principle focuses on the relationship of the transplant team to the organ seller. As Carl Elliott so eloquently explained: a physician as a moral agent decides "not simply whether a subject's choice is reasonable or morally justifiable, but whether he [the physician] is morally justified in helping the subject accomplish it."[61] In the case of donation, the transplant team physically harms a donor motivated to help save a life. In the case of vending, the transplant team harms a vendor motivated for financial gains. These disparate motivations change the nature of the relationship between transplant team, organ source, and transplant recipient. Although the procedure is the same, the transplant team should refuse to participate in procurement of a vendor's kidney not only because of the injustice of their complicity in organ vending itself, but also because of the social circumstances that led the vendor to consider selling his organ as a solution. By agreeing to procure a kidney from a vendor, the transplant team is complicit in taking advantage of injustice:

> Turning other people's unjust circumstances into profit for oneself isn't morally innocent, even if they consent to and benefit from the exchange.... To take advantage of structural injustices . . . is to become implicated in their perpetuation. One becomes, in a word, complicit.[62]

The risks are the same, but the risk:benefit calculation is not.

13.3 Conclusion

We are sympathetic to Mr. Cranford's willingness in case 13-1 to explore other options to help obtain a kidney for his daughter who suffers from ESRD. At the same time, we must keep in focus that the organ provider (whether vendor or donor) must be treated as a patient. In the 60-plus years since the first living kidney transplant, our understanding of the risks of unilateral nephrectomy has grown considerably. This knowledge should make us even more cautious about procurement from living sources. The solution to our organ shortage should not be based primarily on increasing the number of organs from living persons. Rather, we need to focus on developing alternative treatment options for patients in ESRD: whether by increasing the procurement of deceased donor kidneys, creating organs grown from stem cells, or even xenotransplantation. More importantly, we must also focus on preventing or reducing kidney failure.

Notes

1. Hippen B, Ross LF, Sade RM. Saving lives is more important than abstract moral concerns: financial incentives should be used to increase organ donation. *Ann Thorac Surg.* 2009;88:1053–1061.

2. Shapiro R. Legal issues in payment of living donors for solid organs. *Curr Opin Organ Transplant.* 2002;7:375–379, at p. 375.

3. National Organ Transplantation Act (NOTA), Pub L No. 98–507. Approved October 19, 1984, at 42 USC § 274e. There have been legislative attempts, at the state and federal levels, to permit financial incentives (or at least to remove financial disincentives). See examples described in Satel S, Morrison JC, Jones RK. State organ-donation incentives under the National Organ Transplant Act. *Law Contemp Probl.* 2014;77:217–252.

4. World Health Organization (WHO). WHO guiding principles on human organ transplantation. *Lancet.* 1991;337:1470–1471.

5. World Health Organization (WHO). WHO guiding principles on human organ transplantation. Endorsed by the sixty-third World Health Assembly in May 2010, in Resolution WHA63.22. The WHO is quite clear that:

   > The prohibition on sale or purchase of cells, tissues and organs does not preclude reimbursing reasonable and verifiable expenses incurred by the donor, including loss of income, or paying the costs of recovering, processing, preserving and supplying human cells, tissues or organs for transplantation. (Guiding Principle 5)

6. See, for example, Richards JR. Nephrarious goings on. Kidney sales and moral arguments. *J Med Philos.* 1996;21:357–373; Gill MB, Sade RM. Paying for kidneys: the case against prohibition. *Kennedy Inst Ethics J.* 2002;12:17–45; Matas AJ. The case for living kidney sales: rationale, objections and concerns. *Am J Transplant.* 2004;4:2007–2017; Hippen BE. In defense of a regulated market in kidneys from living vendors. *J Med Philos.* 2005;30:593–626; Cherry MJ. *Kidney for Sale by Owner: Human Organs, Transplantation and the Market.* Washington, DC: Georgetown University Press; 2005; Taylor JS. *Stakes and Kidneys: Why Markets in Human Body Parts Are Morally Imperative.* Hampshire, England: Ashgate Publishing Ltd; 2005; Goodwin M. *Black Markets: The Supply and Demand of Body Parts.* New York, NY: Cambridge University Press; 2006; Matas AJ. Why we should develop a regulated system of kidney sales: a call for action! *Clin J Am Soc Nephrol.* 2006;1:1129–1132; Radcliffe Richards J. *The Ethics of Transplants: Why Careless Thought Costs Lives.* Oxford, England: Oxford University Press; 2012; and Yanklowitz S. Give a kidney, get a check. *The Atlantic.* October 27, 2015.

7. Beauchamp TL, Childress JF. *Principles of Biomedical Ethics.* 5th ed. New York, NY: Oxford University Press; 2001. In the *Principles of Bioethics*, Beauchamp and Childress explicate 4 fundamental principles of bioethics that parallel the principles of the *Belmont Report*. The *Belmont Report* had 3 principles focused on research ethics: respect for persons, beneficence, and justice. Beauchamp and Childress had 4 principles for biomedical ethics more broadly (with a focus on clinical ethics): autonomy, beneficence, nonmaleficence, and justice.

8. Matas, "The case."

9. Hippen et al, "Saving lives."

10. Hippen et al, "Saving lives."

11. Friedman EA, Friedman AL. Payment for donor kidneys: pros and cons. *Kidney Int.* 2006;69:960–962; and Friedlaender MM. The role of commercial non-related living kidney transplants. *J Nephrol.* 2003;16(suppl 7):S10–S15.

12. See, for example, Taylor, *Stakes*; Radcliffe Richards, *The Ethics*; Hippen, "Saving lives."

13. Beauchamp and Childress, *Principles*.

14. Oliver Wendell Holmes, Jr. Liberty Tree. Last accessed August 22, 2021. https://quoteinvestigator.com/2011/10/15/liberty-fist-nose/

15. See, for example, Lawler PA. Is the body property? *The New Atlantis*. Fall 2006:62–72; and Kass L. *Life, Liberty, and the Defense of Dignity: The Challenge for Bioethics*. San Francisco, CA: Encounter Books; 2004.

16. Sandel MJ. *What Money Can't Buy: The Moral Limits of Markets*. New York, NY: Farrar, Straus, and Giroux; 2012.

17. Mackenzie C, Stoljar N. Introduction: autonomy refigured. In: Mackenzie C, Stoljar N, eds. *Relational Autonomy: Feminist Perspectives on Autonomy, Agency, and the Social Self*. New York, NY: Oxford University Press; 2000:3–31.

18. Friedman M. Autonomy, social disruptions, and women. In: Mackenzie C, Stoljar N, eds. *Relational Autonomy: Feminist Perspectives on Autonomy, Agency, and the Social Self*. New York, NY: Oxford University Press; 2000:35–51.

19. Satz D. *Why Some Things Should Not Be for Sale: The Moral Limits of Markets*. Oxford, England: Oxford University Press; 2010, at pp. 200–201.

20. Koplin J. Assessing the likely harms to kidney vendors in regulated organ markets. *Am J Bioeth*. 2014;14(10):7–18.

21. Tong A, Chapman JR, Wong G, Cross NB, Batabyal P, Craig JC. The experiences of commercial kidney donors: thematic synthesis of qualitative research. *Transpl Int*. 2012;25:1138–1149.

22. Crouch RA. Elliott C. Moral agency and the family: the case of living related organ transplantation. *Camb Q Healthc Ethics*. 1999;8:275–287.

23. Aronsohn A, Thistlethwaite JR, Jr, Segev DL, Ross LF. How different conceptions of risk are used in the organ market debate. *Am J Transplant*. 2010;10:931–937.

24. Social Security Amendments of 1972 (Pub L No. 92–603).

25. Barnett W, Saliba M, Walker D. A free market in kidneys: efficient and equitable. *The Independent Review*. 2001;5(3):373–383.

26. Becker GS, Elías JJ. Introducing incentives in the market for live and cadaveric organ donations. *J Econ Perspect*. 2007;21:3–24.

27. Matas AJ, Schnitzler M. Payment for living donor (vendor) kidneys: a cost-effectiveness analysis. *Am J Transplant*. 2004;4:216–221.

28. Hippen, "In defense"; Monaco AP. Rewards for organ donation: the time has come. *Kidney Int*. 2006;69:955–957; Erin CA, Harris J. An ethical market in human organs. *J Med Ethics*. 2003;29:137–138; and Brennan T. Markets in health care: the case of renal transplantation. *J Law Med Ethics*. 2007;35:249–255.

29. Jha V, Chugh KS. The case against a regulated system of living kidney sales. *Nat Clin Pract Nephrol*. 2006;2:466–467; and Rizvi SNS, Zafar M, Ahmed E, et al. Health status and renal function evaluation of kidney venders: a report from Pakistan. *Am J Transplant*. 2008;13:453–476.

30. See, for example, Sandel, *What Money Can't Buy*; and Radin MJ. *Contested Commodities: The Trouble with Trade in Sex, Children, Body Parts and Other Things*. Cambridge, MA: Harvard University Press; 1996.

31. Adams AF, Barnett AH, Kaserman DL. Markets of organs: the question of supply. *Contemp Econ Policy*. 1999;17:147–155.

32. As we discuss in section 13.2.4 Vulnerabilities of Mr. Cranford's Friends, multiple studies have shown significant and sometimes burdensome out-of-pocket expenses experienced by living kidney and living liver donors. See, for example, Rodrigue JR, Schold JD, Morrissey P, et al. Predonation direct and indirect costs incurred by adults who donated a kidney: findings from the KDOC [Kidney Donor Outcomes Cohort] study. *Am J Transplant.* 2016;16(7):1973–1981; McCormick F, Held PJ, Chertow GM, Peters TG, Roberts JP. Financial costs incurred by living kidney donors: a prospective cohort study. *Am J Transplant.* 2015;15(9):2387–2393; Przech S, Garg AX, Arnold JB, et al. Financial costs incurred by living kidney donors: a prospective cohort study. *J Am Soc Nephrol.* 2018;29(12):2847–2857; and DiMartini A, Dew MA, Liu Q, et al. Social and financial outcomes of living liver donation: a prospective investigation within the Adult-to-Adult Living Donor Liver Transplantation Cohort Study 2 (A2ALL-2). *Am J Transplant.* 2017;17(4):1081–1096. The transplant community has advocated for policies that would make donation financially neutral, but they have not yet been fully adopted in all parts of the world. See, for example, Hays R, Rodrigue JR, Cohen D, et al. Financial neutrality for living organ donors: reasoning, rationale, definitions, and implementation strategies. *Am J Transplant.* 2016;16(7):1973–1981. There is broad worldwide variability regarding reimbursement policies. See Sickand M, Cuerden MS, Klarenbach SW, et al. Reimbursing live organ donors for incurred non-medical expenses: a global perspective on policies and programs. *Am J Transplant.* 2009;9(12):2825–2836.
33. Matas et al, "The case."
34. Adams et al, "Markets of organs"; and Ghods AJ, Savaj S. Iranian model of paid and regulated living-unrelated kidney donation. *Clin J Am Soc Nephrol.* 2006;1:1136–1145.
35. See, for example, Satel S. Organs for sale. *The American.* November/December 2006. Last accessed August 22, 2021.https://sallysatelmd.com/articles/2006/organs-for-sale/; Matas, "the case"; and Radcliffe-Richards J, Daar AS, Guttmann RD, et al. The case for allowing kidney sales. *Lancet.* 1998;351:1950–1952.
36. Danovitch GM. The doctor-patient relationship in living donor kidney transplantation. *Curr Opin Nephrology Hypertens.* 2007;16:503–505; and Delmonico FL, Surman OS. Is this live-organ donor your patient? *Transplantation.* 2003;76:1257–1260.
37. Frade IC, Fonseca I, Dias L, et al. Impact assessment in living kidney donation: psychosocial aspects in the donor. *Transplantation Proceedings.* 2008;40:677–681; and Johnson EM, Anderson JK, Jacobs C, et al. Long-term follow-up of living kidney donors: quality of life after donation. *Transplantation.* 1999;67:717–721.
38. Goyal M, Mehta RL, Schneiderman LJ, Sehgal AR. Economic and health consequences of selling a kidney in India. *JAMA.* 2002;288:1589–1593; and Zargooshi J. Quality of life of Iranian kidney "Donors." *J Urol.* 2001;166:1790–1799.
39. Goyal et al, "Economic," and Zargooshi, "Quality of life."
40. Sandel, *What Money Can't Buy.*
41. Theoretically, utilitarianism could allow for significant harm to one individual if it were to provide significant benefit to a large number of individuals. That is, it could allow 1 adult to sacrifice himself to serve as a multi-organ donor for 10 individuals on the waitlist for financial gain to his next of kin. Worse yet, it might justify human

lotteries in which individuals were sacrificed to maximize the well-being of 10 individuals per sacrifice!

42. John Rawls. *A Theory of Justice*. Cambridge, MA: Belknap Press of Harvard University Press; 1971.

43. Rawls, *A Theory*.

44. Rawls, *A Theory*.

45. Rawls, *A Theory*; and Veatch RM, Ross LF. *Transplantation Ethics*. 2nd ed. Washington, DC: Georgetown University Press; 2015.

46. Rivera-Lopez E. Organ sales and moral distress. *J Applied Philos*. 2006;23(1):41–52

47. Rivera-Lopez, "Organ sales," at p. 50.

48. Klarenbach S, Gill JS, Knoll G, et al. Economic consequences incurred by living kidney donors: a Canadian multi-center prospective study. *Am J Transplant*. 2014;14:916–922, at p. 917 (mentions to tables were removed).

49. Rodrigue JR et al, "Direct and indirect," at p. 873 (references omitted).

50. Przech et al, "Financial costs" ; and Barnieh L, Kanellis J, McDonald S, et al. Direct and indirect costs incurred by Australian living kidney donors. *Nephrology*. 2018;23:1145–1151.

51. Hays et al, "Financial neutrality"; McCormick F, Held PJ, Chertow GM, Peters TG, Roberts JP. Removing disincentives to kidney donation: a quantitative analysis. *J Am Soc Nephrol*. 2019;30:1349–1357; and Capron AM, Delmonico FL, Danovitch GM. Financial neutrality in organ donation. *J Am Soc Nephrol*. 2020;31:229–230.

52. Moniruzzaman M. Against a regulated market in human organs: ethical arguments and ethnographic insights from the organ trade in Bangladesh. *Hum Organiz*. 2018;77:323–334, at p. 327.

53. Tong et al, "The experiences."

54. Matas et al, "The case," at p. 2010.

55. See, for example, Boulware LE, Troll MU, Wang NY, et al. Public attitudes toward incentives for organ donation: a national study of different racial/ethnic and income groups. *Am J Transplant*. 2006;6:2774–2785; Kranenburg L, Schram A, Zuidema W, et al. Public survey of financial incentives for kidney donation. *Nephrol Dial Transplant*. 2008;23:1039–1042; Leider S, Roth AE. Kidneys for sale: who disapproves, and why? *Am J Transplant*. 2010;10:1221–1227; van Buren MC, Massey EK, Maasdam WC, et al. For love or money? Attitudes toward financial incentives among actual living kidney donors. *Am J Transplant*. 2010;10:2488–2492.

56. See, for example, Sadler H, Davison L, Carroll C, et al. The living, genetically un-related, kidney donor. *Semin Psychiatry*. 1971;3(1):86–101; Fellner CH, Schwartz SH. Altruism in disrepute: medical versus public attitudes toward the living organ donor. *N Engl J Med*. 1971;284(11):582–585; Gade DM. Attitudes toward human organ transplantations: a field study of 119 people in the greater Detroit area. *Henry Ford Hosp J*. 1972;20(1):41–50; Landolt MA, Henderson AJZ, Barrable WM, et al. Living anonymous donation: What does the public think? *Transplantation*. 2001;71(11):1690–1696; Spital A. Public attitudes toward kidney donation by friends and altruistic strangers in the United States. *Transplantation*. 2001;71(8):1061–1064; Stiller CR, Lindberg MC, Rimstead D, et al. Living related donation. *Transplant Proc*.

1985;17(6 suppl 3):85–100; Toronyi E, Alfoldy R, Jaray J, et al. Attitudes of donors towards organ transplantation in living related kidney transplantations. *Transpl Int.* 1998;11(suppl 1):S481–483; and Landolt MA, Henderson AJ, Gourlay W, et al. They talk the talk: surveying attitudes and judging behavior about living anonymous kidney donation. *Transplantation.* 2003;76(10):1437–1444.

57. OPTN (Organ Procurement and Transplantation Network) National Data. Last updated August 19, 2021, last accessed August 22, 2021. https://optn.transplant.hrsa.gov/data/view-data-reports/national-data/.

58. Tong et al, "The experiences," at p. 1147.

59. Ghods and Savaj, "Iranian," at p. 1141.

60. Muzaale AD, Massie AB, Wainwright J, McBride MA, Wang M, Segev DL. Long-term risk of ESRD attributable to live kidney donation: matching with healthy non-donors. *Am J Transplant.* 2013;13(suppl 5):204–205; and Mjoen G, Hallan S, Hartmann A, et al. Long-term risks for kidney donors. *Kidney Int.* 2014;86:162–167; and Maggiore U, Budde K, Heemann U, et al. Long-term risks of kidney living donation: review and position paper by the ERA-EDTA DESCARTES working group. *Nephrol Dial Transplant.* 2017;32:216–223.

61. Elliott C. Doing harm: living organ donors, clinical research and *The Tenth Man. J Med Ethics.* 1995;21:91–96, at p. 95.

62. Malmqvist E. Taking advantage of injustice. *Soc Theory Pract.* 2013;39:557–580, at p. 567.

PART 5
DECISION-MAKING AND RISK THRESHOLDS

PART 5
DECISION MAKING AND RISK
THRESHOLDS

14

Candidate Criteria for Living Versus Deceased Donor Liver Grafts

Same or Different?

Case 14-1: The case is reprinted verbatim from Branislav Kocman et al from Zagrab Croatia.[1]

Our patient first presented at the age of 46 years with adenocarcinoma of the left colon and a large synchronous liver metastasis. Notably, both her CEA [carcinoembryonic antigen] and CA- [Carbohydrate antigen]19-9 at presentation, as well as postoperatively, were within normal limits. She underwent left hemicolectomy and right hepatectomy. Pathology revealed Dukes D stage adeno-carcinoma of the colon with positive regional lymph nodes. After an uneventful postoperative course, she was treated with Folfox. Twenty months later, computerized tomographic (CT) scans revealed several secondary metastases in the remaining liver, and she underwent atypical resection for 6 liver metastases. Five months later, multiple new secondary tumors were present with diffuse liver involvement and no possibility for further resection. Her CEA and CA19-9 were 1 µg/L [normal = <2.5 µg/L] and 7.93 kIU/L [normal = 0–37 kIU/L], respectively. Taking into account the patient's age, her good general condition and the possibility of treatment with new immunosuppressive agents that also have antineoplastic properties, LT [liver transplantation] was considered as a radical but potentially curative treatment. Because the current Croatian allocation system would not allow a patient with unresectable colorectal metastases to the liver to receive a cadaveric liver graft, the possibility of an LDLT [living donor liver transplantation] was presented to the patient and her family. Her husband agreed to be the donor. He was evaluated under standard protocol for living donors, and the patient's evaluation included additional work-up in search of possible extrahepatic disease. . . . No extrahepatic tumor sites were found, and after the approval of the Institutional Ethics Committee, the decision was made

The Living Organ Donor as Patient. Lainie Friedman Ross and J. Richard Thistlethwaite, Jr, Oxford University Press.
© Oxford University Press 2022. DOI: 10.1093/oso/9780197618202.003.0014

to proceed with the transplantation . . . standard LDLT of the right liver lobe was performed. . . . The postoperative course was uneventful and the patient was discharged home 3 weeks after transplantation. . . . At the time of writing, 5 years after the transplantation, she was alive and disease free.

Case 14-2: (A hypothetical case).

Molly is 20 years old who had her first liver transplant as an older adolescent after a failed suicide attempt by ingesting acetaminophen. She currently lives at home, does not work, and is currently not attending college because of her mental health issues. She has a history of severe depression and anxiety and has had multiple suicide attempts/gestures both before and subsequent to her liver transplant for acetaminophen toxicity. She tried in-patient drug rehabilitation once but left before treatment was completed. She has an outpatient psychiatrist and therapist whom she sees frequently. On the day of admission, she was found minimally responsive by her parents who called 9-1-1. They had been at a wedding the night before, assumed Molly was asleep, and had not checked in on her until the morning when she was very difficult to arouse. Her drug screen on admission was positive for acetaminophen, marijuana, and a trace amount of benzodiazepines. Her acetaminophen level was 200 mg/L at admission and the team began N-acetylcysteine. Her liver function tests are quite abnormal and her immunosuppression medication levels are undetectable. She is diagnosed with acute liver failure (ALF).

   It is not clear whether her liver will recover. In the emergency room, she is somnolent but arousable. At one point, she tearfully apologizes to her parents, states she wants to live, and is ready for intensive inpatient psychiatric treatment. The transplant team is consulted. After their evaluation, including a psychiatric consultation, the transplant team discusses Molly's case. Consistent with their center's policy, the transplant team decides she is not a deceased donor liver transplant candidate because of her multiple previous suicide attempts and the risk for future attempts despite the intense professional help she has already received. Molly's father, Mr. B, is a college-educated professional who understands that his daughter is a high-risk candidate but offers to donate part of his liver. He understands that the surgery exposes him to risk and that the likelihood of long-term graft and patient survival are low but argues, "I have no choice."

14.1 Eligibility for Waitlisting

We now explore whether living donor liver transplant (LDLT) is morally permissible when the candidate is not eligible for a deceased donor liver transplant (DDLT) because of clinical or psychosocial exclusion.

There are widely variable eligibility criteria waitlisting a candidate in end-stage organ failure for a deceased donor organ. James Levenson and Mary Ellen Olbrisch documented medical, psychosocial, and financial reasons why transplant programs either refused to evaluate or refused to list a patient for a deceased donor transplant.[2] Most notable was the degree of variability between centers and between organs (with stricter criteria at all centers for heart transplant compared to liver transplant, with kidney transplant having the least strict criteria). A more recent study in 2011 also found wide variability in provider opinions regarding the importance of various medical, psychosocial, and financial issues.[3]

Patients in end-stage organ failure may not be eligible for liver transplantation because they are too well. For example, candidates with a MELD score below 15 should not be listed for a liver transplant (although there are exceptions for certain conditions[4]) because they do not get a survival benefit and may even be harmed by transplantation (lower 1-year survival post-transplant compared with remaining on the waitlist[5]).

At the other extreme are cases where a candidate is judged too ill or otherwise fails to meet the criteria for a deceased donor organ. In the 2013 Practice Guideline by the American Association for the Study of Liver Diseases and the American Society of Transplantation for the "Evaluation for Liver Transplantation in Adults," the authors enumerated a number of medical and psychosocial exclusion criteria.[6]

There are 2 caveats about the exclusion criteria. First, in some cases, patients who are excluded because they meet 1 of the exclusion criteria could still benefit from a liver transplant. For example, even if a patient is noncompliant and therefore highly likely to lose the organ in a shorter time frame than a more compliant candidate, the patient may benefit from the improved quality of life in the short term. While there is no universal consensus about what minimum life expectancy post-liver transplant should be expected to justify undergoing transplantation, most programs cite an expected 5-year survival between 50 and 70%.[7] Of note, the Organ Procurement and Transplant Network (OPTN)/United Network for Organ Sharing (UNOS) does not dictate to transplant centers what decision should be made, but does require each center to have their own policies on deceased donor transplant eligibility and can review a center's records to assure consistency in policy application. Thus, for example, it is important to distinguish the case 14-2 of Molly who has developed ALF secondary to a repeated suicide attempt from the case of Jane who presented in ALF in chapter 10, which was caused by an unintentional ingestion. Jane meets the inclusion criteria for status 1 liver allocation whereas Molly does not, based on her center's criteria for acceptance for deceased donor transplantation. This has implications for both the candidates and the donors. If Jane were to need a liver transplant and the decision was made to use a living donor graft from her father, she would be eligible for a DDLT if a graft became available while her father was still undergoing the work-up and Jane would be eligible for re-listing as status 1 in the case of acute graft failure. Molly would not be eligible for a DDLT. Our aim in this chapter is to ask whether the fact that Molly is not eligible for a deceased donor graft should preclude her from being a recipient of a living donor graft.

Second, the exclusion criteria are not static but change with evolving therapies, changing social attitudes, and outcome data. For example, candidates with cirrhosis from alcoholic liver disease were traditionally excluded from the liver deceased donor waitlist if they had not proven a certain period (usually 6 months) of sobriety, even though the 6-month rule, as it became known, was not based on evidence.[8] Even after they had proven sobriety, some theorists and transplant professionals wanted to place them lower on the waitlist on the grounds that they needed to accept some responsibility for their situation.[9] Others argued that alcoholism is a disease and should be treated no differently than any other disease.[10] This latter position was strengthened by the fact that outcomes were not really different from patients receiving liver transplants for other causes.[11] French data from 2011 showed how well some patients with acute chronic alcoholic liver disease do with a liver transplant.[12] Early on, some transplant centers elected to perform transplants on selected patients with alcohol use disorder even if they do not meet a pre-set time period of sobriety, and more programs have moved in this direction. A survey published in 2019 found that:

> only 43% of the programs required a specific period of abstinence before transplant for alcoholic liver disease and only 26% enforced 6-month abstinence policy. For patients with AAH [acute alcoholic hepatitis], 71% programs waived the 6-month abstinence requirement and considered

psychosocial factors, such as family support, patient's motivation, or commitment to rehabilitate. Few programs used validated instruments to assess risk of relapse in AAH patients.[13]

As Jaiming Zhu and colleagues concluded, "Policies regarding alcohol use have become more flexible particularly toward patients with AAH."[14]

14.2 Waitlist Exclusion for DDLT: The Case of Non-Hepatic Cancer With Liver Metastases

Colorectal carcinoma (CRC) is one of the most common cancers in western countries. Approximately 15%–25% of these patients have distant metastases at the time of diagnosis, most commonly to the liver. Another 25%–50% of these patients will develop liver metastases within 3 years of diagnosis.[15] Colorectal liver metastases (CRLM) are currently the most frequent indication for liver resection in western countries.[16] Most patients with CRLM, however, have unresectable disease and a median survival of 6.9 months.[17] Attempts at liver transplant for CRLM in the 1980s met with dismal results,[18] and liver transplantation for liver cancer was indicated only for primary tumors of the liver (eg, hepatocellular carcinoma [HCC]).[19] Even liver transplantation for HCC had poor results until guidelines about size and number (the "Milan Criteria") were developed.[20] Criteria have loosened to allow for liver transplantation for some nonprimary liver cancers that only metastasize to the liver, such as "carcinoid tumors, neuroendocrine tumors, and gastrinomas."[21]

In 2013, liver transplant teams in Norway reported on a prospective DDLT study in patients with CRLM named the SEcondary CAncer (SECA-1) study that was conducted between November 2006 and March 2011:

> . . . a total of 25 eligible patients were put on the waiting list for liver transplantation. One patient who developed ascites and lung metastases on chemotherapy was withdrawn from the list. Three other patients did not undergo transplantation because of metastatic lymph nodes in the hepatic ligament on frozen section taken during the perioperative staging procedure. A total of 21 patients underwent liver transplantation according to the study protocol. No patients were lost to follow-up.[22]

The 21 study participants in the SECA-1 study were transplanted with a deceased donor graft with a 1-, 3- and 5-year survival rate of 95%, 68%, and 60% although many have developed and are living with recurrent disease.[23] Although CRLM has not been classified as an indication for DDLT, and patients with CRLM would not get a deceased donor liver graft in most countries, Norway is unique in having an excess of deceased donor livers.[24] The Oslo group is also experimenting with a deceased donor split-liver technique to provide a small-for-size (left lateral segment) liver graft for patients with CRLM. They have developed the RAPID strategy (resection and partial liver segment 2–3 transplantation with delayed total hepatectomy) in which candidates with CRLM undergo partial hepatectomy (to remove as much of the cancer as feasible) and supplement the patient's liver function with a left lateral segment deceased donor transplant while most of their non-resected liver remains in place. When the orthotopic liver has grown sufficiently, the remainder of the patient's native liver is removed.[25] A similar protocol is being implemented in Germany, but in Germany the left lateral segment is being obtained from a living donor.[26] Full lobe (left or right) LDLT for CRLM is being done in a few institutions in the United States (US) and in countries that do not allow listing on the deceased donor list for this condition (case 14-1).[27]

14.3 Waitlist Exclusion After Suicide Attempt

In the US, suicide is the 10th leading cause of death.[28] There are many more suicide attempts than actual suicides, and men are more likely to actually die. Part of the reason is the method of suicide attempt: males are more likely to commit suicide with firearms, whereas women are more likely to attempt suicide by drug overdose.[29]

Liver allocation policies often exclude patients who need a liver transplant due to a suicide attempt. In 1993, James Levenson and Mary Ellen Olbrisch reported that a recent suicide attempt was an absolute (17.4%) and relative (63.0%) contraindication to liver transplantation.[30] More specific to our case (case 14-2), respondents thought that patients with multiple suicide attempts should be an absolute (41.3%) and relative (45.7%) contraindication to liver transplantation.[31] Molly's affective disorder would also be seen as a relative contraindication to liver transplantation by 63.0% of respondents although none thought it was an absolute contraindication.[32] Almost 2 decades later, Katharine Secunda and colleagues found that only 2 of 246 (0.8%) of respondents thought a first suicide attempt was an absolute contraindication (and another 131 or 53.3% a relative contraindication) but 108/245 (44.1%) of respondents thought it should be an absolute contraindication (and another 127 or 51.8% a relative contraindication) when the patient had 2 or more suicide attempts.[33] This diversity of opinion is also seen in a study by Catherine Crone and Andrea DiMartini that provided 5 vignettes to psychiatrists, psychologists, and social workers involved in liver transplant evaluations.[34]

The most common acute drug overdose used in suicide attempts is acetaminophen (also known as Tylenol in the US and Paracetamol internationally). In a study from 7 European countries between 2005 and 2007, 600 cases of ALF leading to registration for transplantation were identified from the liver transplant registries and hospital records. Of these, 114 involved overdoses, and 111 of the 114 involved Paracetamol.[35] Although many patients with ALF recover spontaneously, if the liver failure continues to worsen, a liver transplant may be needed quite acutely. Because a deceased donor liver graft may not become available, LDLT may be an option. In case 14-2, the transplant team does not want to list Molly for a deceased donor organ, but her father steps forward to state that he is willing to serve as a living donor. Should he be allowed to donate if the team will not waitlist her for a deceased donor? That is, should the criteria for LDLT be the same as the criteria for deceased donor liver transplantation?

14.4 Should Criteria for Candidates Be the Same for Living and Deceased Donor Grafts?

There is no consensus in the US regarding whether and when to permit living organ donation when the candidate is ineligible (or of low priority) for a deceased donor organ. One argument against holding candidates with a potential living donor to the same standard as candidates who are awaiting a deceased donor organ is that deceased organs are a public good and living donor grafts are a private good. In most countries, the demand for deceased donor organs greatly outpaces supply, and it is morally appropriate to create transparent criteria for inclusion, exclusion, and allocational prioritization. To be fair, the focus of the criteria should be on whether the candidate can benefit from a transplant.[36] To the extent that there are thresholds about how much benefit a candidate should be expected to accrue, the criteria should be applied fairly and transparently across conditions. For example, if patients with hepatocellular carcinoma are eligible for a liver transplant if they have a 50% 5-year life expectancy, then patients with amyloidosis should also be expected to have a 50% 5-year survival. Developing and consistently applying professional guidelines that are based on such empirical evidence as estimated 5-year survival helps avoid intentional or unintentional discrimination in allocation.

One problem with the private versus communal good argument is that the lines are more blurred than they may seem. LDLT entails not merely a private good (the living donor graft) but also uses many public resources—from operating rooms and intensive care unit beds to professional time at the bedside, all finite resources that might have benefitted another patient more.

Yong Kwon and colleagues, however, argue it is time to develop allocation policies that permit a double standard:

> For those who have living donors, different selection criteria based on their specific disease, not based on the principle of utilization should be used to evaluate their candidacy. These patients should not be denied of a lifesaving liver transplant opportunity if they have fully disclosed and consented living donors who are aware of the risk of the surgery as well as the expected survival benefits of the recipients. Furthermore, from a regulatory standpoint, our current outcome-based regulatory and recredential process will need to be revised such that these living donor liver transplant outcomes are evaluated independently and separately from the deceased donor outcome.[37]

British guidelines specifically permit a double standard for both living donor kidney transplantation (LDKT) and LDLT. In both the third and fourth editions of the United Kingdom *Guidelines for Living Donor Kidney Transplant*, the guidelines state:

> In particular, when a potential recipient is considered unsuitable for inclusion on the deceased donor waiting list but a planned living donor transplant is considered an acceptable risk, the donor must not feel under any "obligation" to donate.[38]

The British *Guidelines for Living Donor Liver Transplant* also support the double standard, particularly when there is lack of evidence regarding long-term outcomes:

- There is a lack of evidence about the long-term outcomes for recipients of liver transplants in some diseases e.g. acute alcoholic hepatitis, cholangiocarcinoma, solitary colorectal liver metastases. In these cases, experienced centres may wish to consider adult recipients for LDLT, with appropriate protocols, patient information and phased introduction. (Not graded)
- In diseases where long term outcomes are unclear due to lack of evidence or reproducibility of results, LDLT may offer an opportunity for ethically approved research studies within the UK, but LDLT should only be performed under that condition. (Not graded).[39]

The guidelines also specifically acknowledge the role of LDLT when DDLT is not available to the patient in end-stage liver disease:

> LDLT in the UK may be most advantageous for patients with conditions where access to DDLT is limited due to lack of liver failure or other prioritisation systems (e.g. restricted organ resources).[40]

Our framework supports such a policy.

14.5 The Living Donor Ethics Framework

14.5.1 Respect for Persons

In case 14-2, the main argument in support of the father's request to donate a part of his liver to his daughter is respect for persons: the competent patient has the right to consent to donate a liver lobe. If the donor both judges the benefits to outweigh the risks and gives a voluntary and informed consent, then the donor should be permitted to donate. Likewise, the case report of case 14-1 states that the husband donor "was evaluated under standard protocol for living donors."[41] While the case is from Croatia, in the US this would mean, at a minimum, that he went through an extensive medical and psychological work-up by the living donor advocate team (LDAT) who also ensured that his consent was voluntary and that he was not under "undue pressure."

Living donor consent may not be fully voluntary, particularly when there is no therapeutic alternative. When no alternative exists, the use of the phrase "has no choice" emphasizes medical vulnerability—the presence of a serious health-related condition in the intended recipient for which there are no satisfactory or timely remedies. The living donor may feel "compelled" to donate.

Does this mean that the donor did not act voluntarily? Elliot and Crouch argue that the reason we interpret the parental phrase "had no choice" as coercive or at least nonvoluntary is that we employ "a picture of agency that identifies freedom with independence." They explain:

> The moral commitments associated with intimacy, such as loyalty and devotion, are seen as "coercive" because they motivate a person to actions that a completely independent person would not take. Thus parents who risk their own lives to donate organs to a child are not acting freely, because they are bound by moral and emotional ties to the child.[42]

Instead, they argue:

> If we are ever to get straight about the nature of voluntariness, we must recognize that moral and emotional commitments are not exceptional, are not constraints on freedom, but are rather a part of ordinary human life. More specifically, they are a part of ordinary *family* life that we must take seriously if we want to understand how family members can make free choices about organ donation.[43]

Medard Hilhorst, a medical ethicist from the Netherlands, explores why the utterance "has no choice" does not mean that the decision was not voluntary. He claims that in the context of personal relations, general ethical concepts "seem to lose their unambiguous, self-evident, ordinary meaning."[44] He cites "utterances that detect moral intuitions that are authentic and double-edged at the same time."[45] For example, he cites a parent who states,

> I felt I had no choice, but it gave me a good feeling that I could donate and help my child; I took responsibility, I didn't feel like a victim of the situation; I took an active part in the process.[46]

That is, although the parent claims that he "had no choice"; which suggests coercion, the parent in this example also acknowledges that the situation was empowering in that it allowed him/her to take responsibility.

This is not to deny that the father may feel a significant degree of internally imposed pressure. At the first conference on ethics and transplantation

in 1966 sponsored by the CIBA Foundation, the attendees distinguished between justified and unjustified pressure to donate.[47] David Daube, a British
legal scholar discussed that the type of pressure one feels regarding donating
to a loved one may be both internally and externally derived. He argued that
the pressure created by familial obligations and self-expectations is permissible because it "belongs to the normal burden and dignity of social exist-
ence."[48] In 1989, justifying the first parent-child living liver donation in the
US, John Lantos and Mark Siegler of the MacLean Center for Clinical Medical
Ethics at the University of Chicago similarly argued that the psychological or
internal coercion "created by the donor's own feelings of guilt because the patient may die without donor participation" needs to be balanced "by positive
emotional responses to donation, such as feelings of loyalty, responsibility,
love, or duty toward a family member."[49] Like Daube, they concluded that
this type of pressure does not invalidate consent because "The need to balance selfishness and altruism is a universal feature of an individual's relationship with his or her family."[50]

Despite strong bonds and a sense of "no choice," the empirical data show
that family members are able to refuse. In the early 1970s, before chronic
dialysis had become routine, Simmons and colleagues found that some
family members refused to serve as a living donor, even to the detriment of
family relationships.[51] In the 1980s, when children were dying because no
liver grafts were available (deceased donor organs were allocated based on
size and split liver techniques were only being developed[52]), the University
of Chicago proposed removing part of an adult's liver (anticipated to most
likely be a parent, but not excluding other relatives) to be used as a graft
for a child.[53] Larry Goldman, the psychiatrist working with the University
of Chicago transplant team, documented that in the first 20 cases, at least 1
parent opted out which shows that at least some parents can say no.[54]

We know virtually nothing about the spouse in case 14-1 except that
"he agreed to be the donor" when the option was proposed with the whole
family present, including the candidate (his wife).[55] In case 14-2, Mr. B
seems to be acting autonomously as he volunteered without being asked.
Have we done due diligence to empower these potential donors to make a
decision that best reflects their interests and needs? In 14-1, we do not know
if the spouse met with the team privately and was given the opportunity
to back out. In 14-2, we know nothing of the father's other obligations—
does he have a spouse and other (minor) children? Who will look after them
if something were to happen to him? The donor LDAT, the team focused

on the donor's well-being, is charged with not merely getting the donor to authorize the procurement, but to incorporate a relational conception of autonomy in which the transplant team empowers the donor to reflect on his values and make decisions in a bidirectional shared decision-making process that reflect the donor's interests broadly construed.[56] This entails exploring the donor's self-regarding interests as well as his other-regarding interests, and his interests that are relationally intertwined with the potential candidate, which is consistent with "the idea that donors make decisions as socially embedded agents."[57] Only then can autonomy be understood as accommodating "the strong bonds between donor, recipient, and other closely involved persons."[58]

14.5.2   Beneficence

If living donation is permitted when a candidate is ineligible for a DDLT, is there some recipient benefit threshold below which it would be morally problematic to permit living donation?

The argument to prohibit donation when the candidate is not eligible for deceased donor is based on the principle of nonmaleficence. If the recipient is a high-risk candidate, the likelihood of success is lower. Some data show that donor benefit depends in part on the success of the transplant, and that donor quality of life decreases if the graft fails and/or if the recipient dies.[59] Other studies show that recipient outcome has no or minimal effect.[60] A robust consent discussion requires that the donor contemplate his or her response to a failed transplant, and that recipient risk status may impact the decision whether to donate. This is part of the lawsuit filed against the Lahey Clinic by Lorraine Hawk, whose husband Paul died while donating part of his liver to his brother-in-law Tim Wilson. Tim had both end-stage liver disease and liver cancer. Lorraine sued the Lahey Clinic because she believes that her husband did not give a fully informed consent. She states that she and her husband were not aware that Tim was not given standardized exception points (possibly not listed) for a deceased donor organ because his cancer was too large. Lorraine asserts that if her husband had known that Tim's prognosis for long-term survival was low, he might not have offered to be a donor. Of note, although Paul died peri-operatively, his liver graft was transplanted successfully into Tim who died less than 1 year after the transplant from recurrent disease.[61]

In cases 14-1 and 14-2, if there are reason to think that the recipients would experience acute graft failure, it would be immoral to proceed, even if the husband in 14-1 and the father in 14-2 consent to the procurement. It would also be immoral if the likelihood of long-term success were quite low.[62] In both cases, if the likelihood of benefit were similar to the benefit accrued for other conditions in terms of graft and patient survival, and if the living donors gave an informed and voluntary consent, then it would be ethical to proceed with LDLT.

14.5.3   Justice

Justice as fairness seeks to determine whether it is fair for a candidate to be eligible for a living donor graft when ineligible for a deceased donor organ. A serious concern is whether the ineligibility represents a fair selection of transplant candidates because some of the criteria vary widely between centers and are quite subjective.[63] For example, transplant programs include psychosocial evaluations to determine which candidates will be good stewards of an organ, but not listing a candidate due to stewardship concerns may represent unconscious discrimination based on race/ethnicity or socio-economic factors.[64] Psychosocial evaluations must be made more consistent, more transparent, and employ culturally competent measures.

Even if the transplant program decides that the likelihood of benefit does not justify a deceased donor liver graft, living donors may have a different risk:benefit benchmark, and may be willing to donate to an emotionally related individual even if the candidate is not assessed to be a "good candidate."[65] Since a patient in end-stage liver disease who undergoes LDLT does not take a scarce public resource (deceased donor graft), the question remains whether to permit different standards for LDLT and DDLT. Some may question whether it is fair that some people get a chance at life because they happen to have an emotionally related individual willing to be a donor and others do not. While unfortunate, this is not unfair.[66] As we have noted, living donor grafts are private goods to some extent and are not (or at least should not be) subject to the same equity and efficiency allocation rules that apply to deceased donor grafts.[67]

There are limits to this argument. Although a living liver graft is a private resource, living donor transplantation requires many public resources which at least partly muddies the distinction that living donor grafts are beyond the public domain and do not require any resource oversight.[68] Rather, one can argue that a living donor candidate should be held to the same standards as a deceased donor candidate. It would be the natural impulse of a transplant program to feel a strong commitment to continue to try to save a living donor graft recipient whose graft fails acutely or early in the postoperative period to the best of their abilities by retransplantation. Thus, a patient with early graft failure, who did not meet a center's criteria for receiving a DDLT at the time he was accepted for and underwent a LDLT, could be listed in the highest MELD category based on his failed transplant liver and receive a DDLT for which he otherwise would not have been eligible. Such use of a deceased donor liver would be unfair to others who do not meet the criteria for DDLT who are not listed, and unfair to all patients on the DDLT waitlist who are denied the chance to get the organ or at least be elevated on the waitlist. This is not a hypothetical concern, as 13.2% of all living donor grafts failed in the first 90 days in the Adult to Adult Living Liver Transplant (A2ALL) cohort.[69]

It would be unfair if recipients who are ineligible for a deceased donor graft, based on agreed-upon inclusion and exclusion criteria, were to become eligible if their living graft fails quickly, and then they are listed for re-transplantation with a deceased donor graft (for which they were ineligible). It is important to note that, for all causes where an individual was ineligible for a DDLT before receiving a LDLT, removal of the original liver does not remove the risk(s) that made the individual ineligible for a deceased donor graft in the first place. Nonetheless, to not re-transplant the candidate who now has a failing transplant will be difficult for many transplant teams. For those transplant teams that are unwilling to take a patient to the operating room for an LDLT if they know there is no safety net for the recipient with early graft failure, they should refuse to perform the LDLT.[70] As moral agents, hospital teams can refuse to perform LDLT in patients ineligible for DDLT, but justice demands that all candidates ineligible for DDLT be treated equally with regard to deceased donor grafts and not let some have access to these grafts through the back door. Candidates ineligible for a DDLT who undergo a LDLT should not be eligible for DDLT because of acute graft failure.

14.5.4 Vulnerabilities

In cases 14.1 and 14.2, the husband and father are medically vulnerable because their intended recipient has a serious health-related condition for which there are only less satisfactory alternative remedies. Medical vulnerability means, however, that, in both cases, the potential donors need a separate health care team that will allow them to focus on their own needs and interests. The LDAT can help the donor consider the decision in a holistic context. The LDAT should help potential donors explore the value of donation to the donor himself and what it means in the context of both a good and bad outcome for both the donor and the recipient. The LDAT must inform and reassure potential donors that they can say no and that others have done so, empowering parents to realize that there is a choice.

Both donors are medically vulnerable because their candidate needs a liver transplant and is not eligible for deceased donor liver transplants. The donor in case 14-2 is even more medically vulnerable than the donor in case 14-1 because the liver graft is needed quite emergently. Still, we believe that LDLT is morally permissible even when the recipient does not qualify for a DDLT provided that: (1) the living donors are informed, motivated, voluntarily consenting, and aware that they have the right to withdraw; and (2) the risks and benefits fall within a standardized written protocol to which all potential living donors for candidates are held.

The donor in case 14-1, in contrast, may have greater deferential vulnerability if the case proceeded as it was described:

Because the current Croatian allocation system would not allow a patient with unresectable colorectal metastases to the liver to receive a cadaveric liver graft, the possibility of an LDLT was presented to the patient and her family. Her husband agreed to be the donor....[71]

Ii is ethically problematic if the recipient candidate patient was present when the possibility of LDLT was first presented to the family. It places a lot of pressure on the family members to respond to the team's request. The family, particularly the spouse, may feel compelled to offer to undergo the work-up. The LDAT in case 14-1 must explore with the spouse whether he is donating freely without undue pressure, offer him multiple opportunities to opt out, and should declare him ineligible if he is found to be donating under duress.[72] The father in case 14-2 was in a less deferentially vulnerable position as the case is described because he offered to donate and it was the team that struggled with whether to proceed.

14.5.5 Special Relationships Create Special Obligations

Are double standards morally permissible? In both cases 14-1 and 14-2, the recipient candidate is not eligible for DDLT and the patient's only chance for long-term survival is LDLT. We believe it is ethical for candidates to circumvent their ineligibility with a living donor graft if all 3 moral agents—the living donor, the potential recipient, and the transplant professionals—all believe that the benefits outweigh the risks and all understand and accept that there will be no safety net in case of early graft failure. The transplant professionals are moral agents who must decide not only whether the donor and recipient are providing a voluntary and informed consent but also that they themselves are willing to help the donor-recipient pair. As Carl Elliott explains:

> Finally, it is important to realize that the doctor is not a mere instrument of the patient's wishes. Analyses of living organ donation and risky clinical research are often simplified needlessly by a failure to acknowledge outright that the doctor is also a moral agent who should be held accountable for his actions. If a patient undergoes a harmful procedure, the moral responsibility for that action does not belong to the patient alone; it is shared by the doctor who performs it. Thus a doctor is in the position of deciding not simply whether a subject's choice is reasonable or morally justifiable, but whether he is morally justified in helping the subject accomplish it.[73]

Morally, the transplant team should refuse to perform the procedures, despite the consent of the potential donor and candidate, if (1) the transplant will not significantly extend or improve the candidate's life; or (2) the lack of a safety net (no ability to urgently get a deceased donor liver if the partial liver transplant from the donor fails acutely) poses too much moral distress on the transplant professionals.

Transplant programs need a transparent protocol clearly stating under what conditions they will offer living donor organ transplants in the case of a candidate being ineligible for DDLT and ineligible for an emergency deceased donor graft if the living donor graft fails acutely. Some transplant programs may decide against offering this option. To avoid unintended bias, transplant programs should develop written criteria for donor risk and recipient benefit thresholds for LDLT and hold all living donor-recipient pairs to the same threshold to ensure a fair and equitable process.

14.6 Conclusion

In case 14-1, the patient with CRLM is currently stable and may respond for some period of time to adjuvant therapies. The living donor work-up should be done properly, allowing the husband to take some time to reflect upon his decision.

In the case of 14-2, Molly is diagnosed with ALF due to 1 of many suicidal attempts. Her liver function is not correcting spontaneously and is not improving despite aggressive medical therapy. The transplant team does believe that transplantation can provide benefit at acceptable risk. Although the recipient has been determined to be outside the center's criteria for a DDLT, the team determines that she is an acceptable candidate for an LDLT. Based on her father's unsolicited volunteering, the LDAT should start a full donor work-up on the father immediately, even before it is known if his daughter's current liver will recover from the drug toxicity.

Within limits, it is ethically permissible that healthy adults provide living organ grafts in situations where the candidate is ineligible for deceased donor graft. These limits should require some reasonable likelihood of recipient success, and a reasonably low likelihood of donor harm. Different transplant professionals will differ as to how much increased likelihood of risk and how much decreased likelihood of benefit exists in any given case. If the transplant professionals involved in any given case believe that the benefit-to-risk ratio justifies proceeding, then it is permissible to do so as long as the donor clearly knows and accepts that a DDLT will not be available as a backup should the LDLT fail. Transplant professionals should ensure that the potential donor realizes that he has a choice and can say no at any point in the process and that the reasons for withdrawing will be kept confidential. Through bidirectional discussions, the LDAT empowers donors to make a decision that best reflects their interests and needs, all things considered.

Notes

1. Kocman B, Mikulic' D, Jadrijevic S, et al. Long-term survival after living-donor liver transplantation for unresectable colorectal metastases to the liver: case report. *Transplant Proc.* 2011;43:4013–4015.
2. Levenson JL, Olbrisch ME. Psychosocial evaluation of organ transplant candidates: a comparative survey of process, criteria, and outcomes in heart, liver, and kidney transplantation. *Psychosomatics.* 1993;34:314–323.

3. Secunda K, Gordon EJ, Sohn MW. National survey of provider opinions on controversial characteristics of liver transplant candidates. *Liver Transpl.* 2013;19(4):395–403.

4. See section 9.5 Specific Standardized MELD or PELD Score Exceptions. This section enumerates candidates eligible for MELD or PELD score exceptions or extensions that do not require evaluation by the NLRB (National Liver Review Board). This includes candidates with the following diagnoses: (1) cholangiocarcinoma (CCA); (2) cystic fibrosis; (3) familial amyloid polyneuropathy; (4) hepatic artery thrombosis (HAT); (5) hepatopulmonary syndrome; (6) metabolic disease; (7) portopulmonary hypertension; (8) primary hyperoxaluria; and(9) hepatocellular carcinoma (HCC). See Organ Procurement and Transplantation Network (OPTN) Policies. Last updated 7/14/2020. https://optn.transplant.hrsa.gov/media/1200/optn_policies.pdf.

5. Merion RM, Schaubel DE, Dykstra DM, Freeman RB, Port FK, Wolfe RA. The survival benefit of liver transplantation. *Am J Transplant.* 2005;5:307–313; and Berg CL, Merion RM, Shearon TH, et al. Liver transplant recipient survival benefit with living donation in the MELD allocation era. *Hepatology.* 2011;54:1313–1321. Of note, others set MELD at 12. See, for example, Schaubel DE, Guidinger MK, Biggins SW, et al. Survival benefit-based deceased-donor liver allocation. *Am J Transplant.* 2009;9:970–981.

6. Martin P, DiMartini A, Feng S, Brown R Jr, Fallon M. Evaluation for liver transplantation in adults: 2013 Practice Guideline by the American Association for the Study of Liver Diseases and the American Society of Transplantation. *Hepatology.* 2014;59(3):1144–1165. Last accessed August 23, 2021. https://www.aasld.org/sites/default/files/2019-06/141020_Guideline_Evaluation_Adult_LT_4UFb_2015.pdf. Table 4, p. 70.

7. See for example, Mazzaferro V, Sposito C, Coppa J, et al. The long-term benefit of liver transplantation for hepatic metastases from neuroendocrine tumors. *Am J Transplant.* 2016;16:2892–2902; and National Health Services Blood and Transplant (NHSBT). Policy POL 195/7: Liver transplantation: selection criteria and recipient registration. Last updated and approved March 2018. Last accessed August 23, 2021. https://nhsbtdbe.blob.core.windows.net/umbraco-assets-corp/9440/pol195_7-liver-selection-policy.pdf

8. Marroni CA, Fleck AM Jr. Fernandes SA, et al. Liver transplantation and alcoholic liver disease: history, controversies, and considerations. *World J Gastroenterol.* 2018;24(26):2785–2805.

9. See for example, Moss AH, Siegler M. Should alcoholics compete equally for liver transplantation? *JAMA.* 1991;265:1295–1298; Glannon W. Responsibility, alcoholism, and liver transplantation. *J Med Phil.* 1998;23(1):31–49; Brudney D. Are alcoholics less deserving of liver transplants? *Hastings Cent Rep.* 2007;37(1):41–47; and Veatch RM. *Transplantation Ethics.* 1st ed. Washington, DC: Georgetown University Press; 2001.

10. See for example, Cohen C, Benjamin M, Committee of the Transplant and Health Policy Center. Alcoholics and liver transplantation. *JAMA.* 1991;265:1299–1301; Veatch RM, Ross LF. *Transplantation Ethics.* 2nd ed. Washington, DC: Georgetown

University Press; 2015; and Tonkens R. Wickedness, moral responsibility, and access to transplantable livers. *Cambridge Q Healthc Ethics*. 2018;27(1):62–74.

11. Marroni et al, "History and controversies."

12. Mathurin P, Moreno C, Samuel D, et al. Early liver transplantation for severe alcoholic hepatitis. *N Engl J Med*. 2011;365:1790–1800.

13. Zhu J, Chen P-Y, Frankel M, Selby RR, Fong T-L. Contemporary policies regarding alcohol and marijuana use among liver transplant programs in the United States. *Transplantation*. 2018;102:433–439, at p. 433.

14. Zhu et al, "Contemporary policies," at p. 433.

15. Kocman et al, "Long-term survival," at p. 4013; see also Chotai P, Matsuoka L. Reassessing the role of liver transplantation for patients with metastatic colorectal cancer to the liver. *Curr Opin Organ Transplant*. 2019;24(2):118–120.

16. Andres A, Oldani G, Berney T, Compagnon P, Line P-D, Toso C. Transplantation for colorectal metastases: on the edge of a revolution. *Transl Gastroenterol Hepatol*. 2018 Sep 26;3:74. doi:10.21037/tgh.2018.08.04

17. Manfredi S, Lepage C, Hatem C, et al. Epidemiology and management of liver metastases from colorectal cancer. *Ann Surg*. 2006;244:254–259; and Kopetz S, Chang GJ, Overman MJ, et al. Improved survival in metastatic colorectal cancer is associated with adoption of hepatic resection and improved chemotherapy. *J Clin Oncol*. 2009;27(22):3677–3683.

18. Mühlbacher F, Steininger R, Gnant M, et al. Is orthotopic liver transplantation a feasible treatment for secondary cancer of the liver? *Transplant Proc*. 1991;23(1 pt 2):1567–1568.

19. Hibi T, Itano O, Shinoda M, Kitagawa Y. Liver transplantation for hepatobiliary malignancies: a new era of "transplant oncology" has begun. *Surg Today*. 2017;47(4):403–415.

20. Mazzaferro V, Regalia E, Doci R, et al. Liver transplantation for the treatment of small hepatocellular carcinomas in patients with cirrhosis. *N Engl J Med*. 1996;334:693–700.

21. See Kocman et al, "Long-term survival," at p. 4103 (references omitted).

22. Hagness M, Foss A, Line P-D, et al. Liver transplantation for nonresectable liver metastases from colorectal cancer. *Ann Surg*. 2013;257(5):800–806, at p. 801.

23. Hagness et al, "Nonresectable," at p. 801.

24. See, for example, Kocman et al, "Long-term survival"; Gorgen et al, "The New Era"; Simoneau E, D'Angelica M, Halazun KJ. Liver transplantation for colorectal liver metastasis. *Curr Opin Organ Transplant*. 2019;24(2):175–181; and Glinka J, Ardiles V, Pekoli J, et al. Liver transplantation for non-resectable colorectal liver metastasis: where we are and where we are going? *Langenbeck's Arch Surg*. 2020;405:255–264.

25. Line P-D, Hagness M, Berstad AE, Foss A, Dueland S. A novel concept for partial liver transplantation in nonresectable colorectal liver metastases: the RAPID concept. *Ann Surg*. 2015;262(1):e5–9.

26. Königsrainer A, Templin S, Capobianco I, et al. Paradigm shift in the management of irresectable colorectal liver metastases: living donor auxiliary partial orthotopic liver transplantation in combination with two-stage hepatectomy (LD-RAPID). *Ann*

Surg. 2019;270(2):327–332; and Rauchfuß F, Nadalin S, Königsrainer A, Settmacher U. Living donor liver transplantation with two-stage hepatectomy for patients with isolated, irresectable colorectal liver-the LIVERT(W)O-HEAL study. *World J Surg Oncol.* 2019;17:11.

27. See, for example, Kocman et al, "Long-term survival"; Gorgen et al, "The New Era"; Simoneau et al, "Liver transplantation"; and Glinka et al, "Liver transplantation."

28. Centers for Disease Control and Prevention. WISQARS™—Web-based Injury Statistics Query and Reporting System. Leading Causes of Death Reports, 1981–2018. https://webappa.cdc.gov/sasweb/ncipc/leadcause.html

29. This is discussed in Rhodes R, Aggarwal S, Schiano TD. Overdose with suicidal intent: ethical considerations for liver transplant programs with citations. *Liver Transpl.* 2011;17:1111–1116, at p. 1111. Of note, acetaminophen-induced ALF is more common and severe in women. See Rubin JB, Hameed B, Gottfried M, Lee WM, Sarkar Acetaminophen-induced acute liver failure is more common and more severe in women. *Clin Gastroenterol Hepatol.* 2018;16:936–946.

30. Levenson and Olbrisch, "Psychosocial evaluation," at p. 318.

31. Levenson and Olbrisch, "Psychosocial evaluation," at p. 318.

32. Levenson and Olbrisch, "Psychosocial evaluation," at p. 318.

33. Secunda et al, "National survey," at p. 399.

34. Crone C, DiMartini A. Liver transplant for intentional acetaminophen overdose: a survey of transplant clinicians' experiences with recommendations. *Psychosomatics.* 2014;55:602–612.

35. Gulmez SE, Larrey D, Pageaux G-P, et al. Liver transplant associated with paracetamol overdose: results From the seven-country SALT Study. *Br J Clin Pharmacol.* 2015;80:599–606.

36. Mellinger JL, Volk ML. Transplantation for alcohol-related liver disease: is it fair? *Alcohol.* 2018;53:173–177.

37. Kwon YK, Etesami K, Genyk Y. Should living donor liver transplant selection be subject to the same restrictions as deceased donor transplant? *Curr Opin Organ Transplant.* 2020;25:47–51, at p. 50.

38. Joint Working Party of the British Transplantation Society and the Renal Association. *United Kingdom Guidelines for Living Donor Kidney Transplantation.* 3rd ed. May 2011. https://bts.org.uk/wp-content/uploads/2016/09/19_BTS_RA_Living_Donor_Kidney-1.pdf, at p. 36. The wording is slightly different in the 4th edition. See The British Transplantation Society and the Renal Association. *Guidelines for Living Donor Kidney Transplantation.* 4th ed. March 2018 https://bts.org.uk/wp-content/uploads/2018/07/FINAL_LDKT-guidelines_June-2018.pdf, at p. 41.

39. Joint Working Party of the British Transplantation Society and the British Association for the Study of the Liver. *Living Donor Liver Transplantation.* July 2015. https://bts.org.uk/wp-content/uploads/2016/09/03_BTS_LivingDonorLiver-1.pdf, at pp. 13–14.

40. Joint Working Party of the British Transplantation Society and the British Association for the Study of the Liver, *Living Donor Liver Transplantation,* at p. 45.

41. Kocman, "Long-term survival," at p. 4014.

42. Crouch RA, Elliott C. Moral agency and the family: the case of living related organ transplantation. *Camb Q Healthc Ethics.* 1999;8:275–287, at p. 277.
43. Crouch and Elliott, "Moral agency," at p. 278.
44. Hilhorst MT, Kranenburg LW, Busschbach JJV. Should health care professionals encourage living kidney donation? *Med Health Care Philos.* 2007;10:81–90, at p. 88.
45. Hilhorst et al, "Should health care," at p. 88.
46. Hilhorst et al, "Should health care," at p. 88.
47. Wolstenholme GEW, O'Connor M, eds. *Ethics in Medical Progress: With Special Reference to Transplantation.* Boston, MA: Little, Brown and Company; 1966.
48. Wolstenholme and O'Connor, *Ethics in Medical Progress,* at p. 198 citing David Daube.
49. Siegler M, Lantos JD. Commentary: ethical justification for living liver donation. *Camb Q Healthc Ethics.* 1992;1:320–325, at p. 323.
50. Siegler and Lantos, "Ethical justification," at p. 324.
51. Simmons RG, Marine SK, Simmons RL. *Gift of Life: The Effect of Organ Transplantation on Individual, Family and Societal Dynamics.* New Brunswick, NJ: Transaction Books, 2002.
52. Alonso EM, Whitington PF, Broelsch CE, Emond JC, Thistlethwaite JR. "Split liver" orthotopic liver transplantation. *Pediatr Res.* 1989;25:107.
53. Singer PA, Siegler M, Whitington PF, et al. Ethics of liver transplantation with living donors. *N Engl J Med.* 1989;321:620–622.
54. Goldman LS. Liver transplantation using living donors. Preliminary donor psychiatric outcomes. *Psychosomatics.* 1993;34(3):235–240.
55. Kocman et al, "Long-term survival," at p. 4014.
56. This conception of relational autonomy is richly explored in Mackenzie C, Stoljar N, eds. *Relational Autonomy: Feminist Perspective on Autonomy, Agency, and the Social Self.* New York, NY: Oxford University Press; 2000; and Entwistle VA, Carter SM, Cribb A, McCaffery K. Supporting patient autonomy: the importance of clinician-patient relationships. *J Gen Intern Med.* 2010;25(7):741–745. For a thorough discussion about shared decision-making, see Epstein RM, Gramling RE. What is shared in shared decision making? Complex decisions when the evidence is unclear. *Med Care Res Rev.* 2013;70(1 suppl):94S–112S.
57. Biller-Andorno N. Voluntariness in living-related organ donation. *Transplantation.* 2011;92(6):617–619, at p. 618.
58. Knibbe ME, Maeckelberghe EL, Verkerk MA. Confounders in voluntary consent about living parental liver donation: no choice and emotions. *Med Health Care Philos.* 2007;10:433–440.
59. Watson JM, Behnke MK, Fabrizio MD, McCune TR. Recipient graft failure or death impact on living kidney donor quality of life based on the living organ donor network database. *J Endourol.* 2013:27:1525–1529; Jin SG, Xiang B, Yan LN, et al. Quality of life and psychological outcome of donors after living donor liver transplantation. *World J Gastroenterol.* 2012;18:182–187; and Kim-Schluger L, Florman SS, Schiano T, et al. Quality of life after lobectomy for adult liver transplantation. *Transplantation.* 2002;73:1593–1597.

60. Clemens K, Boudville N, Dew MA, et al. *Am J Transplant*. 2011;11:463–469; and Verbesey JE, Simpson MA, Pomposelli JJ, et al. Living donor adult liver transplantation: a longitudinal study of the donor's quality of life. *Am J Transplant*. 2005;5:770–777.

61. Kowalczyk L, Globe staff. Donor's death shatters family, stuns surgeons. *The Boston Globe*. February 02, 2014. Last accessed August 23, 2021. https://www.bostonglobe.com/lifestyle/health-wellness/2014/02/02/death-living-liver-donor-calamity-for-two-families-and-lahey/q9iRF9nHyQdewWjvlTgmRI/story.html

62. We do not specify what is "quite low." Actual thresholds need to be determined by broad stakeholder consensus.

63. See, for example, Levenson and Olbrisch, "Psychosocial evaluation"; Duerinckx et al, "Psychological care"; Levenson JL, Olbrisch ME. Psychosocial screening and selection of candidates for organ transplantation. In: Trzepacz PT, DiMartini AF, eds. *The Transplant Patient: Biological, Psychiatric and Ethical Issues in Organ Transplantation*. Cambridge, England: Cambridge University Press; 2000: 21–41; and Duerinckx N, Timmerman L, Van Gogh J. Predonation psychosocial evaluation of living kidney and liver donor candidates: a systematic literature review. *Transpl Int*. 2014;27(1):2–18.

64. Studies document the lack of consistent referral, evaluation, and listing practices for deceased donor liver transplantation, particularly with respect to racial and ethnic minorities and those of lower socioeconomic status. See, for example, Jesse MT, Abouljoud M, Goldstein ED, et al. Racial disparities in patient selection for liver transplantation: an ongoing challenge. *Clin Transplant*. 2019;33(11):e13714; and Mathur AK, Ashby VB, Fuller DS, et al. Variation in access to the liver transplant waiting list in the United States. *Transplantation*. 2014;98(1):94–99.

65. Molinari M, Matz J, DeCoutere S, El-Tawil K, Abu-Wasel B, Keough V. Live liver donors' risk thresholds: risking a life to save a life. *HPB*. 2014;16:560–574; and Popp FC, Eggert N, Hoy L, et al. Who is willing to take the risk? assessing the readiness for living liver donation in the general German population. *J Med Ethics*. 2006;32(7):389–394.

66. Daniels N. *Just Health: Meeting Health Needs Fairly*. New York, NY: Cambridge University Press; 2008, at pp. 13–14; Engelhardt HT Jr. *Health care allocations: responses to the unjust, the unfortunate, and the undesirable*. In Shelp E, ed. *Justice and Health Care*. Boston, MA: Kluwer; 1981:121–137; and Nagel T. Justice and nature. *Oxford J Leg Studies*. 1997;17:303–321.

67. Kwon et al, in "Should living," come to the same conclusion.

68. The British living donor liver transplant guidelines clearly articulate this tension:

> . . . There is scope for the wider UK transplant community, including patient groups, to debate the practical and moral issues that arise and to agree whether it is appropriate to have different criteria for transplantation depending on whether or not a living donation is available, and whether to use the additional NHS (National Health Services) resource of a donor operation in such circumstances.

Joint Working Party of the British Transplantation Society and the British Association for the Study of the Liver. *Living Donor Liver Transplantation*, July 2015, at p. 49.

69. Olthoff KM, Merion RM, Ghobrial RM, et al. Outcomes of 385 adult-to-adult living donor liver transplant recipients: a report from the A2ALL Consortium. *Ann Surg.* 2005;242:314–323, at p. 314.

70. A related question, which goes beyond the focus of this book, is what should happen if the transplant is successful but now 10 years have transpired and the liver graft is failing: should the patient now be eligible for a DDLT?

71. Kocman et al, "Long-term survival."

72. In the article, Kocman et al state that "Her husband agreed to be the donor." Given the brevity with which the case is described, it is not clear whether this means that the transplant team asked him to serve as a living donor or whether he consented to be evaluated. We believe that it is important that he donates voluntarily, free from undue influence, and being asked to serve as a living donor could make him quite vulnerable. Later on, Kocman et al state that "He was evaluated under standard protocol for living donors." In the US, this would mean that he would meet with an LDAT, possibly a psychologist and/or social worker, to again ensure that this is what he wanted to do. If he was not acting freely, the LDAT should inform him that his reluctance would not be shared with his family, but that the team would not proceed with the work-up or donation.

73. Elliott C. Doing harm: living organ donors, clinical research and *The Tenth Man*. *J Med Ethics*. 1995;21:91–96, at p. 95.

15

Dealing With Uncertainty

APOL1 as a Case Study

Case 15-1: A survey question from the American Society
of Transplantation regarding APOL1 testing of living donors.
"If you were informed that a potential 30 yo live donor carried 2 high-risk APOL1 polymorphisms, would you exclude the donor specifically based upon this finding? (Y/N)."[1] This question was part of a five-question survey created by a committee of the American Society of Transplantation (AST). It was distributed "to AST/American Society of Nephrology transplant nephrology fellowship directors, to high-volume transplant centers, and to selected smaller programs based on geographic and volume diversity" in advance of a meeting of experts in the study of APOL1 and renal disease and kidney transplantation in December 2015.[2]

15.1   Introduction

Although the incidence of end-stage renal disease (ESRD) is known to be 3 to 5 times higher in Blacks than in Whites, theories abound whether the cause of this disparity is biologic or environmental or a combination of both.[3] Recent research suggests that having 2 apolipoprotein L1 (APOL1) risk alleles may explain much of the excess rate of ESRD in Blacks compared with European Americans.[4]

APOL1 G1 and G2 alleles are common genetic variants in the Black community (about 39% of Blacks carry either G1 or G2 and 12% carry 2 copies, ie, G1/G1, G1/G2, or G2/G2).[5] Having at least 1 copy of either allele protects against African sleeping sickness. Having 2 copies of either G1 or G2 or 1 copy of both predisposes to kidney failure. Parsa et al found that carrying 2 APOL1 risk alleles was associated with higher rates of ESRD and with

The Living Organ Donor as Patient. Lainie Friedman Ross and J. Richard Thistlethwaite, Jr, Oxford University Press.
© Oxford University Press 2022. DOI: 10.1093/oso/9780197618202.003.0015

progression from chronic kidney disease (CKD) to ESRD in both diabetic and nondiabetic individuals.[6] Importantly, many individuals with 2 APOL1 risk alleles do not develop ESRD. This has led some to theorize a "2-hit" hypothesis—that individuals with 2 APOL1 risk alleles only develop ESRD if there is a second hit—an environmental exposure, another health condition, or another genetic factor.[7]

Importantly for the transplant community, deceased donor kidney grafts from donors with 2 APOL1 risk alleles have worse graft survival. Reeves-Daniel et al found that the risk of early graft failure in Black deceased donor kidneys carrying 2 APOL1 risk alleles is greater than the risk observed for most other traits including race, human leukocyte antigen (HLA) matching, and panel reactive antibodies (PRA).[8] In this study, Black deceased donor kidneys with fewer than 2 APOL1 risk alleles had similar kidney graft function with European American deceased donor grafts.[9] However, a follow-up study found that Black deceased donor grafts with fewer than 2 APOL1 risk alleles had intermediate graft survival between White deceased donor grafts and Black deceased donor grafts with 2 APOL1 risk alleles, suggesting ApoL1 risk status may not explain all of the increased kidney graft loss observed with Black deceased donor kidneys.[10] There are data to show that recipients who receive Black living donor grafts do not do as well recipients who receive living donor grafts from other racial/ethnic groups.[11] However, no data exist regarding graft survival from Black *living* donors based on the number of donor APOL1 risk alleles.[12]

The good news for kidney transplant recipients with 2 APOL1 risk alleles is that recipient genotype does not appear to impact posttransplant clinical outcomes adversely, that is, all the risk comes from the genotype of deceased donor kidney and not that of the recipient. A retrospective analysis of 119 Blacks who underwent kidney transplants (living and deceased) found that almost half (48.7%) carried 2 APOL1 risk alleles, but found no difference in living and deceased donor allograft survival at 5 years posttransplant compared to Blacks who did not carry 2 risk alleles.[13]

Although the mechanism of APOL1 and kidney disease is uncertain, transplant data support a cell-based expression explanation, not a circulating protein explanation.[14] The current leading hypothesis is that APOL1 is expressed in podocytes. The expression of the G1 and G2 variants leads to podocyte injury which is magnified in the presence of other adverse host factors.[15] For example, the odds ratio of a Black individual with 2 APOL1 risk alleles, developing lupus nephritis-associated nephropathy, hypertension-associated

ESRD, idiopathic focal segmental glomerulosclerosis—associated nephrop-athy, or HIV-associated nephropathy are 2.4, 7.3, 16.9, and 29.2, respectively compared to a Black individual without 2 risk alleles.[16] Freedman urges caution in drawing conclusions based on the kidney transplant data,[17] but current empirical data and mechanistic hypothesis place the transplant com-munity at a policy crossroads regarding whether to test or screen potential living kidney donors for APOL1, and whether and how to discuss APOL1 test results with prospective donors and recipients.

15.2 Apolipoprotein L1 and Living Donors

The scientific and medical communities do not know whether kidneys from living donors with 2 APOL1 risk alleles have an increased risk of graft failure compared to those from living donors with 0 or 1 risk allele. It is also un-known what impact the unilateral nephrectomy has on living donor clinical outcomes. Current data indicate that living donors are at low but increased risk of developing ESRD,[18] particularly young Black male donors.[19] What we don't know is whether unilateral nephrectomy places the Black donor with 2 APOL1 risk alleles at greater risk than donors who have fewer than 2 APOL1 risk alleles. Given this uncertainty, how the data should impact transplant programs' discussions with potential Black living donors is controversial.

Four options exist. The first is to remain silent about APOL1 risk alleles and renal failure and wait for more data.[20] The potential donor is not in-formed about the risks nor the possibility of testing. The second option is to counsel about what is known and unknown about the association of race, APOL1, and subsequent renal failure. The potential donor is informed about the possibility of genetic testing for APOL1 but the clinician is neutral about testing, claiming that her inability to interpret test results precludes doing such testing until further data are collected. If pressed, testing could be or-dered with the caveat that it is not clear how the information should be used. The third option is to provide counseling and offer voluntary genotyping of prospective living donors of African ancestry as part of the living donor workup.[21] If testing is performed, the potential donor and members of the living donor advocate team (LDAT; the health care providers focused on donor well-being and donor motivation) should engage in a thorough dis-cussion about the uncertain meaning of donor APOL1 status for the long-term well-being of the donor and its implication for graft survival in the intended recipient. The fourth option would be to mandate APOL1 testing for all prospective living donors of African ancestry as part of the living donor workup and counseling.[22]

The problem with waiting for more data, the first option, is that collecting the data from future studies will be time consuming, expensive, and may never occur. The history of sickle cell trait (SCT—carriers of 1 hemoglobin S allele) is a case in point. Like APOL1 gene variants, SCT is protective against an endemic African disease (malaria). Like APOL1 gene variants, SCT is also associated with renal health risks. For over 30 years, we have known that individuals with SCT have increased risk of hyposthenuria and albuminuria.[23] Most recently, Naik et al used 5 large, prospective, US population-based studies to evaluate SCT and kidney disease and found that "Among Blacks in these cohorts, the presence of SCT was associated with an increased risk of CKD, decline in eGFR [estimated GFR], and albuminuria, compared with noncarriers."[24]

Whether donation accelerates subsequent reductions in GFR in individuals with SCT and/or whether living donors with SCT are at increased risk of developing ESRD are unknown because data have not been collected systematically. As a result, there is no uniform policy about screening donors for SCT. Reese and colleagues surveyed transplant centers in 2007 and found that 83% (113 of 137) of responding transplant centers had no policy, although 34% (46 of 135) screened living donors for SCT in practice.[25] Importantly, 37% (39 of 105) of centers reported excluding donors known to have SCT always or most of the time.[26] The problem with such variability is that programs that exclude donors with SCT are either discriminating against these donors unfairly or are appropriately excluding high-risk donors and others are being too cavalier. In the case of SCT, the lack of data has resulted in arbitrary and inconsistent policies and practices by transplant centers. The analogy of APOL1 and SCT is imperfect, but serves as a warning that benign neglect may not be benign.

For APOL1, the ethical justification for the first option, remaining silent and waiting for more definitive APOL1 data, is nonmaleficence—to avoid harm.[27] Currently, the usefulness of knowing one's APOL1 genotype is minimal. There are no effective preventions or treatments for APOL1-associated nephropathies, and no medications (as exist for other conditions like hypertension) that have been shown to slow the progression of renal disease in those with 2 APOL1 risk alleles.[28] Some physicians fear that the uncertain information as well as the uncertainty concerning how to use the information may increase anxiety without concomitant benefit.[29] To avoid the negative consequences of incomplete knowledge, some physicians may prefer to avoid this discussion.[30]

This argument has 2 problems. First, to elect nondisclosure based on concerns that patients will become anxious or make bad decisions is paternalistic. It fails to show respect for the potential donor as a person with decisional capacity who can best decide for herself what is the best course of all action given the uncertainty. Second, uncertainty is ubiquitous in medicine and ignoring uncertain information fails to give prospective donors information they might potentially use in their decision-making. This fails to respect their right to make an informed decision.

The second option is to talk generically about race, APOL1, and ESRD and to acknowledge that testing is possible, but to remain neutral about testing (eg, to order it only if requested). This requires that transplant professionals share with potential donors what is known and unknown about health risks on living kidney donors. We know from recent studies that living donors have a small increased risk of ESRD (Blacks > Whites).[31] Black donors also need to know that should they have 2 APOL1 risk alleles, then they are at increased risk of developing ESRD, whether or not they donate.[32] Unknown is whether unilateral nephrectomy increases this risk (ie, acts as a second hit) or whether the decreased baseline GFR caused by the unilateral nephrectomy hastens the occurrence of ESRD if other clinical, genetic, or environmental factors exist. This is a crucial discussion point, especially for young healthy potential living-related donors whose recipients have familial diseases that caused their renal failure (eg, hypertension).[33]

The ethical justification for counseling about race and APOL1, but being neutral about testing, is based on autonomy—the competent prospective donor has the right to information and then to decide for herself whether the benefits of testing and making transplant decisions based on the results outweigh the risks. The problem with this approach is that APOL1 and its implications for kidney health in the context of kidney transplantation are complex. Patients may find it useful to be aware of the professional controversy about APOL1 status on long-term health risks in their decision-making calculations. They may want to know what their own physicians think and why. Not offering a recommendation is not necessarily respectful of autonomy. Early modern genetic counseling in the 1960s and 1970s focused on reproductive decision-making and was based on a model of nondirective counseling (ie, counseling without making any recommendations).[34] With the move to genetic counseling for disease risk, there has been a growing consensus that nondirectiveness may not be appropriate or even possible.[35] This approach to autonomy ignores a more bidirectional understanding of autonomy that goes beyond the traditional notion of autonomy and the right to make decisions by oneself without interference, to a more robust relational conception of autonomy that includes the health care team's role in empowering patients to make more deliberated decisions that better reflect their considered and informed preferences and values.[36] That is, while this option respects a narrow (negative) conception of autonomy, it inadequately embraces the principle of respect for persons as actualized through a relational autonomy approach.

The third option is to provide counseling to all living donors of African ancestry about APOL1, to offer genotyping both to help the donor make an informed decision about her own kidney health, as well as her willingness to donate and its possible meaning for graft survival in the recipient. Testing is optional. Respect for the potential donor's autonomy, understood relationally, is best operationalized in a shared decision-making process in which health care professionals and patients actively discuss the current state of medical knowledge (and ignorance) to help the patient make an informed decision that best reflects her considered preferences and values.[37] Donors who elect to undergo testing as well as pre- and posttest counseling can make an informed decision about how to use this information in a way consistent with their own assessment of the risks and benefits of donating. Such an approach is respectful of the patient as person.

The fourth option is to mandate genetic testing of all prospective Black donors. To be done ethically, this would also require pre- and posttest counseling. The ethical justification for making testing mandatory is to be sure that all donors have as much information as possible in order to make an informed decision. The problem is that the policy is premature: it is unknown whether living donors with 2 high-risk alleles are at greater risk from unilateral nephrectomy. It is unknown whether a recipient who receives living donor graft with 2 risk alleles has a worse outcome than other recipients who receive living donor grafts with fewer risk alleles. Given the ambiguity, some donors might not want to be tested to prevent both themselves and the transplant program from knowing the result and making arbitrary decisions as in the case of SCT. A mandatory testing program would take this option away from them. It also highlights the second problem with mandatory testing: we still don't know what should be done with the information.

The mandatory fourth option can be operationalized in three ways. The first way is to rely on each transplant center to decide what to do with test results. This could lead to arbitrary practices, as in the case of SCT, and would not lead to better understanding of donor risks. A second possibility is to require screening of all Black potential living donors at all centers. All prospective donors would be counseled about their results and would be empowered to decide about donation using a shared decision-making process.[38] This approach only differs from option 3 in that all donors must agree to testing. This may deter some from donating merely to remain ignorant of their APOL1 status and its uncertain significance. It may also result in some potential donors choosing not to donate based on their APOL1 status, despite the uncertainty. This may be a safe solution, but it also may be an over-reaction and harm both those recipients whose wait is extended and those donors who truly wanted to donate.

The third possible way to operationalize the fourth option is to combine mandatory testing with a policy to exclude all individuals with 2 risk alleles from donation. This approach could be justified on the principle of nonmaleficence or first do no harm to potential donors and their recipients. It is strengthened because having 2 APOL1 alleles is also associated with other health problems such as atherosclerotic cardiovascular disease.[39] The problem with the nonmaleficence argument is that the principle should not be evaluated separately from other competing values and moral principles. Prohibiting living donors with 2 high-risk alleles from donating on the grounds that unilateral nephrectomy may accelerate the development of ESRD ignores the harms of excluding all donations from individuals with 2 risk alleles. This includes the harm of not allowing an individual to serve as a living donor for a loved one despite the uncertainty of whether the nephrectomy actually increases the donor's personal risk of ESRD. It also ignores the harm to the recipient whose wait is prolonged without this living donor, the harm of decreasing the total number of Black donors based on uncertain data, and the harm of exacerbating the wait on the deceased donor waitlist.[40] (This is discussed further in section 15.3.) Even if there is an increased risk of developing ESRD in donors with 2 high-risk alleles, the overall risk will still be low. It may be a risk that prospective donors are willing to take and many transplant professionals may be willing to tolerate. Because of these facts, the policy fails to respect the individual's autonomy and the process of shared decision- making.[41] It might lead some potential donors to refuse testing in order to protect their ability to donate, even if they want the information.[42]

We support the third option: education and voluntary testing with pre- and posttest counseling. The informed consent process should address what is known about APOL1 for donor health (increased risk of ESRD in Blacks), what is unknown (whether donation increases or accelerates the risk), and what is known and unknown about APOL1 for recipient health (while deceased donor kidneys with APOL1 appear to have worse graft outcomes, the effect of living donor APOL1 status on kidney graft survival is unknown).

Prior to testing, transplant teams should explore with prospective donors whether test results might change their willingness to donate. The decision belongs to the donor.[43] Competent adults have the right to take some incremental risks if they do so knowingly and voluntarily. Some donors with 2 APOL1 risk alleles may elect to withdraw because of this information; other donors may be willing to proceed. There are no data to say which decision best promotes the potential living donor's interests, even for potential young Black male donors who have the highest risk of postdonation ESRD.[44]

15.3 Disclosure to Recipients

The living donor advocate team should explore whether the potential living donor is willing to share her APOL1 status with her intended recipient. Donor and recipient work-ups are currently performed separately with only minimal sharing of information. Nondisclosure by the transplant program unless both potential donor and recipient approve disclosure is meant to protect the privacy of both donor and recipient. The OPTN policy handbook states what is to be shared. Recipients must be told that living donors are required to undergo screening for a list of transmissible diseases,[45] but that "there is no comprehensive way to screen potential deceased and living donors for all transmissible diseases."[46] Some donor-specific information must be shared with candidates. This includes donor increased risk of transmitting HIV, hepatitis B and C, and/or malignancy.[47] In contrast, no specific recipient health information must be shared with the donor. Rather the policy reads:

Any transplant candidate may have an increased likelihood of adverse outcomes (including but not limited to graft failure, complications, and mortality) that:

- Exceed local or national averages
- Do not necessarily prohibit transplantation
- Are not disclosed to the living donor.[48]

Although donors and recipients may share additional information with each other outside the clinical encounter, both must consent before transplant professionals can share more in the clinical encounter.

Under current OPTN policies, donors are not required to share their APOL1 status. Donors may want to keep their APOL1 status private so as not to create anxiety for their recipient (anxiety about the donor's well-being and/or about its potential impact on recipient graft outcome). However, transplant recipient candidates, if informed about APOL1 and its significance in kidney disease, may want to know their prospective living donor's APOL1 genotype and may obtain this information if the prospective living donor agrees. If their prospective donor has 2 APOL1 risk alleles, this then allows candidates to look for a different potential living donor, either because they are unwilling to expose their loved ones to the possible increased risk of ESRD or because they are unwilling to expose themselves to the risk of undergoing a transplant with a living donor graft that has a potentially poor outcome. Unfortunately, these candidates may not have other eligible living donor candidates.[49] Living donors are often family members, and first-degree relatives of individuals in ESRD are more likely to have APOL1 risk alleles. In 1 study of Black patients in ESRD, 23% and 46% of relatives of Black transplant candidates with ESRD had 2 or 1 risk variants compared with 12% and 39% of the general Black population.[50] If there are no other potential living donors, then the recipient candidate who knows that the living donor has 2 APOL1 risk alleles must decide if he wants the living donor transplant with unknown consequences for both himself and his donor, or if he would rather wait for a deceased donor kidney. Currently, deceased donor kidneys are not screened for APOL1 clinically such that if the candidate is offered a Black deceased donor kidney, the recipient's graft may still end up having 2 APOL1 alleles, and it is known that deceased donor grafts with 2 APOL1 alleles have lower graft survival. The candidate can take some comfort knowing that the transplant does not put the deceased donor at any risk. The candidate can choose to reject all Black deceased donor grafts, but this could mean a very long wait on dialysis, and the rejection of what frequently would be an excellent graft given that the risk of a Black donor having 2 APOL1 high-risk alleles is only about 12%.

15.4 Community Attitudes

Several research teams have examined the attitudes of Blacks about APOL1 testing. In 2017, Carol Horowitz and colleagues tested 26 Black adults for APOL1 variants, and conducted in-depth interviews about their beliefs and attitudes toward genetic testing and kidney disease. The researchers explain:

> While most knew someone close to them with kidney disease, were concerned they would develop kidney disease, and knew Blacks had increased kidney disease burden, few knew there was a connection between hypertension and kidney disease. None had heard of APOL1 or a genetic test that revealed an increased risk for kidney problems. Yet, they rapidly integrated their new knowledge of APOL1 into subsequent discussions about ways to protect their kidneys and described how genetic risk was similar to other risks they associate with kidney problems, such as unhealthy lifestyle and stress.[51]

A major strength of this study was that the participants actually were tested for APOL1 as part of the research and regardless of their results, they thought the results could:

> ... motivate them and their providers to take actions to improve hypertension care and protect their kidneys, rather than causing stress or decision regret. They nearly universally felt genetic testing for people of African ancestry holds more promise than peril, providing opportunities to improve health.[52]

A major limitation of this study, however, is that the participants were highly educated and this group is known to have positive views of genetic testing.[53] Several participants were concerned, however, that "their providers would not understand genetics well enough to explain it."[54] Their concern was not far off at the time, although in 2020, APOL1 has become better known in the nephrology and transplant community.

Ebele Umeukeje and colleagues provide more data about the public's attitude about APOL1 testing, having conducted focus groups with 39 Black participants in Jackson, Mississippi; Nashville, Tennessee; and Seattle, Washington.[55] They found that participants expressed "unanimous support for offering testing to living donors (95%), and considerable but strongly contested support for mandatory testing of living donors (73%)."[56] Some argued that participants needed, and perhaps had a right to, this information to make truly informed decisions about whether to accept the kidney. Others argued that "mandatory testing would violate people's autonomy and rights and possibly lead to negative outcomes, such as deterring potential donors and shrinking the pool of available kidneys."[57] Concerns about privacy breaches and discrimination in health care, life insurance, and employment was expressed at all 3 sites.[58]

A study by Elisa Gordon and colleagues at Northwestern University (Chicago) involved semi-structured interviews of 23 Black living donors and found that most (87%) would have been willing to undergo APOL1 testing before donating, most (61%) would have donated even if they had 2 high-risk alleles, most thought APOL1 genetic testing was useful to make informed decisions, but most feared that APOL1 testing could be used to discriminate against Blacks as donors or with respect to wider health care issues.[59]

15.5 Evolution of Professional Knowledge, Attitudes, and Practice

The first step in the rapid adoption of APOL1 testing in the clinical transplant arena was a meeting in December 2015 convened by the AST with representatives from other governmental organizations.[60] To better understand current perceptions about APOL1 testing in the transplant setting, the AST conducted a five-question survey (see case 15-1) that was distributed to 92 centers, 83 of which responded. Respondents included 43 of the 50 highest-volume kidney transplant centers. Despite this, the survey revealed limited knowledge and experience:

> Only two-thirds were aware of the clinical availability of a test for APOL1 gene variants, and of these, <20% had used the test clinically. Among respondents who had used APOL1 testing, most had used it in the setting of living donor evaluation. Of those aware of but not using APOL1 testing, the most common reason selected was "data was too preliminary." Interestingly, when respondents were asked whether the presence of two APOL1 risk alleles would in and of itself exclude a potential 30-year-old living kidney donor, two-thirds [52 of 78] indicated that it would.[61]

Based on the survey and the conference, the consensus conclusion was that potential donors should be informed about the availability of APOL1 testing, that screening should be voluntary, and that the results should be considered as just 1 more factor. A donor with 2 high-risk alleles should not be automatically excluded.[62]

Next, in late 2018, the National Institutes of Health funded the APOL1 Long-Term Kidney Transplantation Outcomes Network (APOLLO) Network.[63] The APOLLO Network will prospectively assess both the effects of APOL1 nephropathy risk variants in living kidney donors with recent African ancestry and recipient outcomes after deceased and living donor kidney transplantation using Black grafts stratified by the number of APOL1 risk alleles. To do this, organ procurement organizations (OPOs) and HLA genotyping centers in the United States (US) and Puerto Rico will attempt to collect blood and DNA from all Black, Afro-Caribbean, Hispanic Black, and African deceased kidney donors for APOL1 testing.[64] The original study had planned to collect living donor follow-up for only a few years but extended the follow-up time in response to criticisms. The APOLLO Network also approved an ancillary study to evaluate outcomes involving 1,100 Black living donors who donated between 2001 and 2005.[65] The first aim of the Living Donor Extended Time Outcomes (LETO) study is:

> [t]o determine in a nationally representative sample whether Black living kidney donors with 2 APOL1 renal-risk variants are at higher risk of developing clinically significant chronic kidney disease (estimated glomerular filtration rate <45 ml/min/1.73m2) approximately two decades after donation.[66]

The LETO investigators will also seek to perform other genetic tests on these living donors to determine if there are any "independent (or APOL1 interactive) gene variants that are associated with an increased risk of clinically significant chronic kidney disease (estimated glomerular filtration rate <45 ml/min/1.73m2) in Black living kidney donors" and/or with graft survival in the recipients of these living donor kidney grafts.[67]

Prior to the funding of the APOLLO study, Gordon and colleagues queried members of the AST, the American Society of Transplant Surgeons, and the American Society of Nephrology regarding their practices for testing or screening Black donor candidates for APOL1.[68] Of 5177 potential respondents they got 383 usable responses (7%). Most (69%) respondents thought that potential living donors should be informed about the option of APOL1 testing. Most (66%) agreed that potential donors needed to know to decide about their own risks from a unilateral nephrectomy and 33% thought that candidates needed to know to prevent recipients from accepting a living donor graft that might have shorter graft survival.[69]

In 2017, Amit Garg and colleagues, in collaboration with the United Network for Organ Sharing (UNOS), surveyed US transplant programs regarding the practices used to assess kidney health in living kidney donor candidates. They found that "ApoL1 genotyping is obtained routinely or selectively by 45%; half of these programs use the high-risk genotype as an absolute exclusion criterion."[70] In September 2018, Tristan McIntosh and colleagues queried nephrologists and transplant surgeons at 63 transplant centers in the US that currently performed at least 10 Black living donor transplants per year according to 2015 UNOS data. They found that 16 (48%) were offering APOL1 testing and another 6 (18.2%) were considering adding it. In response to the question, "How often do centers encourage potential living organ donors who are black or of West African ancestry, to take part in APOL1 genetic testing," only 9 (28.1%) said never although most (25 or 78.1%) did not support mandatory testing.[71]

The data from Gordon et al, Garg and colleagues, and McIntosh and colleagues show that clinical practice changes were being made before the APOLLO study began. This will complicate getting data about both the living donors and their recipients across a broad range of APOL1 genotypes. Many living donors with high-risk alleles are already being excluded from donating despite the fact that we do not know the impact of unilateral nephrectomy on these donors, nor the expected survival of living donor grafts with 2 high-risk alleles.

15.6 Conclusion

In 2016, APOL1 testing was not being performed routinely in the clinical transplant setting. A search of the Genetic Testing Registry in June 2016 listed only 10 laboratories certified to do clinical ApoL1 testing worldwide, the cost was approximately $400, and turnaround was 1 week or longer.[72] By 2019, Wake Forest University was getting results in less than 4 hours.[73] In August 2021, the Genetic Testing Registry now counts 39 laboratories worldwide,[74] at similar or lower cost.

We believe that living donor transplant programs are ethically obligated to educate and counsel Black living donors and their potential recipient candidates about APOL1. We support voluntary APOL1 testing of prospective living donors of African ancestry as part of the living donor work-up.[75] With the donor's consent, the results should also be disclosed to their recipient so that each can make an informed, voluntary decision.

More information is needed regarding the risk of unilateral nephrectomy both for those with 2 APOL1 risk alleles and only 1 APOL1 risk allele who may be at some additional risk. We need to determine whether there are any interactions between APOL1 and other genes known to cluster in the Black community (eg, SCT), as well as gene-environment interactions. Finally, psychosocial and ethical information must be collected to determine how the wider Black community will respond to the genotyping of prospective donors and whether it will have an adverse or discriminatory impact. Although the Genetic Information Nondiscrimination Act of 2008 protects against health insurance discrimination,[76] protection from discrimination in other areas of life is less certain.[77] Current data are inadequate to justify mandatory testing, but, at a minimum, a donor registry that collects long-term follow-up information is needed.[78] The OPTN already collects some living donor data and mandates the collection of 2 years of living donor follow-up data.[79] The OPTN should add a field into their registry for APOL1 test results. SCT testing of living donors has provided a clear lesson; unless there is a coordinated effort to determine the effects of APOL1 on living donor health, outcomes, and living donor kidney graft survival, data will not be systematically collected, and policies and practices will be arbitrary and inconsistent.

Notes

1. Newell KA, Formica RN, Gill JS, et al. Integrating APOL1 gene variants into renal transplantation: considerations arising from the American Society of Transplantation Expert Conference. *Am J Transplant.* 2017;17:901–911, at p. 905.
2. Newell et al, "Integrating," at p. 904.
3. Hsu CY, Lin F, Vittinghoff E, Shlipak MG. Racial differences in the progression from chronic renal insufficiency to end-stage renal disease in the United States. *J Am Soc Nephro.* 2003;14:2902–2907; and Choi AI, Rodriguez RA, Bacchetti P, Bertenthal D, Hernandez GT, O'Hare AM. White/black racial differences in risk of endstage renal disease and death. *Am J Med.* 2009;122:672–678.

364 DECISION-MAKING AND RISK THRESHOLDS

4. Genovese G, Friedman DJ, Ross MD, et al. Association of trypanolytic ApoL1 variants with kidney disease in African Americans. *Science.* 2010;329(5993):841–845; Foster MC, Coresh J, Fornage M, et al. APOL1 variants associate with increased risk of CKD among African Americans. *J Am Soc Nephrol.* 2013;24:1484–1491; Parsa A, Kao WH, Xie D, et al. APOL1 risk variants, race, and progression of chronic kidney disease. *N Engl J Med.* 2013;369:2183–2196; and Palanisamy A, Reeves-Daniel AM, Freedman BI. The impact of APOL1, CAV1, and ABCB1 gene variants on outcomes in kidney transplantation: donor and recipient effects. *Pediatr Nephrol.* 2014;29:1485–1492.
5. Genovese et al, "Association."
6. Parsa et al, "ApoL1."
7. Olabisi O, Al-Romaih K, Henderson J, et al. From man to fish: What can Zebrafish tell us about ApoL1 nephropathy. *Clin Nephrol.* 2016;86 (Suppl 1):114–118; Mohan S, Iltis AS, Sawinski D, DuBois JM. APOL1 genetic testing in living kidney transplant donors. *Am J Kidney Dis.* 2019;74(4):538–543; and Shah S, Shapiro R, Murphy B, Menon MC. APOL1 high-risk genotypes and renal transplantation. *Clin Transpl.* 2019;33:e13582. https://doi.org/10.1111/ctr.13582
8. Reeves-Daniel AM, DePalma JA, Bleyer AJ, et al. The APOL1 gene and allograft survival after kidney transplantation. *Am J Transplant.* 2011;11:1025–1030.
9. Reeves-Daniel et al, "The APOL1 gene."
10. Freedman BI, Julian BA, Pastan SO, et al. Apolipoprotein L1 gene variants in deceased organ donors are associated with renal allograft failure. *Am J Transplant.* 2015;15:1615–1622.
11. Actually, the data show:

> the 5-year living donor graft survival was lower for black recipients than for any other racial/ethnic group, at 82.0% compared with 92.3% for Asian, 89.9% for Hispanic, and 85.7% for white recipients (Figure KI 83).

> Hart A, Smith JM, Skeans MA, et al. OPTN /SRTR 2017 Annual data report: kidney. *Am J Transplant.* 2019;19(Suppl 2):19–123. Figure KI 83.

The PDF can be found at: https://onlinelibrary.wiley.com/doi/epdf/10.1111/ajt.15274. Last accessed August 23, 2021.

> Although the data only discuss the race of the recipients, one can assume that donor-recipient race are concordant. According to Reese and colleagues, "[d]ata from the United Network for Organ Sharing during the 15-year period 1995–2009 show that 95% of white living kidney donors gave to white recipients and 96% of black living kidney donors gave to black recipients." Reese PP, Nair M, Bloom RD. Eliminating racial disparities in access to living donor kidney transplantation: how can centers do better?" *Am J Kidney Dis.* 2012;59:751–753, at p. 751.

12. A National Institutes of Health (NIH) study has been funded to retrospectively evaluate living donor well-being. The Living Donor Extended Times Outcome (LETO) study is a supplement to the APOLLO (APOL1 Long-term Kidney Transplantation Outcomes) Network. AIM 3 of LETO is focused on living donor well-being: "To determine the impact of donor APOL1 renal-risk variants and other novel genetic risk

factors on graft survival and recipient outcomes in a nationally representative sample of living donor kidney transplant recipients from African American living donors." Hsu C-Y, Lentine KL, Park M. Living donor extended time outcomes (LETO) study. Aim 3. Last accessed August 23, 2021. https://grantome.com/grant/NIH/R01-DK120 551-01. Both LETO and APOLLO are discussed in more detail in section 5.

13. Lee BT, Kumar V, Williams TA, et al. The APOL1 genotype of African American kidney transplant recipients does not impact 5 year allograft survival. *Am J Transplant.* 2012;12:1924–1928. doi:10.1111/j.1600-6143.2012.04033.x

14. Quaggin SE, George AL Jr. Apolipoprotein L1 and the genetic basis for racial disparity in chronic kidney disease. *J Am Soc Nephrol.* 2011;22:1955–1958; Pollak MR, Genovese G, Friedman DJ. APOL1 and kidney disease. *Curr Opin Nephrol Hypertens.* 2012;21:179–182; and Madhavan SM, O'Toole JF. The biology of APOL1 with insights into the association between APOL1 variants and chronic kidney disease. *Clin Exp Nephrol.* 2014;18:238–242.

15. Lan X, Jhaveri A, Cheng K, et al. APOL1 risk variants enhance podocyte necrosis through compromising lysosomal membrane permeability. *Am J Physiol Renal Physiol.* 2014;307(3):F326–F336.

16. Genovese et al, "Association"; and Freedman BI. APOL1 and nephropathy progression in populations of African ancestry. *Semin Nephrol.* 2013;33:425–432.

17. Freedman, "APOL1 and nephropathy."

18. Mjøen G, Hallan S, Hartmann A, et al. Long-term risks for kidney donors. *Kidney Int.* 2014;86:162–167; and Muzaale AD, Massie AB, Wang MC, et al. Risk of end-stage renal disease following live kidney donation. *JAMA.* 2014;311:579–586.

19. Mjøen et al, "Long-term risks."

20. Ojo A, Knoll GA. APOL1 genotyping of African American deceased organ donors: not just yet. *Am J Transplant.* 2015; 15:1457–1458; and Freedman BI, Julian BA. Should kidney donors be genotyped for APOL1 risk alleles? *Kidney Int.* 2015;87:671–673.

21. Lee et al, "The APOL1 genotype"; Cohen DM, Mittalhenkle A, Scott DL, Young CJ, Norman DJ. African American living-kidney donors should be screened for APOL1 risk alleles. *Transplantation.* 2011;92:722–725; and Riella LV, Sheridan AM. Testing for high-risk APOL1 alleles in potential living kidney donors. *Am J Kidney Dis.* 2015;66:396–401.

22. This can be done at the national level by modifying Organ Procurement and Transplantation Network (OPTN) policies. Hereinafter referred to as OPTN Policies. This could be included under Policy 14.4: Medical Evaluation Requirements for Living Donor, specifically Table 14-5: Requirements for Living Donor Medical Evaluations. Last updated 6/17/21; last accessed 8/23/21. https://optn.transplant.hrsa.gov/media/1200/optn_policies.pdf

23. Sears DA. The morbidity of sickle cell trait: a review of the literature. *Am J Med.* 1978;64:1021–1036; and Johnson LN. Sickle cell trait: an update. *J Natl Med Assoc.* 1982;74:751–757.

24. Naik RP, Derebail VK, Grams ME, et al. Association of sickle cell trait with chronic kidney disease and albuminuria in African Americans. *JAMA.* 2014;312:2115–2125, at p. 2123.

25. Reese PP, Hoo AC, Magee CC. Screening for sickle trait among potential live kidney donors: policies and practices in US transplant centers. *Transpl Int.* 2008;21:328–331.

26. Reese et al, "Screening."

27. Ojo and Knoll, "APOL1."

28. Cohen et al, "African American"; and Freedman BI, Murea M. Target organ damage in African American hypertension: role of APOL1. *Curr Hypertens Rep.* 2012; 14:21–28.

29. See, for example, Katz J. Why doctors don't disclose uncertainty. *Hastings Cent Rep.* 1984;14(1):35–44; Mischel MH. Uncertainty in illness. *Image J Nurs Sch.* 1988; 20:225–232; and Han PK, Klein WMP, Arora NK. Varieties of uncertainty in health care: a conceptual taxonomy. *Med Decis Making.* 2011;31:828–838.

30. Katz, "Why doctors"; and Eddy DM. Variations in physician practice: the role of uncertainty. *Health Aff.* 1984;3(2):74–89.

31. Muzaale et al, "Risk."

32. Freedman, "APOL1 and nephropathy."

33. Riella and Sheridan, "Testing."

34.. Fraser FC. Genetic counselling. *Am J Hum Genet.* 1974;26:636–661.

35. Chieng WS, Chan N, Lee SC. Non-directive genetic counselling—respect for autonomy or unprofessional practice? *Ann Acad Med Singapore.* 2011;40(1):36–42; and Weil J. Psychosocial genetic counseling in the post-nondirective era: a point of view. *J Genet Couns.* 2003;12:199–211.

36. Mackenzie C, Stoljar N. Introduction: autonomy reconfigured. In: Mackenzie C, Stoljar N, eds. *Relational Autonomy: Feminist Perspectives on Autonomy, Agency and the Social Self.* New York, NY: Oxford University Press; 2000:3–31; and Elwyn G, Frosch D, Thomson R, et al. Shared decision making: a model for clinical practice. *J Gen Intern Med.* 2012;27:1361–1367. The notion of relational autonomy is more fully described in the text in chapter 3, section 3.2 Respect for Persons, corresponding to references 3–8.

37. See, for example, Elwyn et al, "Shared decision making"; Entwistle V, Carter S, Cribb A, McCaffery K. Supporting patient autonomy: the importance of clinician-patient relationships. *J Gen Intern Med.* 2010;25(7):741–745; and Walter JK, Ross LF. Relational autonomy: moving beyond the limits of isolated individualism. *Pediatrics.* 2014;133(suppl 1):S16–S23.

38. Asgari E, Hilton RM. One size does not fit all: understanding individual living kidney donor risk. *Pediatr Nephrol.* 2021;36(2):259–269. Published online Jan 2, 2020. doi:10.1007/s00467-019-04456-8

39. Ito K, Bick AG, Flannick J, et al. Increased burden of cardiovascular disease in carriers of APOL1 genetic variants. *Circ Res.* 2014;114(5):845–850.

40. Mohan S, Iltis AS, Sawinski D, DuBois J. APOL1 genetic testing in living kidney transplant donors. *Am J Kidney Dis.* 2019;74:538–543.

41. Elwyn et al, "Shared decision making"; and Walter and Ross, "Relational autonomy."

42. Mohan et al, "APOL1."

43. An interesting issue is how to address a case where there are 2 or more motivated potential Black living donors. Here, if the donors know each other, it might be useful to get them to agree to share results and to discuss donor selection using the incomplete

knowledge that we have about APOL1 and its implications for graft survival in the recipient and donor outcomes. If they don't know each other, do not want to discuss options as a group, or are willing to let the LDAT decide which donor should proceed, then the LDAT should select who among the motivated donors would have the most favorable risk:benefit ratio.

44. Mjøen et al, "Long-term risks."
45. OPTN Policies. See Policy 14.4: Medical Evaluation Requirements for Living Donor, specifically Table 14-5: Requirements for Living Donor Medical Evaluations.
46. OPTN Policies. See Policy 15.3A (3).
47. OPTN Policies. See Policy 14.3 Informed Consent requirements, specifically Table 14-1: Requirements for Living Donor Informed Consent: "Any infectious disease or malignancy that is pertinent to acute recipient care discovered during the donor's first two years of follow-up care."
48. OPTN Policies. See Table 14-1: Requirements for Living Donor Informed Consent (#7). Last updated 6/17/2021. Last accessed 8/23/21. https://optn.transplant.hrsa.gov/media/1200/optn_policies.pdf.
49. Hidalgo G, Tejani C, Clayton R, et al. Factors limiting the rate of living-related kidney donation to children in an inner city setting. *Pediatr Transplant*. 2001;5:419–424.
50. Freedman, "APOL1 and nephropathy."
51. Horowitz CR, Ferryman K, Negron R, et al. Race, genomics and chronic disease: what patients with African ancestry have to say. *J Health Care Poor Underserved*. 2017;28:248–260, at p. 251.
52. Horowitz et al, "Race, genomics," at p. 254.
53. Horowitz et al, "Race, genomics," at p. 255 citing Taylor JY, Peternell B, Smith JA. Attitudes toward genetic testing for hypertension among African American women and girls. *Nurs Res Pract*. 2013:Article ID:341374. Published 2 Nov 2013; last accessed 8/23/2021. https://www.hindawi.com/journals/nrp/2013/341374
54. Horowitz et al, "Race, genomics," at p. 254.
55. Umeukeje EM, Young BA, Fullerton SM, et al. You are just now telling us about this? African American perspectives of testing for genetic susceptibility to kidney disease. *J Am Soc Nephrol (JASN)*. 2019;30:526–530.
56. Umeukeje et al, "You are just now," at p. 527.
57. Umeukeje et al, "You are just now," at p. 528.
58. Umeukeje et al, "You are just now," at p. 529.
59. Gordon EJ, Amórtegui D, Blancas I, Wicklund C, Friedewald J, Sharp RR. African American living donors' attitudes about APOL1 genetic testing: a mixed methods study. *Am J Kidney Dis*. 2018;72:819–883.
60. Newell et al, "Integrating."
61. Newell et al, "Integrating," at pp. 904–905.
62. Newell et al, "Integrating," at p. 907.
63. Freedman BI, Moxey-Mims M. The APOL1 Long-Term Kidney Transplantation Outcomes Network—APOLLO. *Clin J Am Soc Nephrol*. 2018;13:940–942.
64. Freedman and Moxey-Mims, "APOLLO."
65. Hsu et al, "LETO."

66. Hsu et al, "LETO," Aim 1.
67. Hsu et al, "LETO," Aims 2 and 3.
68. Gordon EJ, Wicklund C, Lee J, Sharp RR, Friedewald J. A national survey of transplant surgeons and nephrologists on implementing apolipoprotein L1 (APOL1) genetic testing into clinical practice. *Prog Transplant*. 2019;29(1):26–35.
69. Gordon et al, "A national survey."
70. Garg N, Lentine KL, Inker LA, et al. The kidney evaluation of living kidney donor candidates: US practices in 2017. *Am J Transplant*. Published online April 28, 2020. doi:10.1111/ajt.15951
71. McIntosh T, Mohan S, Sawinski D, Iltis A, DuBois J. Variation of ApoL1 testing practices for living kidney donors. *Prog Transpl*. 2020;30:22–28.
72. Riella and Sheridan, "Testing."
73. Mena-Gutierrez AM, Reeves-Daniel AM, Jay CL, Freedman BI. Practical considerations for *APOL1* genotyping in the living kidney donor evaluation. *Transplantation*. 2020;104:27–32.
74. In 2020, the Genetic Testing Registry (GTR) now counts 21 laboratories. Genetic Testing Registry (GTR). APOL1. Accessed August 23, 2021. https://www.ncbi.nlm.nih.gov/gtr/all/tests/?term=apol1
75. Riella and Sheridan, "Testing"; and Mena-Gutierrez et al, "Practical considerations."
76. Genetic Information Nondiscrimination Act (GINA) of 2008, Pub L. 110-233, H.R. 493, 110th Congress.
77. Geppert CM, Roberts LW. Ethical issues in the use of genetic information in the workplace: a review of recent developments. *Curr Opin Psych*. 2005;18:518–524; Parkman AA, Foland J, Anderson B, et al. Public awareness of genetic nondiscrimination laws in four states and perceived importance of life insurance protections. *J Genet Couns*. 2015;24:512–521; and Green RC, Lautenbach D, McGuire AL. GINA, genetic discrimination, and genomic medicine. *N Engl J Med*. 2015;372:397–399.
78. A long-term registry is being developed. See Kasiske BL, Asrani SK, Dew MA, et al. The Living Donor Collective: a scientific registry for living donors. *Am J Transplant*. 2017;17:3040–3048. Unfortunately, long-term funding has not been guaranteed (personal communication with Bert Kasiske, June 2020).
79. OPTN Policies. See Policy 18, Data Submission Policy.

16

Questioning the Premise

Is Living Donor Organ Transplantation Ethical?

16.1 Questioning by Transplant Surgeons

We began this book by asserting that the field of living donor organ transplantation is ethical (even if some specific applications are not). However, even in the early years, not all involved in the emerging field of organ transplantation believed that it was an ethical long-term solution. Joseph Murray, the surgeon who performed the first living donor kidney transplant in 1954, stated his position at the CIBA Foundation symposium entitled *Ethics in Medical Progress: With Special Reference to Transplantation* that took place in London in 1966:

> As physicians motivated and educated to make sick people well, we make a
> basic qualitative shift in our aims when we risk the health of a well person,
> no matter how pure our motives. To relieve ourselves of this responsibility
> all clinicians working with kidney transplantation should strive for better
> organ procurement so that the day will come when even the identical twins
> will not require a living donor.[1]

Nor was Murray alone. Thomas Starzl, another early pioneer in kidney transplantation, was criticized at the CIBA symposium for his willingness to procure kidneys from healthy prisoners to perform nonrelated living donor kidney transplants.[2] At a symposium the following year that was published in the *Annals of Internal Medicine* in September 1967, he wrote:

> I have dwelt at some length on the question of organ procurement from
> living volunteers because it is perhaps the most sensitive and limiting issue
> in clinical transplantation. Today, the best prognosis can be offered to the

The Living Organ Donor as Patient. Lainie Friedman Ross and J. Richard Thistlethwaite, Jr, Oxford University Press.
© Oxford University Press 2022. DOI: 10.1093/oso/9780197618202.003.0016

recipient only with the use of such donors, particularly when these are from within the family. In the future it is hoped that the need for living donors will be made obsolete by improvements in immunosuppression, antigen typing, and tissue preservation. Then, organs obtained solely from cadavers could be used with a high expectation of long-term survival.[3]

With the development of azathioprine (Imuran) in the early 1960s and the first polyclonal antilymphocyte globulin in 1967, results of deceased donor kidney transplantation improved. Starzl stopped using living donors for kidney transplantation in 1972. He explained in his memoir:

Although I was one of the first to use the expedient of living kidney do-nation and have never had a donor die, I was shaken by these discussions [of donor death at the Ciba conference at one of the premier transplant centers]. The concept of living donation seemed less and less acceptable to me as the years went by. After the Ciba conference, I tried to avoid the prac-tice without oppressing my colleagues who believed in its probity, and in 1972 I stopped using kidneys from any living donors.[4]

Starzl debated Felix Rapaport, another transplant surgeon, regarding kidney transplantation with living donors in 1996 at the International Congress of the Transplantation Society held in Helsinki. Rapaport pointed to:

the large body of objective data which point to the safety of living-donor kidney transplantation, and to the major benefits which can be accrued by the donor in terms of enhanced feelings of self-esteem and self-worth at the conclusion of this heroic act.[5]

Starzl argued that "in spite of the most stringent precautions to protect the donor, this operation can never be totally safe for the donor."[6]

By 1994, Rapaport had also become less enamored with living donor transplantation. This was due in part to the expansion of living organ donor transplantation to involve living liver, lung, and pancreas donors, each with higher morbidity and mortality than kidney donation. Writing with Starzl, Rapaport also expressed concern that the focus on living donor transplan-tation would occur "at the expense of other equally important therapeutic avenues" most notably the need to "increase retrieval rates of cadaver-organ donation."[7]

16.2 Questioning by Social Scientists, Philosophers, and Theologians

Nonclinicians also viewed living donation as a temporary solution justified because the benefits were thought to outweigh the harms. Two such commentators were the theologians Paul Ramsey and Richard McCormick. Richard McCormick wrote:

> I agree with Ramsey that there must be a thrust away from use of living donors and that such use must be viewed as only transitionally justifiable. Such a statement rests on the altogether reasonable conviction that the causing of harm to the donor is ethically justified only where it is proportionately grounded. Where artificial or cadaver organs will provide the same benefit, there is obviously no proportionate reason for the loss to the living donor.[8]

One question that this risk:benefit perspective leaves open is whether the calculation is done from the perspective of the donor-recipient pair, or whether the risk: benefit calculation must be done individually for both donor and recipient. Early judicial rulings justifying kidney donation by a minor to his or her identical twin reasoned that both parties needed to benefit individually and argued that the donor would benefit psychologically (or at least not be psychologically harmed by being prohibited) from donation.[9] Some participants at the CIBA symposium argued that the benefits to the recipient might legitimately weighed against the risks to the donor,[10] whereas others argued, as we do in chapter 3, that the benefits and risks must be weighed separately for each party.[11]

Benefits to the donor are psychological. Even at the CIBA symposium, attendees described both positive and negative psychological effects of serving as a living donor. Social science data also showed both positive and negative outcomes.[12] Donation was more often viewed positively when there was a good outcome. Significant harms occurred more frequently when the recipient did poorly, which correlated with poor donor quality of life post-donation. But even when the recipient did well, donors described stress created by the request and intrafamilial discord created by refusal.

16.3 Questioning Donor Autonomy

Both clinicians and nonclinicians emphasized a robust informed consent process, although early data showed that donors made their decisions spontaneously, and decisions rarely if ever changed after a potential donor was apprised of the facts.[13] Concerns that donors were not acting fully voluntarily were dismissed by some who argued that "the pressure on the family donor . . . is a pressure consonant with the dignity and responsibility of free life."[14] The CIBA symposium transcript as well as the early social science literature show that donor consent is affected by the gravity of the recipient candidate's health (medical vulnerability). Some programs (like Hamburger's program in France and Murray's program in Boston) incorporated psychologists from the onset.[15] In the US, a living donor advocate (LDA) or a living donor advocacy team (LDAT) focused on donor physical and mental well-being would not become standard until the early 2000s,[16] after the widely publicized death of a living donor.[17]

The LDAT's role is to promote the interests of the donor, to advocate for her rights, and to ensure that the donor receives and understands information about consent, evaluation, donation, and post-donation processes, and to help her exercise her autonomy in a way that is consonant with her reflective preferences.[18] The LDAT ensures that the donor is physically, psychologically, and emotionally healthy enough to donate, and LDAT team members also evaluate donor comprehension, motivation, and voluntariness. Using the language of Kipnis[19] and Goodin,[20] this means that the LDAT is responsible for evaluating all the vulnerability threats that the potential donor may experience and must be able to ensure that the vulnerability threats are adequately addressed, empowering the potential donor to give a voluntary and informed consent.

The role of the LDAT focuses on the competent patient's right to determine what is in her best interest. Using a wider conception of autonomy than the traditional bioethics notion of the right to make decisions without interference, relational autonomy requires acknowledging and addressing donor vulnerabilities in a way that promotes and advances the donor's capacity for autonomy.[21] This does not mean that the LDA(T) should protect potential donors from all risks. The donor's transplant team should respect the donor's right to take health risks if the donor believes them to be outweighed by potential benefits, with the caveat that the LDAT are moral agents who can refuse to participate in an action (approval of the individual to serve as a living organ donor) if they do not believe the donation is medically or psychologically appropriate.

16.4 Are There Limits to Donor Autonomy?

Some commentators limit on the extent to which donors may be harmed by organ donation. Nicola Williams explains:

> although an intended organ donor may not act wrongly by offering his organs to another when to do so is likely to come at great personal cost, the intended recipient/s and indeed the donor physician may act wrongly in accepting such an offer.[22]

Carl Elliott concurs: "a doctor is in the position of deciding not simply whether a subject's choice is reasonable or morally justifiable, but whether he is morally justified in helping the subject accomplish it."[23] The LDA(T) can and should decline to participate in an action (approval of the individual for living donation) that they do not believe is justified.

Challenges to donor autonomy are further justified if alternatives exist. Would living donation still be permitted if (1) there were an adequate supply of deceased donor organ grafts, (2) organs could be grown in vitro, (3) scientists had developed the capacity to create synthetic organs, or (4) the immunologists had developed techniques that would allow xenografts to be used safely and effectively?

Part of the answer to whether living donation would still be permissible when alternative organ sources are plentiful may depend on the quality of the alternatives. Living donor kidneys currently function longer than deceased donor organs. A living donor kidney may reduce the number of repeat transplants a young individual in organ failure will need over a lifetime. An answer may also depend upon the cultural or religious values of living donors and their intended recipients: Some may object to a xenograft or deceased donor organ on moral grounds; others may feel a sense of duty to donate their own organs.

Imagine supply were truly not an issue and alternatives existed that did not pose any novel health risks, that had the potential to obviate the need for immunosuppression, that were expected to last for decades, and that came from sources did that not violate the personal, emotional, or cultural beliefs of candidates in end-stage organ failure and their families. The basic question remains: should we allow individuals to expose themselves to such risks? Murray's conclusion that we would not even allow an identical twin to donate in a world of non-scarcity speaks to his belief that living donor transplantation was (ought to be) a temporary plan.[24]

We come to the same conclusion using our living donor ethics framework (see chapter 3). While respect for persons supports a potential donor's autonomous decision to donate an organ at this time when demand greatly outpaces supply, justice demands not only that the benefits outweigh the risks, but that there is no safer, similarly effective alternative. Once a safe, similarly effective alternative exists, justice demands that we protect people from themselves. It is understandable why an adult may voluntarily risk his life and run into a burning building to save a human life especially if a family member were inside, and some would do so even if they did not know the imperiled person. But it makes no sense to respect the decision of an adult to run into a burning building if there are no persons or other living beings at risk. If there is an abundance of alternative organs, even if a prospective donor wants to donate and screams that the refusal by the LDAT is unacceptably paternalistic, the moral response is to argue that when interventions (kidney transplantation) require the participation of third parties (like transplant professionals) our special obligations to our patients and future patients (prospective donors) demand that we not put them at unnecessary risks. A sufficiently safe and effective alternative to living donor grafts changes the balance on the scales of justice.

16.5 Where Are We Now?

More than 55 years since the CIBA symposium (and more than 65 years since the first successful living donor kidney transplant), we are no closer to the goal of adequate organ supply without living donors than we were when Murray did the first long-term successful living donor kidney transplant. If anything, the supply:demand ratio is worse. Demand is much greater than our waitlists suggest. Demand is artificially lowered by structural, financial, and logistical obstacles that exclude many individuals in organ failure from being listed. We create psychosocial barriers to ensure good stewardship because of scarcity. In other illnesses where there is no treatment shortage, we treat everyone in need, including the subset of patients who we expect will not take care of themselves, will not be compliant, and for whom the treatment will fail. But there is a shortage or organs and the supply:demand gap is growing. The number of people who will need organs is growing rapidly due to lifestyle choices: overeating; stressful jobs; underfunded public health and preventive medicine programs; inadequate access to quality foods, health care, and education; poor adherence to medications; and too few rehabilitation programs.

Despite Murray's optimism at the start of the CIBA symposium that living donation was a temporary stopgap, in the final discussion he concluded that the main limitation in organ transplantation for the foreseeable future was and would be a dearth of organs: "I agree that we should concentrate on the cadaver programme as the most pressing problem, but the living donor is always going to be necessary."[25]

Murray was prescient in saying that living donation was not going away any time soon. What he might not have predicted was how willing the transplant community and the public at large would become in exposing healthy individuals to the potential harms of living donation—both with respect to which organs they can donate and to whom. Today, organ transplants using living kidney, liver, lung, pancreas, intestines, uterus, and domino heart donors have been performed successfully. Individuals can donate to family, friends, and strangers, and they can donate directly or participate in paired exchanges and domino chains. Social scientists study ways to further promote living donation and to maximize the number of candidates who can benefit from a single Good Samaritan donor through the development of living donor paired exchange and domino chain registries. These activities are proliferating despite our increased understanding of the short- and long-term medical and psychosocial risks of living organ donation.

As we were finishing a draft of this book, Renée Fox died on September 23, 2020.[26] A sociologist by training, she spent 4 decades studying organ transplantation and often collaborated with Judith P. Swazey, a biologist and historian of science and medicine. Their first book, *The Courage to Fail* (1974, second edition 1978) was an examination of the social and cultural significance of therapeutic innovation in the development and improvement of organ transplantation and dialysis. They focused on "[p]roblems of uncertainty, meaning, life and death, scarcity, justice, equity, solidarity, and intervention in the human condition [which] are all evoked by these therapeutic interventions."[27] Their second book, *Spare Parts* (1992), continued to explore these themes but described their "increasingly troubled and critical reaction to the expansion of organ replacement," ending with their decision to leave the field.[28] Their near-to-final words explain their decision to leave the field:

> But we have come to believe that the missionary-like ardor about organ re-placement that now exists . . . and the seemingly limitless attempts to pro-cure and implant organs that are currently taking place have gotten out of hand.[29]

Some of the proposals analyzed in this book substantiate their concerns and underscore the need to find ways to reduce the demand for organs. We support a more robust preventive medicine approach that addresses the underlying factors that cause end-stage organ disease in the first place: medical and lifestyle treatments to reduce obesity, hypertension, diabetes, alcohol use disorder, and smoking. The focus of this book, however, has been to provide a framework that helps to determine the appropriate moral limits of living solid organ donation and to provide a systematic approach for LDATs to evaluate the physical, psychological, and emotional health as well as comprehension, motivation, and voluntariness of donor candidates. We support helping potential motivated individuals make well-informed decisions about some innovative practices that increase the opportunities to serve as living organ donors (eg, kidney paired exchanges and domino chains) while also seeking to rein in a single-minded pursuit to legitimize ethically questionable attempts to increase the supply of living organ grafts (eg, obtaining organs from imminently dying individuals). Our approach requires the transplant community to fully embrace the fact that living organ donors (and prospective living organ donors) are patients. We have special obligations to them. Only when living organ donors are regarded as patients in their own right can the moral limits of living solid organ donation be realized and the living donors be given the full respect that they deserve.

Notes

1. Wolstenhome GEW, O'Connor M, eds. *Ethics in Medical Progress: With Special Reference to Transplantation.* Boston, MA: Little, Brown and Company; 1966, citing Joseph Murray at p. 59.

2. Wolstenhome and O'Connor, at pp. 74–76.

3. Starzl TE. Ethical problems in organ transplantation: a clinician's point of view. *Ann Intern Med*. 1967;67:32–36, at p. 35.

4. Starzl TE. *The Puzzle People: Memoirs of a Transplant Surgeon*. Pittsburgh, PA: University of Pittsburgh Press; 1992, at p. 147.

5. Rapaport FT, Starzl TE. The influence of organ supply and demand pressures upon the "primum non nocere" principle in living-donor transplantation. *Clin Transpl*. 1994;348–349, at p. 348.

6. Rapaport and Starzl, "The influence," at p. 348.

7. Rapaport and Starzl, "The influence," at p. 349. Another surgeon who questioned living donation was Charles Stiller, the head of transplant surgery at the University of Western Ontario. Altman LK. The doctor's world: the limits of transplantation: how far should surgeons go? *The New York Times*. December 19, 1989. Last accessed August 23, 2019.https://www.nytimes.com/1989/12/19/science/the-doctor-s-world-the-limits-of-transplantation-how-far-should-surgeons-go.html

8. McCormick RA. Transplantation of organs: a comment on Paul Ramsey. *Theol Stud*. 1975;36(3):5033–5039, at p. 509.

9. See, for example, *Huskey v Harrison*, Eq. No. 68666 (Mass 1957); *Foster v Harrison*, Eq. No. 68674 (Mass 1957); and *Masden v Harrison*, Eq. No. 68651 (Mass 1957).

10. For example, David Daube, a legal scholar, wondered if the 2 procedures could be viewed as 1 to ensure that the benefits outweighed the risks; see Wolstenhome and O'Connor, *Ethics in Medical*, at p. 208. The surgeon, Michael Francis Addison Woodruff, viewed the risk:benefit ratio as acceptable given that the risks to the donor were minimal and were offset by the significant benefit to the recipient. See Wolstenhome and O'Connor, *Ethics in Medical*, at pp. 18–20.

11. See, for example, the discussion by the nephrologist George E. Schreiner discussing the concept of totality in Wolstenhome and O'Connor, *Ethics in Medical*, at pp. 130–131. More recently this point has been made by Aaron Spital. See, for example, Spital A. Donor benefit is the key to justified living organ donation. *Cambridge Q Healthc Ethics*. 2004;13(1):105–109.

12. See, for example, Simmons RG, Klein S, Simmons RL *Gift of Life: The Social and Psychological Impact of Organ Transplantation*. New York, NY: John Wiley and Sons; 1977, updated and with new material; and Fox RC, Swazey JP. *The Courage to Fail: A Social View of Organ Transplants and Dialysis*. 2nd ed, rev. Chicago IL: Chicago University Press; 1978.

13. See, for example, Fellner CH, Marshall JR. Kidney donors—the myth of informed consent. *Am J Psych*. 1970;126(9):1245–1251; and Fellner CH, Selection of living kidney donors and the problem of informed consent. *Semin Psychiatry*. 1971;3(1):79–85.

14. Wolstenhome and O'Connor, *Ethics in Medical*, citing David Daube at p. 204.

15. Wolstenhome and O'Connor, *Ethics in Medical*, citing Jean Hamburger at p. 14 and citing Joseph Murray at p. 18.

16. Department of Health and Human Services, Part II. Centers for Medicare and Medicaid Services. 42 DFR Parts 405, 482, 488, and 498. Medicare Program; Hospital Conditions of Participation: Requirements for Approval and Re-Approval of Transplant Centers to Perform Organ Transplants. *Fed Regist*. 2007;72:15198–15280. Of note, United Network for Organ Sharing (UNOS)/Organ Procurement

and Transplantation Network (OPTN) modified its bylaws the same year. Appendix B, Section XIII, 2007. Updated in current UNOS/OPTN policy handbook in section 14.2 Independent Living Donor Advocate Requirements. Last revision 6/17/2021; last accessed 8/23/2021.https://optn.transplant.hrsa.gov/media/1200/optn_policies.pdf

17. Grady D. Donor's death at hospital halts some liver surgeries. *The New York Times*. Jan 16, 2002.

18. Steele J. *Living Donor Advocacy: An Evolving Role Within Transplantation*. New York, NY: Springer; 2013; and Rudow DL. The living donor advocate: a team approach to educate, evaluate, and manage donors across the continuum. *Prog Transplant.* 2009;19:64–70.

19. Kipnis K. Vulnerability in research subjects: a bioethical taxonomy. In: *The National Bioethics Advisory Commission. Ethical and Policy Issues in Research Involving Human Participants. Volume II: Commissioned Papers and Staff Analysis*. Bethesda, MD: National Bioethics Advisory Commission; 2001:G1–13; and Kipnis K. Seven Vulnerabilities in the pediatric research subject. *Theor Med.* 2003;24:107–120, at p. 110.

20. Goodin RE. *Protecting the Vulnerable: A Reanalysis of Our Social Responsibilities*. Chicago, IL: University of Chicago Press; 1985.

21. See, for example, Friedman M. Autonomy social disruptions and women. In Mackenzie C, Stoljar N, eds. *Relational Autonomy: Feminist Perspectives on Autonomy, Agency, and the Social Self*. New York, NY: Oxford University Press; 2000:35–51; and Dodds S. Choice and control in feminist bioethics. In Mackenzie C, Stoljar N, eds. *Relational Autonomy: Feminist Perspectives on Autonomy, Agency, and the Social Self*. New York, NY: Oxford University Press; 2000:213–235.

22. Williams NJ. On harm thresholds and living organ donation: must the living donor benefit, on balance, from his donation? *Med Health Care Philos.* 2018;21:11–22, at p. 13.

23. Elliott C. Doing harm: living organ donors, clinical research and *The Tenth Man*. *J Med Ethics* 1995;21:91–96, at p. 95.

24. Wolstenhome and O'Connor, *Ethics in Medical*, at p. 59.

25. Wolstenhome and O'Connor, *Ethics in Medical*, at p. 207.

26. Genzlinger N. Renée C. Fox, founding figure of medical sociology, dies at 92. *The New York Times*. October 1, 2020. https://www.nytimes.com/2020/10/01/health/renee-c-fox-dead.html#:~:text=1%2C%202020-,Ren%C3%A9e%20C.,She%20was%2092

27. Fox and Swazey, *The Courage to Fail*, at p. xvii.

28. Fox RC, Swazey JP, with the assistance of Watkins JC. *Spare Parts: Organ Replacement in American Society*. New York, NY: Oxford University Press; 1992, at the book cover.

29. Fox and Swazey, *Spare Parts*, at p. 204.

Epilogue

Lainie Friedman Ross

This book is over a decade in writing and involves more than 2 decades of ethical reflection on living donor transplantation, 3 decades for my co-author. As we explain in chapter 1, Dick and I first collaborated in 1997 when our colleague Steve Woodle called an ethics consult to discuss the ethical issues that would be raised by kidney paired exchanges. I had come to the University of Chicago in 1994 in both the departments of pediatrics and the MacLean Center for Clinical Medical Ethics. I happened to be taking call that month and it led to the development of a sounding board piece in the *New England Journal of Medicine*,[1] an IRB protocol to actually proceed with a kidney paired exchange, and a life-long collaboration between Dick and myself.

Now Dick had already been involved in a Section on Transplantation Surgery collaboration with the MacLean Center for Clinical Medical Ethics at the University of Chicago. In 1988, Dick and surgical colleagues had collaborated with several ethicists in the MacLean Center, including its director, Mark Siegler, in the development of a novel living liver donor transplantation protocol. They published their ethical analysis in *The New England Journal of Medicine* in 1989,[2] and, with IRB approval, performed 20 cases within the next 2 years which they published in 1991.[3] Alas, our kidney paired exchange program did not have such rapid uptake, the reasons for which we explore in chapter 8.

In 2007, I was awarded a National Institutes of Health (NIH) National Library of Medicine (NLM) grant to explore the ethical and policy issues in living donor transplantation (NLM 1G13LM009096 Ethical and Policy Issues in Living Donor Transplantation (July 1, 2007–June 30, 2010)). I was spurred on by two distinct events. First was the limited discussion of living donors in Robert M. Veatch's 2000 masterpiece, *Transplantation Ethics*.[4] Second was a gnawing concern for the long-term well-being of living donors. As a non-transplant professional, it was clear to me that my transplant colleagues were focused on saving the lives of patients in end-stage organ failure and it was

not clear to me that we had enough concern about the living donors who become patients the moment they appear at a clinic to discuss living donation.
In 2007, with Dick and Mark Siegler, we wrote an essay arguing for the need
for a living donor registry in the *Hastings Center Report*, the premier bioethics journal.[5] And I would spend the next 3 years convincing the Human
Resources Service Administration (HRSA) that I should have access to the
personal health information (PHI) of all the living donors who had subsequently developed end-stage renal disease (ESRD). HRSA and all federal
agencies are allowed to provide PHI for exceptional research purposes and
after a thorough vetting and many protocols arguing for the importance of
the research, I was given access to 325 living donor who had subsequently
developed ESRD. I have since been given access to information about an additional 240 living donors who have developed ESRD, and for over 200 I have
located and collected data, including blood samples.[6] The initial sample collection was funded in 2010 from a pilot grant from the University of Chicago
Clinical and Translational Science Award (CTSA) (UL1 RR024999) and
some core funding in 2021 (UL1 RR002389). Future funding will be used to
study if there are identifiable risk factors that can predict this adverse outcome. I thank our collaborators, Jeffrey Kopp and Cheryl Winkler at the
National Institutes of Health. for their friendship, guidance, and help with
processing and storage of these samples.

My vision in 2007 was to write a single-author book focused exclusively
on living donor transplantation. The outline included many of the chapters
in this book. But what was missing was a framework so that others who
wondered about the ethics of living donor practice and policy would have
the methodology and tools with which to analyze their concerns. I worked
on specific topics during that 3-year grant including (1) arguments against
a living kidney market,[7] (2) arguments about why transplant professionals
should not give a false medical excuse to living donors,[8] (3) arguments about
why transplant programs should not disclose misattributed parentage,[9]
and (4) how different conceptions of risk are used in the market debate.[10]
I also familiarized myself with the Organ and Procurement Transplantation
Network allocation policies for deceased donor organs because policies
about living donors and deceased donors cannot be understood in isolation
from each other as they interact, even if unintentionally.[11] But as the grant
period came to a close, I chose not to collect all of my disparate writings into
a book because I lacked a framework.

In 2013, I decided to apply for a Robert Wood Johnson Foundation (RWJF) Investigator Award in Health Policy to continue my work on ethical and policy issues in living donor transplantation. To be honest, this was not my first application to the RWJF program, having tried to convince them to fund me on my work in pediatrics and genetics. But this time, I came to the grant funding opportunity with Dick as my collaborator and Bob Veatch as our consultant. I was elated when it was funded, especially since a few weeks after the announcement, the RWJ Foundation announced that this cycle was the last one for this granting mechanism.

During our 3-year grant period (March 2014–March 2017), Dick and I developed the framework described in chapter 3 and presented it to the RWJF community to positive review in 2015. Life events, however, kept us from finishing the book in the allotted 3 years. Dick retired in June 2016, and I was distracted by a once-in-a-lifetime opportunity to work with Bob Veatch on revising *Transplantation Ethics*. And, of course, as time progressed, the world of organ transplantation evolved: greater understanding of the long-term risks of kidney donation; the identification of ApoL1 as a risk factor for ESRD in Blacks and its implications for deceased and living Black kidney donors; and the first successful births of healthy infants by uterine transplant recipients (first living donor uterine transplant recipients and then deceased donor uterine transplant recipients).

There are many people to whom we owe a big thanks. We first want to thank our funders, both the NIH and the RWJ Foundation. Next we want to thank the journal reviewers, editors and publishers who provided constructive feedback and published our ideas in the area of living donor transplantation. Five of the articles have been revised from journal articles.

Chapter 3:

- Lainie Friedman Ross and J. Richard Thistlethwaite, Jr. Developing an ethics framework for living donor transplantation. *Journal of Medical Ethics*, 2018;44:843–850. Copyright © 2018 BMJ Publishing Group Ltd & Institute of Medical Ethics. Modified and reprinted with permission from BMJ Publishing Group, Ltd.

Chapter 4:

- Lainie Friedman Ross and J. Richard Thistlethwaite. Gender and race/ethnicity in living kidney donor demographics: preference or disparity?

Chapter 6:

Chapter 9:

Chapter 15:

Other chapters include arguments and cases from previous publications and are cited in the chapters in which they are discussed and are also listed below. We thank our co-authors who helped us explore these ideas and for their friendship over the years.

Chapter 5, which is based on previous work:

- Lainie Friedman Ross, J. Richard Thistlethwaite, Jr., and the American Academy of Pediatrics Committee on Bioethics. Minors as living solid organ donors. *Pediatrics*. 2008;122:454–461.
- Lainie Friedman Ross and J. Richard Thistlethwaite, Jr. Children as living donors. In: Greenberg R, Goldberg A, Rodriguez, Arias D, eds. *Ethical*

Issues in Pediatric Organ Transplantation. New York, NY: Springer; 2016, 3–18.

Chapter 7: The first case comes from an article we published with colleagues:

- Lainie Friedman Ross, Walter Glannon, Michelle A. Josephson, and J. Richard Thistlethwaite, Jr. Should all living donors be treated equally? *Transplantation.* 2002;74:418–421.

This chapter borrows ideas from several other articles as well:

- Walter Glannon and Lainie Friedman Ross. Do genetic relationships create moral obligations in organ transplantation? *Cambridge Quarterly of Health Care Ethics.* 2002;11(2):153–159.
- Lainie Friedman Ross. Solid organ donations between strangers. *Journal of Law, Medicine, and Ethics.* 2002;30(3):440–445.
- Lainie Friedman Ross. All donations should not be treated equally: a response to Jeffrey Kahn's commentary. *Journal of Law, Medicine, and Ethics.* 2002;30(3):448–451.
- Lainie Friedman Ross. The ethical limits in expanding living donor transplantation. *Kennedy Institute of Ethics Journal.* 2006;16:151–172.

Chapter 8: This chapter borrows from many different articles.

- Lainie Friedman Ross, David Rubin, Mark Siegler, Michele A. Josephson, J. Richard Thistlethwaite, Jr., and E. Steve Woodle. Ethics of a paired-kidney-exchange program. *New England Journal of Medicine.* 1997;336:1752–1755.
- Lainie Friedman Ross and E. Steven Woodle. Kidney exchange programs: an expanded view of the ethical issues. In: Touraine JL, Traeger J, Betuel H, Dubernard JM, Revillard JP, and Dupuy C, eds. *Organ Allocation: Proceedings of the 30th International Conference on Transplantation and Clinical Immunology.* Dordrecht, The Netherlands: Kluwer Academic Publishers; 1998:285–295.
- Walter Glannon and Lainie Friedman Ross. Do genetic relationships create moral obligations in organ transplantation? *Cambridge Quarterly of Health Care Ethics* 2002;11:153–159.

- Lainie Friedman Ross and Stefanos Zenios. Practical and ethical challenges to paired exchange programs. *American Journal of Transplantation.* 2004;4:1553–1554.
- Paul D. Ackerman, J. Richard Thistlethwaite, Jr., and Lainie Friedman Ross. Attitudes of minority patients with end stage renal disease regarding abo-incompatible list-paired exchanges. *American Journal of Transplantation.* 2006:6:83–88.
- Lainie Friedman Ross. What the medical excuse teaches us about the donor as patient. *American Journal of Transplantation.* 2010;10:731–736.
- Lainie Friedman Ross, James Rodrigue, and Robert M. Veatch. Ethical and logistical issues raised by the advanced donation program "Pay It Forward" scheme. *Journal of Medicine and Philosophy.* 2017;42:518–536.

Chapter 11 borrows from chapter 18 of *Transplantation Ethics* (2nd ed.). It was the only chapter that Bob and I could not come to consensus and so it is one of the best argued chapters in the book:

- Robert M. Veatch and Lainie Friedman Ross. Voluntary risks and allocation: does the alcoholic deserve a new liver? In: Robert M Veatch and Lainie F Ross, eds. *Transplantation Ethics.* 2nd ed. Washington, DC: Georgetown University Press; 2015.

Chapter 14, in which the case comes directly from an article about a debate between me and Ben Hippen, moderated by Robert Sade. We freely use my arguments from this article:

Benjamin Hippen, and Lainie Friedman Ross, and Robert M. Sade. Saving lives is more important than abstract moral concerns: financial incentives should be used to increase organ donation. *Annals of Thoracic Surgery.* 2009;88:1053–1061.

In addition to the collaborators enumerated above, there are many other colleagues at the University of Chicago in the MacLean Center for Clinical Medical Ethics and in the Department of Surgery, Section on Transplantation who created a supportive environment for us to collaborate. We also want to acknowledge our many colleagues, trainees, and students—both at the University of Chicago but also across the globe—who helped us think about organ transplantation through a broader lens, invited us to share ideas at conferences and over working meals, and argued with us in lecture halls and auditoriums as well as in print. A special thanks to Ann Dudley Goldblatt, who read a complete working draft with the fastidiousness of a Harvard-trained lawyer and the grace of a supportive and loving friend. Our framework is more robust and our arguments sharper because of all of you.

Last but not least we want to thank our families who supported us in this endeavor and were patient with every final draft that we revised.

We dedicate this book to our spouses.

Notes

1. Ross LF, Rubin D, Siegler M, Josephson MA, Thistlethwaite JR, and Woodle ES. Ethics of a paired-kidney-exchange program. N Engl J Med. 1997;336:752–755.

2. Singer PA, Siegler M, Whitington PF, et al. Ethics of liver transplantation with living donors. N Engl J Med. 1989;321:620–622.

3. Broelsch CE, Whitington PF, Emond JC, et al. Liver transplantation in children from living related donors. Surgical techniques and results. Ann Surg. 1991;214:428–437, discussion pp. 437–439.

4. Veatch RM. Transplantation Ethics. Washington, DC: Georgetown University Press; 2000.

5. Ross LF, Siegler M, Thistlethwaite JR Jr. We need a registry of living kidney donors. Hastings Cent Rep. 2007;7(6):1, page following p. 49. https://onlinelibrary.wiley.com/doi/epdf/10.1353/hcr.2007.0091

6. A special thanks to Jennifer Wainright PhD at HRSA. Of note, since then I was able to renegotiate my request, and I received information about several hundred additional living kidney donors who developed ESRD and were on the kidney transplant waitlist.

7. Hippen B, Ross LF, Sade RM. Saving lives is more important than abstract moral concerns: financial incentives should be used to increase organ donation. Ann Thorac Surg. 2009;88:1053–1061.

8. Ross LF. What the medical excuse teaches us about the donor as patient. Am J Transplant. 2010;10:731–736.

9. Ross LF. Good ethics requires good science: why transplant programs should NOT disclose misattributed parentage. Am J Transplant. 2010;10:742–746.

10. Aronsohn A, Thistlethwaite JR Jr, Segev DL, Ross LF. How different conceptions of risk are used in the organ market debate. Am J Transplant. 2010;*10*:931–937.
11. Thistlethwaite JR Jr, Ross LF. Potential inefficiency of a proposed efficiency model for kidney allocation. Am J Kidney Dis. 2008;*51*(4):545–548.

Index

For the benefit of digital users, indexed terms that span two pages (e.g., 52–53) may, on occasion, appear on only one of those pages.